NORMAL ASPECTS
OF
SPEECH, HEARING, AND
LANGUAGE

NORMAL ASPECTS OF SPEECH,

contributing authors

David J. Broad
Speech Communications Research Laboratory at Santa Barbara

Charles E. Cairns
Queens College of the City University of New York

Helen S. Cairns
Queens College of the City University of New York

Raymond G. Daniloff
Purdue University

Theodore J. Glattke
Stanford University Medical Center

Thomas J. Hixon
University of Wisconsin

Fred D. Minifie
University of Washington

Ronald Netsell
University of Wisconsin

Arnold M. Small
University of Iowa

Frederick Williams
University of Texas

HEARING, AND LANGUAGE

Edited By

FRED. D. MINIFIE
University of Washington

THOMAS J. HIXON
University of Wisconsin

FREDERICK WILLIAMS
University of Texas

Prentice-Hall, Inc., Englewood Cliffs, New Jersey

Library of Congress Cataloging in Publication Data

Minifie, Fred D.
   Normal aspects of speech, hearing, and language.

   Includes bibliographies.
    1. Speech—Physiological aspects. 2. Hearing.
3. Language and languages. I. Hixon, Thomas J.,
joint author. II. Williams, Frederick,
joint author. III. Broad, David J.
IV. Title. [DNLM: 1. Hearing. 2. Language.
3. Speech. WV501M665n 1973]
QP306.M617   612'.78   73-2567
ISBN 0-13-623702-9

NORMAL ASPECTS OF SPEECH, HEARING, AND LANGUAGE
Edited by Fred D. Minifie, Thomas J. Hixon, Frederick Williams

© **1973 by Prentice-Hall, Inc., Englewood Cliffs, New Jersey**

Printed in the United States of America

10 9 8 7 6 5 4 3 2 1

Prentice-Hall International, Inc., LONDON
Prentice-Hall of Australia, Pty. Ltd., SYDNEY
Prentice-Hall of Canada, Ltd., TORONTO
Prentice-Hall of India Private Limited, NEW DELHI
Prentice-Hall of Japan, Inc., TOKYO

The editors dedicate this book to JAMES F. CURTIS, Ph.D.,
Professor of Speech Pathology and Audiology
at the University of Iowa,
whose exemplary philosophy of education
and approach to scientific inquiry
has profoundly influenced the study of
normal aspects of speech, hearing, and language.

CONTENTS

PREFACE   xi

1

PERSPECTIVES   *1*

Aim of the Book
A Preview of Acoustic, Physiologic, and Psycholinguistic Aspects
Some Notes about Research

2

ACOUSTICS   *11*

Arnold M. Small

Sound   Electricity   Electroacoustics

3

RESPIRATORY FUNCTION IN SPEECH   *73*

Thomas J. Hixon

Introduction   Respiration for Life Purposes
Respiration for Speech Purposes

4

PHONATION   *127*

David J. Broad

Introduction   The Cartilaginous Framework for Phonation
The Conus Elasticus and the Vocal Ligaments   Laryngeal Sound Production
Respiratory Determinants of Voice   Laryngeal Determinants of Voice
Voice Registers   Intrinsic Laryngeal Muscles
Ancillary Laryngeal Structures   Extrinsic Control of Phonation
Some Unresolved Problems

5

NORMAL ARTICULATION PROCESSES   *169*

Raymond G. Daniloff

Introduction   Vocal Tract   The Sounds of Speech
The Organization of Articulation

6

SPEECH PHYSIOLOGY   *211*

Ronald Netsell

Introduction   Conceptual Framework
Some Physiological Mechanisms

7

SPEECH ACOUSTICS   *235*

Fred D. Minifie

Introduction   Classification of Sounds   Vowels   Consonant Sounds
Impact of Coarticulation on Speech Acoustics
Suprasegmental Aspects of Speech Production   A Caution
A Point of View

8

ELEMENTS OF AUDITORY PHYSIOLOGY   *285*

Theodore J. Glattke

Introduction   The External and Middle Ear Structures
The Inner Ear Structure   Mechanical Action in the Cochlea
Some Morphological and Electrical Characteristics of Neurons
Innervation Patterns of the Auditory System
Some Behavioral Consequences of Lesions in the Auditory System
The Efferent Auditory System   Summary

9

PSYCHOACOUSTICS   *343*

Arnold M. Small

Introduction   Psychophysical Procedures   Auditory Sensitivity
Masking   Loudness   Beats and Subjective Tones   Binaural Effects
Adaptation and Fatigue   Pitch

10

LANGUAGE   *421*

Charles E. Cairns/Frederick Williams

Speech Compared with Language   Linguistic Theory

11

LINGUISTIC PERFORMANCE   *457*

Frederick Williams/Helen S. Cairns

Introduction   The Cognitive Approach
The Learning Theory Approach   A Sociolinguistic Approach

INDEX   *497*

PREFACE

This book is written for undergraduate students who have had limited formal preparation for understanding the processes involved in human speech communication. The advice given to each contributor was to assume no previous experience with the topic by the reader—assume only that he has a grasp of the English language and a desire to learn. In one sense, this book has been written out of frustration—not the normal everyday frustration, but that special brand known only to teachers who have attempted to offer courses for which there are no adequate reference materials available. Several of the contributors to this book have taught basic courses dealing with various aspects of normal human speech communication, only to find that the textual material available was limited in one sense or another. Therefore, this book was prepared to provide an introduction to the total process of human speech communication, including: the physiological aspects of speech production and reception, the acoustical aspects of speech production and transmission, the psychophysics of sound reception, the nature of language, and the language rules used by talkers and hearers.

The complex nature of the material in this book required multiple authorship to provide comprehensive coverage of the topic. The need to limit this book to a single volume and our own biases have restricted even this coverage of the topic. Certainly we would like to have included in this volume a number of other chapters.

The second distinguishing feature of this book is the final section dealing with language. Most introductory texts which deal with normal speech production or sound reception do not include descriptions of the language processes. As a group of contributors, we feel that a comprehensive understanding of human speech communication cannot be achieved without an awareness of the linguistic factors which mediate our responses at all levels. The inclusion of the final portion of this book should assist the beginning student in developing an understanding of the language components influencing his ability to produce or perceive human speech.

The original manuscript was read in its entirety by Dr. William Tiffany. His careful critiques were most helpful in making final modifications on the copy and in retaining a uniformity of style throughout the book.

There are many other persons to whom the authors of this book are indebted, but because of the nature of contributed volumes and the manner in which they are put together, the adequate recognition of our indebtedness would be much too complex to attempt here. These people know that they have helped, directly or indirectly, in the preparation of this book. We are most grateful for your assistance and only wish it were possible to make special mention of each of you.

We have leaned heavily on the body of information available in the literature in order to provide "our" interpretations. In many cases we have cited the work of others for we fall heir to a rich history. Much of the strength of this book is dependent upon the excellent work which we reference. If there are inaccuracies in our references, or weaknesses in our interpretation, we assume full responsibility.

FRED D. MINIFIE
THOMAS J. HIXON
FREDERICK WILLIAMS

NORMAL ASPECTS
OF
SPEECH, HEARING, AND
LANGUAGE

1
PERSPECTIVES

AIM OF THE BOOK

This book is an introduction to subject matter areas usually included under the more general label *speech and hearing science*. The materials in this volume are designed to provide fundamental perspectives of the scientific study of normal speech production and hearing behaviors in humans. The perspectives developed by the contributors incorporate selective theory, research, and research strategies from a variety of disciplines, but chiefly from physiology, acoustics, psychology, and linguistics. This knowledge forms a basis for subsequent understanding of the abnormal—that is, disorders of speech and hearing.

Some of the facets of contemporary study of speech and hearing science undoubtedly date back to antiquity. However, until the 1930s and the research application of the vacuum tube amplifier, which opened the way for definitive studies of acoustical phenomena, most of the scientific interest in speech was in physiological processes. This omits from consideration the

This chapter was jointly prepared by the editors.

linguists' long-time interests in speech because most of what we now call speech science evolved somewhat separately from such concerns. And perhaps unfortunately so.

After World War II, advances in electronic instrumentation, Federal support of graduate training and research programs in speech, and advances in other fields with interests in speech, contributed to the rapid growth of research and theory in the acoustic and physiologic aspects of speech and hearing. In the last decade speech scientists have increasingly tried to incorporate variables of language and language performance into their considerations of the processes of speech production and perception. The contemporary view of speech and hearing science, in the editors' opinions at least, divides generally into what we call the *psycholinguistic, physiologic,* and *acoustic* aspects of normal speech, hearing, and language. Figure 1-1 presents a schematic view of these aspects, as well as how some of the typical topics of speech and hearing relate to them.

Note first how the three aspects are interrelated to the study of speech production and perception processes. In speech production, we assume that every utterance starts with some type of linguistic planning as a cognitive process. Eventually the utterance is articulated, which implies the existence

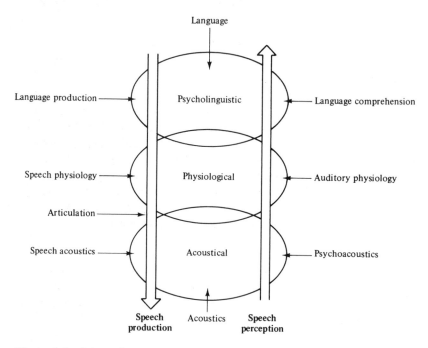

Figure 1-1 Schematic representation of the oral-verbal communication process.

of psychological controls over physiological and acoustical processes. Perception implies the reverse of this sequence. Acoustic phenomena stimulate the auditory mechanism and thereby give rise to a physiological process of converting acoustic energy into neural energy. As a cognitive process, the patterns of neural energy are interpreted by the brain. Thus, although we may sometimes study only the acoustic details of individual speech sounds, very detailed aspects of audition, or some small facet of speech physiology, we envisage all such details as a part of the overall processes of speech production, perception, or both.

There is hardly a topic of traditional study in speech and hearing that does not interrelate the psychological, physiological, and/or acoustical aspects of the overall processes. Psychoacoustics, for example, attempts to correlate variations in acoustic characteristics with variations in perceptual behaviors. Acoustical phonetics represents, in part, a relation between variations in the dynamics of speech physiology with changes in the acoustic patterns of speech.

The basic representation of the three aforementioned aspects of speech can also be used to interrelate many of the topics concerning disorders of speech and hearing. Figure 1-2 illustrates how aphasia can be associated to cognitive processes involved in the psychological aspects of speech planning

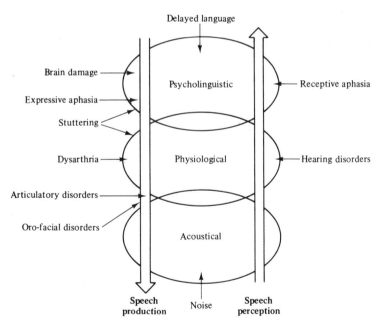

Figure 1-2 Disorders of speech, hearing, and language as viewed within an overall model of human oral-verbal communication.

or perception. Oro-facial problems, for example, relate primarily to the physiological level, as do most organic disorders. Even problems of noise, when viewed in terms of acoustical phenomena, may be assessed relative to their perceptual consequences. Here, too, what we know of theory and research strategies in terms of the larger aspects of the speech and hearing processes can be used in the definition, study, and even the remediation of disorders.

One of the major challenges in attempting to draw from, and to interrelate, materials from psychology, physiology, and acoustics is that these areas are characterized by different theoretical materials and research methods. The extent of agreement among scientists upon accuracy of theory is yet another variant factor. The science of acoustics, for example, makes available for us fixed and agreed-upon theory since the phenomena of acoustics are governed rather directly by natural laws. Given knowledge of the geometric qualities of a tube, we can predict quite accurately the effects upon a sound wave introduced into it. In fact, if our predictions are not borne out in a study, we usually question our instruments before we question the theory. At the other extreme are theories of the psychological components of speech and hearing processes. What generalizations we do have in this area are subject to so many intervening conditions and are so elusive of direct study that we have theories in major competition with one another. We even have major disagreements on what should be required of theory in this area.

The reason for mentioning these contrasts at this point is that the student of speech and hearing is faced not only with the challenge of acquiring fundamental knowledge of the psychological, physiological, and acoustic aspects of speech, but he or she will also have to learn something of the *ways of knowing* these aspects. We will return to this topic in the final portion of this chapter.

A PREVIEW OF ACOUSTIC, PHYSIOLOGIC, AND PSYCHOLINGUISTIC ASPECTS

There are many ways to approach the science of speech and hearing. In the present volume it is assumed that an initial understanding of the basic parameters of sounds is one of the best starting points. Such knowledge permits an understanding of the relations between these parameters and physiologic operations of human production and reception mechanisms. This, in turn, provides a basic framework for considering the psycholinguistic theories of the cognitive behaviors in speech production and perception.

Acoustic Aspects

Acoustics is a branch of physics dealing with the generation, transmission, and modification of sound waves. Understanding the methods by which sound waves are measured and described is necessary for the study of acoustics. Sound characteristics such as frequency, amplitude, wave form, and duration are seen not only as physical phenomena, but also in terms of measurement strategies and instrumentation. In particular, the detailed study of acoustics requires knowledge of electronic instrumentation which has provided the basis for most of the advances in this area. This involves the study of electroacoustics, which is essentially a consideration of the analogs between acoustic and electrical phenomena. The use of sound tape recorders and wave analysis instruments such as the sound spectrograph are instances of acoustic energy patterns being converted to electrical ones as a method of recording, display, and analysis.

A further major area in the study of acoustics is of *resonance*, or the study of environmental phenomena affecting sound waves. Some of the physical laws of resonance which we associate with air columns are used in the description of dynamic resonance phenomena during speech production. In fact, such laws form the basis of our theories of speech acoustics.

Psychoacoustics is a study of the relationship between acoustic characteristics and human auditory perception of these characteristics. For example, at a most basic level there are identifiable associations between acoustic variations of sound frequency and changes in the perceptual awareness of pitch. Similarly, there are relations between acoustic alterations of intensity and perceptual variations of loudness. Like the study of acoustics, psychoacoustics requires an understanding of research methods. Here the challenge is to combine in one area of study, the research methods of the physics of sound and those of the psychology of perception. Thus the researcher in psychoacoustics must be as knowledgeable of instrumentation for varying and measuring sound characteristics as he is with often quite different techniques such as psychological scaling. Although psychoacoustics traditionally deals with the normal hearing processes, it, of course, provides us with a basis for theorizing about disorders of hearing.

Physiological Aspects

In those chapters of this book which deal with speech production, the major emphasis is on speech physiology rather than on a speech anatomy. Strictly speaking, physiology pertains to the functions of the structures of the living organism, whereas anatomy is a study of the structures themselves. Physiology, then, implies a dynamic view of the organism and, as applied to speech, concerns the dynamic functioning of those structures which have to do with speech production and perception. Although we must constantly bear in mind that speech production is an overall interconnected process, for convenience sake we may divide it into arbitrary areas of study. One such division is to focus separately upon processes of *respiration, phonation,* and *articulation.* Given a view of these component processes, one can then integrate them into an overall view of *speech physiology.* At the same time, the study of speech physiology is a necessary precursor to, and an integral part of, the study of *speech acoustics.* Similarly, there is a physiologic view of the auditory mechanism, which itself divides into functional substructures.

Respiration is viewed as the energy source for speech. More specifically, respiratory activity is a physical process of pumping air, the movement of which eventually is transformed into acoustic energy.

Like the study of acoustics, the study of respiratory physiology uses concepts and measurement techniques of physics. Respiration as it relates to speech production is often misunderstood on two accounts. One of these is that the physiological process of respiration is far more complex than is found in many descriptions in the speech and hearing literature. Second, little attention has traditionally been given to the coordination of respiration required for speech as it is superimposed upon respiration required for life purposes. How the organism coordinates speech and breathing is an exceedingly complex topic, and much of the contemporary research into the physiology of speech respiratory activity focuses upon it.

Phonation is a physiologic process whereby the energy of moving air in the vocal tract is transformed into acoustic energy within the *larynx.* Much of the study of phonation involves a consideration of the mechanical, aerodynamic, and physiological activity in the larynx and how all of these relate to the acoustic parameters of voicing. The evolution of research instrumentation has played a particularly significant role in research into the physiological aspects of phonation. The challenge has been to obtain a detailed picture of the dynamics of laryngeal physiology during the production of the different sounds of speech.

Articulation has long been an area of speech and hearing study. However, it has only been in the last decade that researchers have adequately focused on dynamic articulatory processes. Many students will be familiar with the schemes of using place and manner to designate articulatory positions for consonants, and tongue position and height for classification of vowel sounds. Contemporary research has led us away from such static views of articulation and into such concepts as dynamic co-articulation, where we attempt to determine the influence of phonetic environments upon articulatory sequences. Much of the contemporary research into the dynamics of articulation has been dependent upon sophisticated instrumentation and research strategies. As a consequence, the contemporary student of speech and hearing will again find himself studying as much about research strategies as he will about articulation itself. A detailed view of the physiological processes of articulation is complemented by research in speech acoustics.

Speech acoustics is a way of describing all of the consequences of speech articulation, beginning with the generation of sound sources within the vocal tract, and the modification of those sounds by dynamically changing resonance patterns which result from dynamic changes in vocal tract size and shape. Much of the research challenge in speech acoustics is to conjoin what we know about the acoustic parameters of speech with what we know about articulatory physiology. In particular, the most recent trends in research have attempted to equate sequences of speech acoustic patterns with the sequential patterns of articulatory processes. This work, like so many other aspects of speech and hearing research, requires the joint use of research strategies from both acoustics and physiology.

Speech physiology as an overall topic of study represents the integration of such processes as speech respiration, phonation, and articulation. Further, we are often interested in the consequences of these integrated components of speech physiology upon the acoustical patterns of speech. Although we may look at many of the individual and detailed processes of speech production, a combination of these processes leads to more major concepts than simply the sum of the parts. There are many types of contemporary research which focus upon the interrelation among the detailed processes, rather than on the processes themselves. Thus, for example, we may be concerned with the relationship between particular aspects of respiratory activity and articulatory activity. Or we may be interested in the manner by which a phenomenon such as co-articulation interrelates constituent processes involved in speech production. Modern concepts of speech physiology also emphasize the dynamic view of speech production. Thus, speech physiology is more than simply a discussion of structures and their functions. It is an overall operational view of how speech sounds are produced.

Auditory physiology is approached with the same point of view as speech physiology. Here our concern is with a description and explanation of the characteristics and capabilities of the auditory system in converting acoustic energy into neural energy. Auditory physiology divides quite readily into consideration of the outer, middle, and inner ear, as well as the auditory nervous system, with attention given to the functions of each. Although theories of audition are among the oldest in the scientific study of human communication, we still have problems in determining precisely how neural coding of auditory stimulation takes place. The extreme delicacy and small size of the auditory structures account, in large measure, for our present state of uncertainty. However, given a basic understanding of auditory physiology, the student is in a position to make comparisons among theories of the hearing process.

Psycholinguistic Aspects

While much of the science of speech and hearing has traditionally centered upon physiologic and acoustic aspects of speech production and speech perception, it has been increasingly recognized that adequate theorizing about these processes requires that attention be given to the nature of language as well as to what we call language performance. In the broadest sense, speech and hearing behaviors *are* language performances. The processes of speech production and perception involve among other things, the language user's ability to associate sounds with meanings. When we attempt to theorize about the nature of the relationship between sounds and meaning, we can benefit greatly from an understanding of contemporary linguistic theory. Similarly, we can try to consider how these interactions enter into the process of language behavior, and this is the focus of contemporary psycholinguistics.

Language, in generative linguistic theory, is viewed as the knowledge one would have in order to associate sounds and meanings. Apart from the details of behavior, we call this knowledge *linguistic competence*. A *generative grammar* represents abstract descriptions of competence in terms of systems of phonological, syntactic, and semantic rules. Although these rules are not descriptions of the behaviors involved in the creation or understanding of sentences (any more than the rules of arithmetic are a psychological model of how we add two plus two), they do enable us to pose a number of generalizations about what must be required of the behavioral processes of speech production and perception.

Language performance is an attempt to see in behavioral terms the cognitive aspects of how humans create and understand sentences. Although there has been theorizing in this area for many years, the development of generative grammar has stimulated many fresh insights about language behavior. Much of this theorizing is known under the contemporary label of psycholinguistics. Given that linguistics poses for us an abstract description of relationships between sounds and meanings, theories in psycholinguistics attempt to define the way humans perform these relationships in the creation and the understanding of sentences. Also, incorporated within theories of language performance are considerations of the development of language in children.

SOME NOTES ABOUT RESEARCH

When we speak of the *science* of speech and hearing, we imply that our knowledge has such qualities as objectivity, accuracy, consistency, and contributes to overall generalizations of description and explanation called *theory*. In the most practical view, we want assurance that our generalizations fit what we are describing or explaining.

Most of the research in speech and hearing science is regularly reported in scholarly journals.[1] The format of articles in these journals usually reflects the steps in the strategy for scientific research. For example:

(1) *Problem:*   a statement of the rationale for the research; a problem stated in the form of a question or hypothesis.

(2) *Method:*   description of the materials or instrumentation used in the investigation; description of the persons (*subjects*) studied, if humans are involved; description of the procedures undertaken in applying the materials or instrumentation to the subjects to gather data.

(3) *Results:*   a report of the interpretation of the data in terms of answering the question or testing the hypothesis.

(4) *Discussion:*   the interpretation of the results in terms of applicable theory; suggestions for improving the study; suggestions for further research.

In its most ideal conception, research is a formal undertaking, and most journal articles try to reflect this. In practice, however, research proceeds in many forms, and ideas sometimes start with hunches as well as from the results of carefully planned, long-range research programs. Most reports of research emphasize two points: a generalization about something and the rationale for this generalization. Simply understanding journal reports of research is not sufficient; we must be able to evaluate them critically. A good scientific statement reflects its origin and suggests its verification. Often we are as interested in a researcher's claim of the truth of a generalization as we are in his grounds for arguing its truth. These grounds are the business of research.

Again speaking very practically, research involves inductive reasoning from facts to generalizations, deductive reasoning from generalizations to facts, as well as combinations of the two.

A *fact* is the report of a specific observation. Some examples are: "This page is printed in black ink." "The spirogram indicated that 3,000 cc of air was exchanged." "The length of subject B's ear canal is 2.3 cm." Facts are not generalizations; they are specific reports. "The sun rises every morning" is not a fact, but "The sun rose this morning" is. In research, we usually call facts, *data*, or *datum* when referring to one report. In speech science, data are often in the language of measurement. That is, we use numbers as data, or reports of our observations. We can check facts or data by comparing

---

[1] For example: *The Journal of Speech and Hearing Research* and *The Journal of the Acoustical Society of America.*

them with observations. If exactly the same observations yield the same facts, then we say that the data (or measurements) are consistent or *reliable*. If we use different methods of measurement so that one can check the other, we are testing *validity*, or whether a measure reflects what it claims to report.

Science would not progress much if all we had were bodies of data. We need to relate facts to generalizations. We do this by strategies of induction and deduction. If, for example, we were interested in ear canals, data could only provide us with as many individual lengths as we would have the resources to measure. To make a generalization it is possible to calculate an arithmetic mean from a body of data. Thus we might say that "The average length of ear canals in the study was 2.4 cm," and this would be a generalization derived from specific observations. If we then wanted to anticipate the length of ear canals in persons such as those studied, we could use the average as a generalization to predict what measurements we might obtain. This would be a deduction—that is, reasoning to facts from a generalization. A branch of applied mathematics, called *statistics*, gives us mathematical arguments for making the foregoing kinds of arithmetic generalizations. Statistics allows us to reason from a smaller group of observations (a *sample*) to making predictions about what could be expected if a much larger group of observations (a *population*) represented by that sample were measured.

In research we also try to make generalizations about generalizations, and these often reflect what we loosely call *theory*. We are dealing with theory when we try to organize generalizations into some systematic body of principles which enables us to describe or explain a body of facts. We are quite free to theorize all we wish, even in the absence of facts. Thus to call something a "theory" is no stamp of automatic approval. The arguments which support a theory are as important as the theory itself. Theories provide ways of putting together already verified generalizations and lead to further untested generalizations. When we set out to test new generalizations, we typically call them *hypotheses*. Experimental methods of research provide us with the most productive framework for testing generalizations. In experiments we directly manipulate one phenomenon (e. g., variations in acoustic frequency) while observing its consequences upon another phenomenon (e. g., variations in perceived pitch). Our anticipated relation between these phenomena is the hypothesis, and the results of an experiment, by providing facts for our generalization, allow us to accept or reject the hypothesis.

As you examine the chapters of this volume, most all generalizations that you encounter will stand somewhere between a body of facts and a body of theory. As a serious student, you not only have the burden of interpreting what is said about speech and hearing phenomena, but also the burden of judging whether what is said stands somewhere between facts and theory. Ultimately, this latter knowledge may be the most important that you will take away from this book.

2

ACOUSTICS

Arnold M. Small

SOUND

Sound may be defined in several ways. For example, it can be considered as that quantity which, when present, may give rise to the sensation of hearing. While this is important it represents a very narrow definition of sound. In this chapter we will consider sound in a broader context; that is, not only as a stimulus for hearing, but as a physical quantity. In studying sound we will find it convenient to consider three separate processes as outlined in Figure 2-1. This figure shows a sound source, for example, a tuning fork, a loudspeaker, or a human vocal system from which sound is transmitted. Sound travels away from the source through a sound conducting medium which, for our purposes, is most often air. Finally, the sound reaches a receiver which may be the human auditory system or perhaps a physical measuring device. Each of these processes is important and will be discussed in this chapter.

Vibration

Sound may be thought of simply as vibration. Anything that can vibrate has the potential of serving as a sound source. In order for a medium to transmit

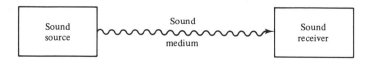

Figure 2-1 Schematic diagram of segments of a sound chain consisting of a source, a medium, and a receiver.

a sound wave (Figure 2-1) it is necessary that it be composed of a substance that is capable of vibration. Similarly, if a receiver is to detect a sound wave in a medium, it must respond to vibration. What is vibration?

Generally we think of *vibration* as consisting of repetitive linear motion; that is, motion that regularly repeats itself and travels in a straight line. For example, the motion of the tines of a tuning fork, the movement of a pendulum on a clock, or the motion of a plucked guitar string all represent vibration. As a matter of fact, vibratory motion need not be periodic; that is, regularly repeating, as in the examples just given, but can also be aperiodic or nonrepetitive. However, let us first consider periodic vibration.

Periodic vibration

Given that the vibration or movement of an object may be periodic we might ask, "exactly what course of motion is followed by the vibrating object?" By definition, we know that its motion must repeat itself, but in what way or what form does it repeat itself? Consider that the motion consists of moving in a straight line from A to B and back again over and over as in Figure 2-2. Now, what possible ways are there that the object can traverse this path? For example, it might move rapidly from A to B and then slowly from B to A, or it might move slowly from A to B and rapidly from B to A, or it might move from A to half-way between A and B, pause for a moment then move on to B and then back to A. Within our definition of periodic motion there are absolutely no restrictions on the way in which the motion can occur providing it does, in fact, repeat itself. Thus there are an infinite number of ways in which one can get from A to B and back again within the framework of periodic vibration. In order to help clarify the situation and at the same time provide ease in discussing the matter, let us consider one particular type of

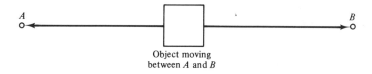

Object moving
between A and B

Figure 2-2 Diagram of repetitive linear motion.

periodic motion. It turns out that this particular motion is simple from a mathematical standpoint and, as we will see, it is a fundamental type of motion upon which we can build for future discussion.

Simple harmonic motion. Simple harmonic motion, often abbreviated SHM, can be defined as the linear projection of uniform circular motion. In order to better understand what this means, consider the example illustrated in Figure 2-3. If on a circle we define a point, the point (A in this case) can be considered to move around that circle at a uniform speed. In other words, it covers the same distance each unit of time. Now, consider a straight line drawn next to the circle. Let's identify this straight line by calling it XY, that is, the line is defined by end points X and Y. Now, let us trace the path of point A on the circle as it moves with uniform circular velocity. At its original, arbitrary position we see that the projection of point A on line XY is given by point B. As point A moves around the circle in counter-clockwise fashion, we see that after it has moved to position A' its corresponding position on line XY is given by B'. Now, as point A continues to move to position A'' its projection on line XY is given by point B''. Thus as point A continues to go through its uniform circular motion, we can find its corresponding position on line XY. What we have described is the linear projection

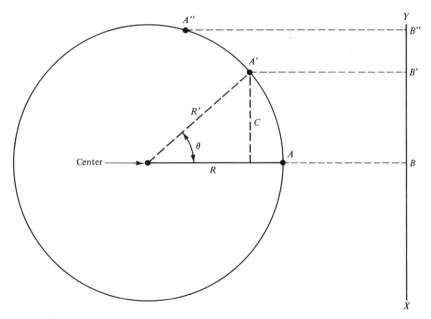

Figure 2-3 Illustration of simple harmonic motion (SHM). Point A moves with uniform circular velocity and its linear projection, B, executes SHM.

(on line XY) of the uniform circular motion being described by point A. You can see from this description that although point A may move the same distance with each unit of time, its projection, point B, on line XY does not necessarily move a corresponding distance. In general, point B moves further when A is on the left and right sides of the circle than it does when A is at the top or bottom. As a matter of fact, we can describe the motion of B on line XY as being initially rapid as it approaches Y, then slowing down. Finally, the motion actually stops momentarily and then reverses slowly, builds up speed, moves with a maximum speed as it passes through position B, slows down as it approaches X, stops, reverses direction, and repeats the cycle. In order to talk a little more easily about this motion it is convenient to assign certain descriptive terms to the figures shown in Figure 2-3. Let us connect the center of the circle to the initial point A with a line which we will call R (radius). As point A revolves along the circle, line R of course will follow, much in the same fashion as a spoke on a wheel. Now, at each moment in time as A moves and R also moves, A and R will assume a new position. Let us assume that at a particular moment in time point A has advanced to position A' and that a line R' connects that point with the center of the circle. R and R' form a certain angle as they converge at the center of the circle. Let us call this angle θ. As A continues to move around the circle, θ increases in size. By the time A goes all the way around the circle and comes back to the original point, θ will have increased from zero to 360 degrees.

By definition then, uniform circular motion, and hence SHM, repeats itself everytime θ goes through 360°. The angle θ refers to the relative *phase* of the SHM. If, for example, the angle θ is equal to 90° then the phase of the SHM is 90° relative to its starting point. The *amplitude* or size of the SHM is given by the maximum excursion of the linear projection on line XY. This is related to the length of R in our circle diagram. The longer R becomes, the larger the circle, and the larger the amplitude of movement in the linear projection. The time taken to complete one revolution (360° of circular motion) or one cycle in terms of SHM, is referred to as the *period* of SHM. The number of cycles completed in any unit of time is equal to the *frequency* of SHM. For example, if point A revolves around a circle in 0.1 sec, point B on line XY goes from B to Y to X and back to B again in 0.1 sec. If it takes 0.1 sec to accomplish this once, then it follows that in 1 sec we can do it ten times. The frequency of motion is then 10 cycles per sec. If the period is expressed in seconds, then the frequency (number of cycles completed each second) is expressed in a unit called a *hertz* (Hz). In our example, the frequency is 10 Hz. The relation between frequency (f), and period (T) may be expressed as:

$$f = \frac{1}{T} \quad \text{or in the example} \quad 10 \text{ Hz} = \frac{1}{.1 \text{ sec}}$$

Thus SHM is completely defined by the three parameters, phase, amplitude, and frequency (or period).

Let us go one step further in Figure 2-3 and drop a perpendicular line *C* from point *A'* to line *R*. Line *C* will clearly change in size as the angle *θ* changes. In fact, this relation can be expressed as:

$$C = (R) (\text{sine } \theta)$$

This relation is from elementary trigonometry and simply says that in a right triangle we can determine the length of *C* if we know the length of *R* (or *R'*) and the angle *θ*. (The value of sine *θ* is conveniently tabled and is defined as the ratio of the length of the side opposite *θ* to the length of the hypotenuse.) In our particular case *θ* is changing as a function of time. Table 2-1 illustrates the way *θ* and *C* would vary as a function of time if the period of the SHM was 1 sec and the radius of the circle was 1 inch (for convenience the period is subdivided into twelve parts).

If the values shown in Table 2-1 are plotted, we obtain the graph shown in

Table 2-1 Evaluation of sine function if *R* = 1 in. Illustrates relation between elapsed time, fractional parts of a cycle, degrees of phase, and length of line *C*. See Figures 2-3 and 2-4 for graphical representation of this material.

	Fractional part of cycle												
	0	1/12	2/12	3/12	4/12	5/12	6/12	7/12	8/12	9/12	10/12	11/12	12/12
t (sec)	0	1/12	1/6	1/4	1/3	5/12	1/2	7/12	2/3	3/4	5/6	11/12	1
θ (degrees)	0	30	60	90	120	150	180	210	240	270	300	330	360
C (inch)	0	0.5	0.87	1	0.87	0.5	0	−0.5	−0.87	−1	−0.87	−0.5	0

Figure 2-4. The vertical scale indicates the value of *C*, the displacement of the SHM, for each value of time indicated on the horizontal scale. The result of plotting displacement as a function of time is referred to as *waveform*. This particular waveform is called a *sine wave* since it comes from a relation which contains a sine function. Any waveform which is a sine wave or a sine wave with a different starting phase is termed a *sinusoid*. We can readily see the features of the sine wave in Figure 2-4 which correspond to the excursions of point *B* on line *XY* and the circular motion of point *A* on the circle in Figure 2-3.

Combination of sinusoids. SHM and the sine wave, although simple in one sense of the word, are by no means common in everyday life. Most of the sounds that we hear are complex sounds in that their vibrations consist of more than one sine wave. Let us see how it is possible to construct a complex wave using single sine waves as building blocks. In Column (*a*) of Figure 2-5 we see a sine wave labeled (1), it has an amplitude of one unit. We also see a sine wave labeled (2) which is identical to (1) with respect to all three parameters of SHM, namely amplitude, frequency, and starting phase. The question is, what will happen when we combine (1) with (2)? The answer

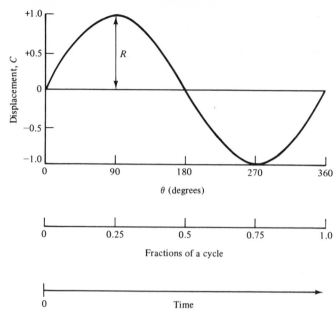

Figure 2-4 SHM as a function of time—a sine wave. Values of C were obtained from Table 2-1. The displacement, C, represents the position of point B of Figure 2-3 for each moment in time as A revolves. The time taken to complete 360° is the time required for A to make one complete revolution. The maximum displacement is the radius, R, of the circle of Figure 2-3.

Figures 2-5 Combination of sinusoids of the same frequency. In (a), (b), and (c) sinusoids (1) and (2) are combined to form sinusoid R. The amplitude of (1) and (2) are identical, but have a phase difference of 0, 90, and 180° in (a), (b), and (c), respectively.

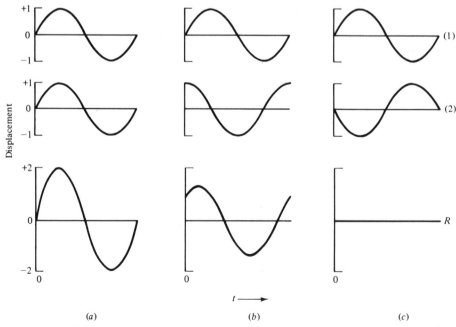

is given by resultant sine wave, R. This resultant is obtained in the following way. For each point on the time axis, starting with time equal to zero, the instantaneous displacement of (1) is added to the corresponding instantaneous displacement of (2). This sum is plotted on the graph labeled R. We see that when we have two sine waves each of unit amplitude, the resulting waveform is a sine wave of the same frequency, the same phase relation, but with an amplitude of two units.

Consider a different situation which is shown in Column (b) of Figure 2-5. Sine wave (1) is identical to that shown in Column (a) while (2) differs from (1) only in starting phase, there being a 90° phase difference between (1) and (2). In our previous example in Figure 2-3 then, (2) would start at Y and (1) would start at position B. What happens when we add these two sinusoids together? The answer is given by R which is obtained in exactly the same way as that of R in Column (a). Instantaneous values of displacement for each sinusoid are obtained for corresponding points in time. They are added together algebraically and plotted to form R. In this case the resulting wave (R) differs in amplitude and phase from the two original sinusoids but has the same frequency.

Consider a third case as shown in Figure 2-5(c), which differs from example (b) only in that the second sinusoid, rather than having a phase difference of 90°, has a phase difference of 180°. In this case R consists of a straight line of value zero. This is the obvious outcome because the two sinusoids are identical in every respect except phase. At every instant in time the displacement of the two waveforms is identical but opposite in sign, thus when these two values are added algebraically the result is zero.

Although we have considered only three examples, the principles outlined in these illustrations hold for the combination of any pair of sinusoids regardless of their frequency, amplitude, or phase. More generally, these same principles hold for the combination of any number of sinusoids. Consider the example shown in Figure 2-6. In this case sine wave (1) is identical to those we have discussed previously, but (2) has a somewhat different amplitude and has a frequency three times as great as (1). The resultant is obtained in the same way as we have discussed previously and is shown as R_{1+2}. Such a waveform is known as a *complex waveform*. Any waveform which is not sinusoidal is, by definition, complex.

Next add to waveform R_{1+2} a third waveform with a frequency five times that of (1). Resultant R_{1+2+3} is obtained from this combination of waveforms (1), (2), (3). You can see that R_{1+2+3} is taking on a rather squarish shape and, in fact, if we continue to add sinusoids whose frequencies are odd numbered multiples of the frequency shown in (1) then eventually we will end up with a waveform shown as $R_{1+2+3+\cdots+n}$. Such a waveform is referred to as a *square wave* and is another example of a complex waveform.

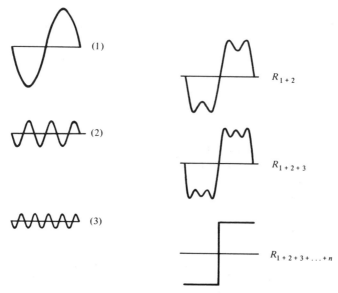

Figure 2-6 Combination of sinusoids of different frequency showing the synthesis of a complex wave from simple sinusoids. In this example (2) and (3) have frequencies of three and five times that of (1). R is the resultant with R_{1+2} representing the combination of (1) and (2); R_{1+2+3} representing a combination of (1), (2), and (3); and $R_{1+2+3+\cdots+n}$ representing a theoretically infinite number of odd numbered multiples of the frequency shown in (1).

In this illustration sinusoid (1) is called a *fundamental frequency* and sinusoids (2) and (3) are the fundamental frequency's third and fifth *harmonic*, respectively. Harmonics of a given frequency are integral multiples of that frequency $(1, 2, 3, \ldots, n)$. For example, for frequencies of 100, 300, and 500 Hz, 300 and 500 are three and five times 100, and they represent the third and fifth harmonics of 100 Hz. Conversely, the fundamental frequency of a series of sinusoids is their largest common multiple. That is, given the frequencies 300, 450, and 600 Hz, we see that 150 is the largest number that, when divided into these frequencies, will yield an integral dividend. Thus, 300, 450, and 600 Hz are the second, third, and fourth harmonics of a fundamental frequency (first harmonic) of 150 Hz.

Fourier analysis. In the last section we showed that a complex waveform may be synthesized from a number of simple sinusoidal building blocks. Thus, it should come as no surprise that we can do the opposite, that is, take any complex waveform and analyze it into its component sinusoids. This is an extremely powerful technique in that it allows us to take the most complex waveforms and break them down into their simple component parts. Thus we need to understand only the characteristics of sinusoids together with the principles that govern the manner in which they may be combined to have a sufficient store of information to allow us to analyze the most complex waveforms.

This process of analysis is referred to as *Fourier analysis* and is named after a French mathematician who first formalized this process. Thus far we have been primarily considering waveform characteristics. We can express essentially the same information about a sinusoid or a complex wave in another way. On the left side of Figure 2-7 we have plotted a number of waveforms. The first is the familiar sine wave. The waveform, of course, is a plot of displacement as a function of time. On the right side of the graph, corresponding to each of the waveforms, we have a plot of amplitude as a function of frequency. Such a plot is referred to as a *spectrum*. The spectrum of a sinusoid consists of a single vertical line located at the particular frequency which characterizes the waveform. The second waveform is that of a sinusoid whose frequency is three times as great as that shown in (1) and it has a spectrum similar to that shown in (1) except that the line is moved up in

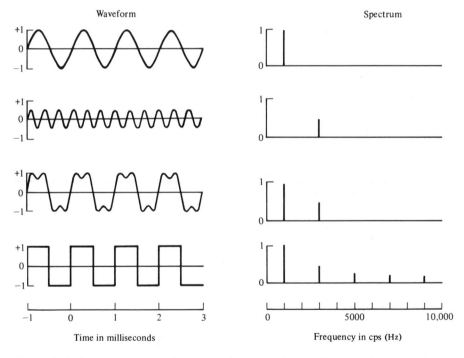

Figure 2-7 Spectra corresponding to various waveforms. The waveforms are those obtained in Figure 2-6 by combining sinusoids whose frequencies were odd multiples of the fundamental.

frequency by a factor of three. The third waveform is the combination of sinusoids (1) and (2) and the spectrum corresponding to this waveform consists of lines at the frequency corresponding to (1) and the frequency corresponding to three times that value. Finally, we have the square waveform which, as you recall, consists of an infinite number of odd integral multiples of the sinusoid shown in (1). Its spectrum consists of lines of particular amplitudes located at one, three, five, seven, and all other odd integral multiples of the frequency of (1). For all periodic waveforms the spectrum will be similar to that shown here; it will consist of discrete lines at various frequencies. Such a spectrum is referred to as a *line spectrum* and is a characteristic of periodic waveforms.

Aperiodic vibration

As indicated earlier, there are basically two kinds of vibrations: periodic, which we have already discussed, and aperiodic. An aperiodic waveform is one that does not repeat itself. Aperiodic waveforms have corresponding spectra which, in contrast to periodic waveforms, consist of a continuous rather than discrete or line spectra. Examples of these spectra will be shown in the sections that follow. There are two kinds of aperiodic vibrations; transient vibrations are those that happen once and only once and random vibrations are those that occur continuously but in such a manner that they never repeat themselves.

Transient vibration. An example of a transient vibration is shown in Figure 2-8. In this figure we see that for all time prior to $t = t_0$ the waveform has a value of 0, but as $t = t_0$ the waveform instantaneously changes to a value $+1$, where it remains. Thus, we have a waveform which never repeats itself and therefore is aperiodic. It occurs once and once only and therefore, by our definition, is a transient.

The spectrum in Figure 2-8 is a continuous distribution of energy which has its maximum value when frequency equals zero and then declines as

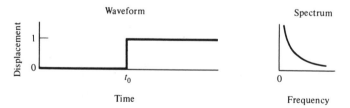

Figure 2-8 Waveform and spectrum of an aperiodic, transient sound. This waveform is known as a step function; a glance at its waveform leaves no doubt as to the basis of the name. The continuous spectrum is characteristic of aperiodic waveforms.

frequency increases. Although the amplitude becomes vanishingly small, it never actually reaches zero amplitude until the frequency is infinitely high. Any transient waveform possesses a spectrum consisting of a continuous distribution of energy as a function of frequency. Such spectra are referred to as *continuous spectra*.

Random vibration. Random vibration is commonly referred to as noise. The waveform of such a vibration is shown in Figure 2-9. We see that the waveform is continuous, but there is no periodicity; the same pattern never repeats itself. If the noise is truly random, that is, knowing the instantaneous value at one point in time does not allow us to predict the instantaneous value at another point in time, then the spectrum will be as indicated to the right of this waveform. Since the noise is not periodic it has a continuous spectrum and, in this case, consists of an equal amount of energy at all frequencies. Noise, in fact, is a general term and what we have shown in Figure 2-9 is merely one particular kind of noise. The noise illustrated is called random noise; at other times it is called *white noise* (by analogy to white light which contains all wavelengths in approximately equal amounts). Sometimes it is called *Gaussian* noise, *wide-band* noise, or *thermal* noise. In all these instances, though different words may be used, reference is being made to the waveform and the spectrum shown in Figure 2-9.

Sound Waves

Sound waves result when the vibrations of a sound source are transmitted through a medium. A medium, in general, is any substance which is capable of undergoing vibration. For the purposes of human sound production and reception, the most common medium is air, consequently our discussion will center on the characteristics of sound waves in air.

There are basically two different types of sound waves and they relate to the geometric configuration of the sound source. If the sound source is a very small point or a sphere, either of which changes diameter, a *spherical sound wave* is produced. If the sound source is a very large flat surface, such as a

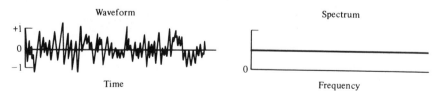

Figure 2-9 Waveform and spectrum of an aperiodic, continuous sound. This is an example of one kind of noise, random noise.

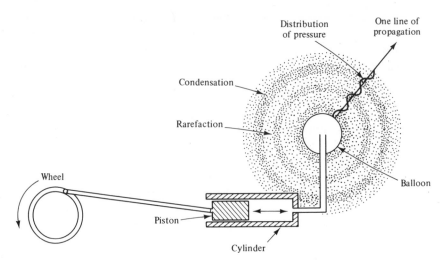

Figure 2-10 A scheme for generating spherical sound waves. Because of the way the air is moved in and out of the balloon, each particle on the balloon's surface will undergo SHM. [*Source: I. J. Hirsh,* The Measurement of Hearing (*New York: McGraw-Hill Book Co., 1952*), *p. 22.*]

wall of a room, then a *plane acoustic wave* is produced. In practice, we seldom have either one of these but rather a combination.

Wave motion

Although a detailed discussion of the characteristics of sound sources will follow later in this chapter, it is necessary to consider some characteristics of the sources in order that we may discuss sound waves themselves. Let us describe a source which is capable of producing spherical waves. We have already indicated that one such source is a pulsating sphere. One way of making a pulsating sphere is indicated in Figure 2-10. First, we attach a long rod to the edge of a rotating wheel (theoretically this rod would be infinitely long). The rod in turn is connected to a piston which is housed in a cylinder. As the wheel turns with uniform circular velocity, the rod moves. This, in turn, moves the piston in and out of the cylinder. From our earlier considerations it should be clear that if the wheel turns with uniform circular velocity the piston will move with SHM. As the piston moves in and out of the cylinder the air in the cylinder is forced through a small tube to a partially inflated balloon. As the piston moves to the right the balloon expands; as the piston moves to the left the balloon contracts. Thus, the stage is set for the generation of a spherical acoustic wave.

Particle displacement. Consider the situation in which the piston moves so as to cause the balloon to expand. In that region of the medium immediately adjacent to the surface of the balloon the air molecules will be swept from their original position and pushed outward as the balloon expands. The air molecules can no longer occupy their original position since that original position is now being occupied by the balloon. As the balloon continues to expand, more and more air molecules are pushed outward; thus during this period of expansion there is a greater than normal number of air molecules in the immediate vicinity of the surface of the balloon. Now the direction of the piston is reversed and the balloon begins to contract. That region of the medium that had been formerly occupied by the balloon contains no air molecules and thus as the balloon continues to contract—even though air molecules find their way quickly into this region next to the surface of the balloon—there are fewer molecules in this vicinity during contraction than there would be if the balloon surface were stationery. Thus, during the contraction phase there are fewer than normal air molecules in the region adjacent to the balloon's surface. As the piston moves in again and the balloon begins to expand, the process is repeated.

If we could follow the motion of a single air molecule during the process just described, we would see that as the balloon surface moves outward, the molecule is pushed outward. Similarly, as the balloon surface contracts the molecule is drawn toward the balloon. Thus, if a point on the balloon's surface is undergoing SHM a particle of the medium adjacent to it will also undergo SHM. We can speak about the movement of this air molecule in terms of its displacement, that is, how far it moves from its original position of rest. As it is moved, however, it interacts with its neighboring molecules in a fashion very roughly analogous to a row of dominos set on end. When one domino falls this causes the adjacent domino to fall and so on down the row. Although air molecules do not necessarily collide, they do exert forces on each other such that when one is displaced it in turn causes a displacement of adjacent molecules. That portion of the medium in which the particles are packed more closely together than normal is termed a region of *condensation*. That portion of the medium in which there are fewer than normal particles is termed a region of *rarefaction*. By means of the particle interaction described, these regions of condensation and rarefaction move outward away from the source as shown in Figure 2-10.

Particle velocity. If a particle of the medium is undergoing simple harmonic motion, its velocity is continuously changing. That is, referring to p. 14 and to Figure 2-11(*a*) and (*b*) we see that when the particle reaches the position of its maximum displacement its velocity is zero. Similarly as the particle passes through the midpoint of its displacement pattern the velocity is maximum. We may, if we wish, specify the magnitude of SHM (or other types of vibration) either in terms of their displacement or in terms of their velocity.

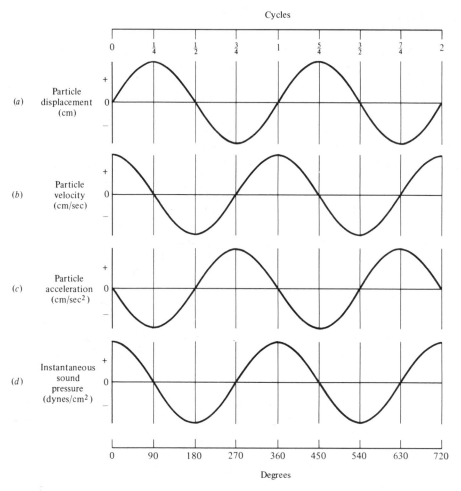

Figure 2-11 Phase characteristics of particle motion in air. The displacement of those particles immediately adjacent to the source will be in phase (0° phase difference) with the source motion. Particle velocity leads displacement by 90° while particle acceleration leads velocity by 90°. Instantaneous sound pressure in phase with particle velocity. [*From I. J. Hirsh,* The Measurement of Hearing (*New York: McGraw-Hill Book Company, 1952*), *p. 22. Reprinted by permission of the author and the publisher.*]

Particle acceleration. To be displaced, a molecule must, of course, be moved from its position of rest. In order for it to move it must change its velocity, which is to say it must be accelerated. Acceleration implies the application of a force, indeed, acceleration is equal to the applied force divided by the mass upon which the force is acting. Acceleration is maximal when velocity is changing most rapidly. In the case of SHM this occurs in the region of greatest displacement. Figure 2-11(*a*) and (*c*) show the relation between particle displacement and acceleration for SHM.

Thus we see that sound waves can be specified by particle displacement and its various time derivatives, i. e., velocity and acceleration. For a particular form of motion, such as SHM, the relations between these measures are fixed as indicated in Figure 2-11. As we will see the choice of which of these three measures we use to specify the magnitude of the sound wave depends in part upon our choice of measuring instruments. Some instruments respond to particle velocity, others to acceleration, still others to aspects of sound wave magnitude we have not yet discussed.

Pressure. As indicated in previous discussion and as shown in Figure 2-10, a disturbance in the medium propagates outward, away from the source. This disturbance can be viewed in terms of the local density of the medium. Those regions in which the molecules are pushed together (condensation) have a greater density than those portions of the medium in which the molecules are less closely packed (rarefaction). Pressure is related to the number of air molecules per unit volume. The larger this number, the greater the pressure. Pressure is also a measure of force divided by the area over which the force is applied, such as lbs/in² or dynes/cm². Because of its condensation and rarefaction phases, a sound wave represents a change above and below atmospheric pressure. Thus, the magnitude of a sound wave may be thought of in terms of pressure variations as well as in terms of particle motion. Figure 2-11(*d*) shows the phase of pressure variations relative to that of various particle motion characteristics.

Energy. The physical concept of energy relates to the capacity for doing work. *Work* is defined in terms of the force applied multiplied by the distance through which it must act. The energy of a vibrating system is the sum of its potential and kinetic energy. The *potential energy* is the work done in moving a mass (perhaps a molecule) from its position of rest. *Kinetic energy* is defined by the product of the mass of a particle multiplied by the square of its velocity. Thus for a particle undergoing SHM, the total energy is given by either the potential energy when the displacement is greatest (at which point it has no velocity), or the kinetic energy when the velocity is greatest (at which point it has no displacement).

Power. The concept of power represents an extension of the idea of energy; specifically *power* is the energy expended per unit time. For example, if energy is expressed in joules, then joules/sec is a measure of power. A *joule* is 10,000,000 ergs. An *erg* is the force, in dynes, required to move an object a distance of 1 cm. A *dyne* is the force required to cause a mass of 1 gm to be accelerated to 1 cm/sec².

Intensity. The term *intensity* is often used to convey the concept of the magnitude of a sound. This in some ways is an improper usage of the term since, in acoustics, intensity refers to a particular aspect of the magnitude. Specifically, intensity is related to energy flow (power) per unit area.

If the energy radiated by the source is constant and if the source, like our balloon, provides a spherical wave, the intensity of the sound wave diminishes as it moves away from the source. Actually it decreases as the square of the distance from the source and this relation is referred to as the *inverse square law*. This relation derives from simple geometry in that the same amount of energy from the source is spread out over an increasingly larger area as the wave moves out from the source.

Decibels. The faintest sound to which the human auditory system can respond is a sound pressure of about 0.0002 dynes/cm². The most intense sound that it can tolerate is approximately 2,000 dynes/cm². This represents a ratio of ten million to one. In order to free ourselves of the inconvenience of dealing with large numbers such as represented by ten million, a short cut notation has been developed which is called the *decibel*. It is principally through the use of logarithms, which are part of the decibel notation, that we avoid the use of large numbers. Table 2-2 illustrates this. In the left column, corresponding to each of these numbers, 10 is raised to some power. That is, the number 100 is equal to 10 multiplied by 10, or 10 raised to the second power; 1,000 is equal to $10 \times 10 \times 10$ or 10^3. From these examples we see that each entry in this column is an indication of the number of times 10 must be multiplied by itself in order to equal the required number. In the right column we have written only those powers that appeared in the middle column, that is, the power to which 10 must be raised in order to equal the number. The numbers in the right column are the *logarithms* of the corresponding numbers in the left column. Thus, we see that a logarithm is the

Table 2-2 Relation between a number, its equivalent representation as a power of 10, and its logarithm$_{10}$.

Number	10 Raised to power	Logarithm$_{10}$
1	10^0	0
10	10^1	1
100	10^2	2
1,000	10^3	3
10,000	10^4	4
100,000	10^5	5
1,000,000	10^6	6
10,000,000	10^7	7

power to which 10 must be raised in order to equal the particular number. Specifically, these logarithms that we have just described are logarithms to the base 10 (written $\log_{10}$). In other words, if 10 is the number that is being raised to a particular power, then 10 is the base of the logarithm. Other bases could be, and are, used in other mathematical applications but since base 10 is used in the decibel notation we will consider only that.

It is clear that we have not included all possible numbers in the left column of Table 2-2; for example, 90 has not been included. We can, however, approximate the value of the logarithm corresponding to the number 90 by noting that 90 lies between 10 and 100 in the left column. This means that its logarithm is between 1 and 2. For the logarithm to be between 1 and 2 it must have some fractional part; it will not be a whole number as are all our entries in the right column. In fact, a logarithm consists of two parts, a whole number portion such as shown in Table 2-2 and which is referred to as the *characteristic*, and a fractional portion called the *mantissa*, which for all the entries in Table 2-2 is 0. The *characteristic* of the logarithm relates to the placement of the decimal point in its corresponding number. In other words, if a logarithim has a characteristic of one, this means it corresponds to a number which has two decimal digits. Fortunately the values of logarithms have been tabled and all we need to do to find the logarithm of a number is refer to a table of logarithms. The tabled value will be the mantissa of the number and we must then, by inspection, assign the characteristic based on the principles that we have just reviewed. For example, if we wish to find the logarithm of the number 90 we examine a table of logarithms, enter the table using the number 9, find the mantissa corresponding to that number, which is the fractional part of the logarithm. By observing that the number 90 has two decimal digits we know immediately that the characteristic is one. Let us now determine the logarithm for the number 900,000. Again enter the same table of logarithms with the number 9, find the mantissa which, of course, is precisely the same one that we found before, and it again forms the fractional portion of the logarithm. The characteristic is fixed by noting that there are six decimal digits in the number indicating the characteristic is 5. Table 2-3 illustrates the process we have just described.

Table 2-3   Use of characteristic and mantissa in specification of $\mathrm{logarithm}_{10}$ of a number.

Number		Mantissa from table	Digits in number	Characteristic	Logarithm to base $_{10}$
9	9×10^0	954	1	0	0.954
90	9×10^1	954	2	1	1.954
900	9×10^2	954	3	2	2.954
9,000	9×10^3	954	4	3	3.954
90,000	9×10^4	954	5	4	4.954
900,000	9×10^5	954	6	5	5.954

Originally a unit called the bel was developed, but it was found to be too large a unit to work with conveniently and therefore, a unit one tenth as large was devised which was known as a decibel (dB). The decibel is defined by the following relations

Energy or Power   Sound Pressure

(1)   No. of dB $= 10 \log_{10} \dfrac{\text{Energy}_1}{\text{Energy}_0}$ (2)   No. of dB $= 20 \log_{10} \dfrac{\text{Pressure}_1}{\text{Pressure}_0}$

Thus although the principles are identical, a different constant is used in each case since pressure is related to the square of sound energy or power. The decibel notation can be used for many things in addition to sound pressure or sound power, but since this is a chapter on acoustics we present decibels in this context.

The decibel has two important characteristics. First, it is a ratio, and for a ratio to have meaning it is necessary that it have some reference value. The referent is indicated by the subscript zero in the equation. The reason for this is clear when we think of a ratio used in more familiar context. If we say "John is twice as tall as," we recognize that the term twice implies a ratio and yet the phrase has no meaning unless we specify who or what John is twice as tall as. If we said "John is twice as tall as Suzie," we have given a reference and we have provided meaning to the ratio. In a similar way a reference should be specified when we speak of decibels. We should always specify the sound power or sound pressure which appears in the denominator of the fraction. In the case of sound pressure there are several standard reference values, one of them is 0.0002 dynes/cm². We may use any sound pressure we wish as the reference as long as we state its value. The other important characteristic of the decibel is that it is basically a logarithm and as such has all the properties of logarithms. For example, if we wish to know the sound pressure of two sounds which are of the same frequency, in phase, and both expressed in decibels relative to some common reference, it might seem that the appropriate thing to do is to add their decibel values. In other words, if we have a sound of 60 dB and another sound of 60 dB, both relative to 0.0002 dynes/cm², we might think that combining these two sounds would produce a sound of 120 dB relative to the same reference. This is simply not so. Logarithms, and hence decibels, do not combine in this fashion. The sum is actually 66 dB.

Although it is possible to compute the decibel values for any given ratio of sound pressure, it is sometimes laborious to do so therefore those who use decibels often find it convenient to use quick approximations. Table 2-4

Table 2-4 Some decibel conversions useful in approximations.

Sound pressure ratio	2:1	10:1
dB	6	20

provides a few key decibel values which can be used to approximate the decibel value for any set of sound pressure ratios. Examples of the approximation procedure are shown in Table 2-5. These examples are self-explanatory except perhaps for noting that ratios less than one are treated as if they were greater than one, but are assigned a negative dB value.

Table 2-5 Sample conversions of sound pressure ratios to dB using relations shown in Table 2-4.

Process	Examples	
Sound pressure ratio	40 to 1	1 to 800
Factor	2 × 2 × 10	2 × 2 × 2 × 10 × 10
Convert to dB, factor by factor	6 + 6 + 20	6 + 6 + 6 + 20 + 20
Combine dB values	+32	−58

Sound transmission

Propagation velocity. As we have noted, a sound wave moves away from the source through the medium. It does so at a certain speed. This speed through the medium is determined solely by characteristics of the medium. It is in no way dependent upon the characteristics of the source. In general the speed of sound, c measured in cm/sec, is given by

$$c = \sqrt{\frac{E}{\rho}}$$

where E is a measure of elasticity of the medium in dynes/cm^2, ρ is the density of the medium in g/cm^3. *Density* is a measure of mass per unit volume. *Elasticity* is the ratio of stress to strain, where *stress* is the restoring force per unit area and *strain* is a measure of the deformation produced by the applied stress. For example, if a wire of length l and cross-sectional area a is clamped at one end and a force F applied to the other as shown in Figure 2-12 the wire stretches (deforms) by an amount d. Thus

$$E = \frac{\text{stress}}{\text{strain}} = \frac{F/a}{d/l}$$

In other materials the manner of the application of the force and measurement of the deformation may vary from the example, but the same principles apply.

Table 2-6 shows the velocity of sound propagation through a number of different media. Also shown are typical elasticity and density figures for each medium. We can see that in air sound travels approximately 1,100 ft/sec. While this seems rapid it is relatively slow compared to the speed of light which is 196×10^6 miles/sec.

Wavelength. If we were able to take a snapshot of a sound wave as it propagates outward from a source we might see something which approximates the situation shown in Figure 2-10, p. 22. Here we see that there are concentric circles of rarefaction and condensation centered about the source.

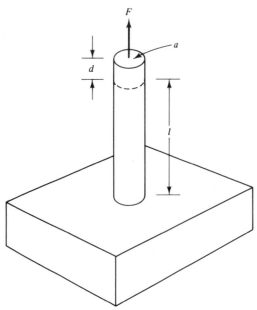

Figure 2-12 Specification of the elasticity of a wire. The wire of cross-sectional area, *a*, is fixed at one end and a force, *F*, applied. The wire originally of length, *l*, elongates by distance, *d*.

This wave motion is in many ways similar to what we can observe in a puddle of water. As a pebble is thrown into the puddle a wave of disturbance in the medium, which in this case is water, moves outward from the source. If the source was not a pebble, but was instead your finger and if your finger was dipped repeatedly into the puddle, then a wave would be formed each time your finger was dipped. Thus, if your finger was dipped periodically, a series of concentric rings, or waves, would form, moving outward away from the source in almost exactly the same manner as shown in Figure 2-10. A quantity which is very useful in describing wave motion, whether that of a sound

Table 2-6 Speed of sound and physical properties of selected materials.

Material	Elasticity	Density	Velocity	
	(dynes/cm²)	gm/cm³	cm/sec($\times 10^4$)	ft/sec
air*	1.4×10^6	1.29×10^{-3}	3.31×10^4	1,087
aluminum	7.1×10^{11}	2.7	51.2×10^4	16,810
copper	11.2×10^{11}	8.9	35.5×10^4	11,660
hydrogen*	1.4×10^6	$.09 \times 10^{-3}$	12.7×10^4	4,165
steel	17.2×10^{11}	7.8	47.0×10^4	15,434
lead	1.38×10^{11}	11.3	11.0×10^4	3,610
water†	0.2×10^{11}	1.0	14.3×10^4	4,695

* normal pressure, 0°C
† 15°C

wave or water wave, is a quantity called *wavelength*. In our puddle example wavelength is given by the distance between two adjacent crests, or two adjacent troughs, or any set of corresponding points on adjacent waves. The same measurements may be made with a sound wave with respect to the distance between adjacent regions of maximum rarefaction, maximum condensation, or intermediate points. Wavelength is a measure of this distance. What factors determine the wavelength of propagated wave motion? In our puddle example these factors may perhaps be seen most clearly. If your finger is dipped at a constant rate, the separation of the adjacent waves will depend upon the speed of wave propagation. The more rapidly the waves move, the further out the first wave will be by the time the second is generated by the second finger dipping. Thus, one factor which determines wavelength is the speed of propagation of the wave. Now, if the speed of propagation is constant, the more rapidly you dip your finger, the more closely spaced the waves will be since the first wave will have had less chance to move away from the source. We can formalize the relations we have just described into the following equation:

$$\lambda = \frac{c}{f}$$

where λ is wavelength measured in cm, c is the velocity of wave propagation in cm/sec, and f is the frequency of the source in Hz. Just to get a feel for the dimension of the wavelength of a sound wave in air, assume that the source frequency is 1100 Hz and recall that the speed of sound in air is about 1100 ft/sec; thus λ in this instance is 1 ft. Wavelength is a function both of media and source characteristics because the speed of propagation depends upon the medium and the frequency depends upon the source.

Acoustic impedance. Acoustic impedance, Z, may be thought of as relating to that characteristic of the medium that impedes the flow of sound waves. It is comprised of two parts, resistance and reactance. The acoustic resistance, R_A, is that part of the impedance that is associated with the dissipation of energy. The reactive portion of the impedance is complex and is that component associated with the effective mass and stiffness of the medium. The following equations define Z and R_A where both are expressed in ohms:

$$Z = \frac{p}{U}, \qquad R_A = \frac{\rho c}{S}$$

where p is the acoustic pressure in dynes/cm^2 on a surface of area S specified in cm^2, U is the volume velocity in cm^3/sec at that surface, ρ is the density of the medium in g/cm^3, and c is the velocity of the wave in cm/sec.

Impedance is a very important concept which aids in providing insight into acoustic phenomena. For example, when a sound wave strikes a wall it is at least partially reflected. It can be shown that the reflection is due to the change of the acoustic resistance of the medium. That is, the acoustic resistance of air is one value, the acoustic resistance of the wall is another value. Thus when a sound wave comes to this change in acoustical resistance, a portion of that wave's energy will be reflected. We will see additional applications of this concept in our discussion of sound sources. For example, in a source comprised of tubes with open and closed ends reflections take place at both ends whether open or closed because these conditions represent a change in acoustic resistance. Another example of a similar kind occurs if a sound source is located in an air medium while the receiver is located under water. The energy reaching the receiver will be much less in this instance than in a situation where the receiver is in the same medium as the source. The two media have different acoustic resistances and consequently a substantial amount of the sound energy is reflected at the boundary between the two media.

Standing waves

If a sound is located within an enclosure, such as a room, some of the sound impinging upon the walls will be reflected. In such a situation all points in the enclosure are acted upon by two sound waves, the direct wave from the source and the reflected wave from the wall. The sound pressure at any given point in the enclosure is simply the sum of the pressures associated with each wave. Although the direct and the reflected waves are themselves moving, the pattern of rarefactions and condensations formed by their interaction is stationary. This stationary pattern is referred to as a *standing wave*. The positions of the regions of rarefaction and condensation are primarily determined by the frequency of the source and the velocity of propagation of the sound wave. If the sound source produces a sinusoidal wave, the enclosure will be filled by alternate regions of rarefaction and condensation which will themselves be sinusoidally distributed between the source and the reflecting surface. It should be added that there may be as many reflected waves as there are reflecting surfaces and consequently very complex standing wave patterns may exist.

Standing waves are particularly important in the practical areas of acoustics such as room acoustics and the production of sound.

Resonance

Resonance is a very general phenomenon occurring in mechanical, electrical, acoustical and other systems. An example of resonance in a mechanical

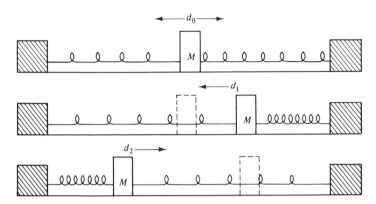

Figure 2-13 Mechanical resonance. Mass, M, initially displaced from its position of rest, d_0, on a frictionless surface oscillates between positions d_1 and d_2. The frequency of oscillation is determined by the mass and the stiffness of the springs connecting the mass to the rigid supports.

system is the continued vibration of an object after initial displacement, such as the vibration of a string of a musical instrument after it is plucked. In a mechanical system, resonance depends on the interaction of stiffness and mass of the vibrating object. This concept is illustrated in Figure 2-13. Assume that we have a mass M resting on a frictionless surface. The mass is connected to two springs each of which in turn is connected to separate rigid supports. Initially the mass is drawn to the right to position d_1 and released, at this point the spring on the left is stretched while the spring on the right is lax. Consequently a force is exerted due to the stiffness of the stretched spring such that the mass is pulled to the left relative to its original position of rest and goes to position d_2. At this point the right spring is stretched and left is lax and consequently the mass is pulled back to the right. The frequency of oscillation, that is, the frequency with which this action is repeated, depends on the stiffness of the springs and the mass involved. A stiff spring is one which shows little deformation (lengthening in this case) as a result of a given applied force. In general, the greater the mass the lower the frequency of vibration. Similarly, the greater the stiffness, the higher the rate of vibration. The frequency of vibration in this case is termed the resonant or natural frequency of the system. Theoretically, these vibrations would continue forever, except that it is impossible to find a frictionless surface along which the mass may slide and, indeed, there is some friction internal to the spring when it provides the restoring action which we have described. As a consequence, energy is gradually dissipated through these frictional forces. After a period of time the oscillations diminish and eventually cease. These forces which act in opposition to oscillation are called *damping forces*. The larger the frictional forces, the more rapidly the oscillations are *damped*.

Air-filled cavities

Resonance of air-filled cavities is of special interest to students of the speech and hearing processes. The speech mechanism depends heavily on such resonance effects for the production of speech sounds. The hearing mechanisms' sensitivity is determined in part by the resonance of the external auditory meatus. Air, or more generally, fluid-filled cavities can be thought of as sound sources or as modifiers of existing sound energy. In the former case energy is delivered to the resonator and it in turn converts that to vibratory motion which, when communicated to a medium, results in a sound wave. In the later case, if a sound wave already exists and impinges upon a resonator, the wave's characteristics may be changed in that energy may be extracted from the wave. The resonant characteristic of air-filled cavities is discussed in detail on p. 45. The properties of air-filled cavities as modifiers of existing sound wave will be described briefly in this section.

Helmholtz resonators. If the dimensions of an acoustical system are small compared with the wavelength of the sound, the motion of the medium in the acoustic system is analogous to that of a mechanical system having the elements of mass, stiffness, and resistance. The simple Helmholtz resonator is an important acoustic system which may be discussed in terms of a simple mechanical analog. Such a resonator is shown in Figure 2-14 and consists of

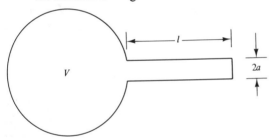

Figure 2-14   Helmholtz resonator. Enclosed volume, *V*, serves as the stiffness element and the medium in the neck of length, *l*, and radius, *a*, as the mass element.

a rigidly enclosed volume *V* communicating with the external medium through a small opening of radius *a* and length *l*. The gas in the opening, which is usually air, is considered to move together as a unit and provides the mass element of the system. The pressure of the air within the cavity of the resonator changes as it is alternately compressed and expanded by the movement of air through the opening. This compressibility provides the stiffness element. At the opening there is radiation of sound into the surrounding medium which leads to the dissipation of acoustic energy and thus provides the resistance element. The resonant frequency, f_0 in Hz, of the Helmholtz resonator is given by the following equation:

$$f_0 = \frac{c}{2\pi} \cdot \sqrt{\frac{S}{l'V}}$$

where S is the area of the neck of the resonator (πa^2) in cm², c is the velocity of sound in cm/sec, l' is the effective length of the neck in cm, and V is volume of the resonator in cm³.

It is important to note that the resonant frequency of the Helmholtz resonator is not dependent upon the shape of the volume but only on the volume itself. It should be added, parenthetically, that standing wave patterns (see p. 32) may develop within the cavity and will contribute their own natural frequencies. The standing wave pattern, however, is not harmonically related to the resonant frequency of the cavity and is dependent upon the dimensions of the cavity rather than the volume.

Also associated with the concept of resonance is sharpness of tuning. Figure 2-15 shows what is known as a *general resonance curve*. Such a curve may be obtained by considering the application of a periodic driving force to a resonant system such as a Helmholtz resonator. The graph shows that if the frequency of the periodic disturbance is far removed from the natural (resonant) frequency of the resonant system, little energy will be transferred from the source to the resonator. On the other hand, as the frequency of the source approaches that of the resonant system, an increasingly large amount of the energy is imparted to the resonant system. The exact form of this

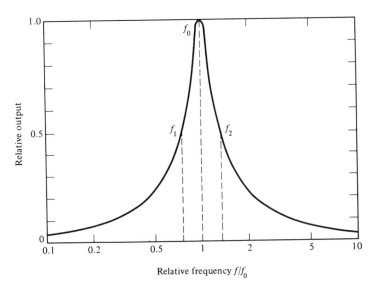

Figure 2-15 General resonance curve. This resonance curve is typical of all resonant systems. For example, in Figure 2-13 if a SHM force was applied to the mass, the displacement of the mass would be greatest when the frequency of the applied force corresponded to the natural resonant frequency, f_0. Relative frequencies f_1 and f_2 are the frequencies at which the amplitude is 0.5 of that at f_0. An index of the sharpness of tuning is the frequency separation of f_1 and f_2. For highly tuned, lightly damped systems f_1 and f_2 are close together.

function depends on the frictional properties of the system; the greater the resistance, the greater the damping and the broader the tuning. In the Helmholtz resonator the resistive component is related to the cross-sectional area of the neck and, in general, the sharpest tuning is obtained with a small opening and a long neck.

Tube resonance. An enclosure may have a configuration which is very different from that of a Helmholtz resonator and still provide evidence of resonance. For example, if we modify the Helmholtz resonator so that its opening has essentially the same diameter as the cavity, but the cavity length becomes very long in respect to the width, we approach the situation in which the cavity is in the shape of a tube or pipe. The resonance characteristics of such enclosures are discussed in connection with the use of a tube or pipe as a sound source on p. 46.

Room Acoustics

It is not possible in this chapter to provide detail with respect to the acoustical characteristics of a large enclosure such as a room. We will make two points, however. First, standing wave patterns will develop if a periodic source and reflective surfaces are present. Standing waves may develop along any dimension of the room for which reflecting surfaces are present. The significance of the presence of standing waves may be considerable in a situation in which one wishes to use a room to test hearing, for example. Sound pressure is likely to be very different at different points in the room.

Another important characteristic is the reverberation time of the room. The *reverberation time* is the time required for the sound generated by an impulsive stimulus, such as the clap of the hand, to decay to some fixed fraction of its original value. If the surfaces of the room are highly reflective with little energy being absorbed, then that sound will continue to bounce off the reflective surfaces for a long time after it is initiated. Under these conditions reverberation time is long. In contrast to this, if the walls absorb a considerable portion of the sound incident upon them, reverberation time will be short. Under this later condition the standing wave patterns would be minimized since the energy loss with multiple reflections would be very large.

There are optimum reverberation times for specific room use. For example, an auditorium which is to be used for lecture purposes requires a shorter reverberation time than does an auditorium to be used for music. In addition to the absorptive characteristics of the room surfaces, reverberation time is also influenced by the volume of the room. For use in speech and hearing studies, room acoustics are important for two reasons: the first has already been mentioned with respect to hearing testing; the second is the influence of room acoustics on the recording of speech samples. It is presumed that when speech samples are recorded on magnetic tape, the obtained recordings reflect the characteristics of the speaker. This is true only to the degree that the room acoustics do not influence the recorded speech. Obviously, if the reverberation time is long the sound reaching the microphone will be that not only directly from the speaker, but a substantial portion will be that reflected from the walls as well. This phenomenon may be a critical consideration in both hearing testing and sound recording.

Sound Sources

Sound sources are objects whose vibratory motion is used as a sound generator. It is possible to classify common sound sources into major categories: strings, bars, membranes or plates, and air columns.

Strings

In our discussion of the vibration of strings we will consider that form of vibration in which the elements of the string oscillate in a plane perpendicular to the line of the string. This form is known as *transverse vibration.* It is that type of string motion with which we are the most familiar, examples of which are seen in stringed musical instruments such as the violin, harp, or piano. In our considerations of the vibrations of strings we will assume that we are dealing with an "ideal" string which a) is perfectly uniform along its length, b) is perfectly flexible, that is, it possesses no stiffness, and c) does not change its length while it is undergoing vibration. A long, thin, tightly-stretched wire held firmly between two massive supports fulfills these conditions quite well. How does such a string vibrate?

For vibration to occur in an actual sound generator such as a string, several conditions must be met. First, energy must be delivered to initiate the vibration and second, if the vibration is to be sustained, it must continue to be delivered at a sufficient rate to compensate for energy loss through damping. Damping, you recall, is the process by which energy is lost in a vibrating system. In some sound sources it occurs through internal frictional forces within the vibration material and dissipates as heat. However, for a string, energy loss occurs mostly due to the interaction with the medium that surrounds the string, usually air, which in fact leads to the production of a sound wave (see p. 23). Second, the system must possess a restoring force, that is, a force which will tend to return the string to its position of rest. For a string the restoring force is the applied tension.

Specifically, how is energy delivered to the string and how is it set into motion? Let us assume that the string is initially displaced (plucked) at some particular spot along its length and then released. Such a situation is shown diagrammatically in Figure 2-16. The position of the bulge in panel (*a*) represents the initial displacement. As the string is released its restoring force

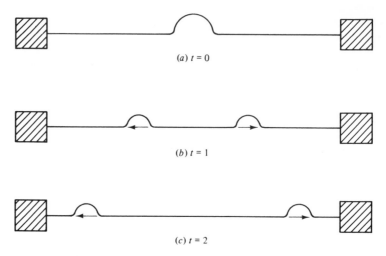

(a) t = 0

(b) t = 1

(c) t = 2

Figure 2-16 Propagation of a transverse disturbance along a stretched string. The initial disturbance occurs at $t = 0$, and as time progresses ($t = 1$, $t = 2$) the original disturbance breaks into separate disturbances and each moves in opposite directions.

causes it to move back toward its position of rest, and in so doing the vibratory motion is initiated. If we could observe the motion of the strings through a slow motion camera, we would see that the initial displacement breaks into two separate motions, each moving with constant speed in opposite directions toward the ends of the strings. This situation is shown in Figure 2-16(*b*) and at a short time later in (*c*). As these displacements reach the end of the string, they are reflected back toward the middle of the string much in the same fashion that an ocean wave, after the striking of a sea wall, is reflected back toward the open ocean. The consequence of this reflection is that the actual amplitude of transverse vibration at any position along the string is the sum of the original displacement plus the reflected motion from both ends of the string. This situation is directly analogous to the generation of standing wave patterns (see p. 32) in a reverberent enclosure. The same principles apply and the results are equivalent. The velocity with which the disturbance from the original displacement moves toward the ends of the string increases as the string tension increases, and decreases as the mass per unit length of the string increases. This velocity, together with the string length determines how long it takes for the string displacement to reach the end, be reflected, return to any given point. This in turn regulates how often a given point on the string "bobs" up and down, which of course, relates to the frequency of vibration. These matters may be formalized in the expression

$$f = \frac{1}{2l} \cdot c = \frac{1}{2l} \cdot \sqrt{\frac{T}{m}}$$

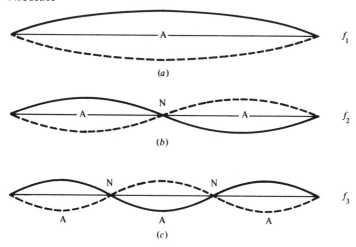

Figure 2-17 Patterns of nodes and antinodes on a vibrating string. The drawing, from top to bottom, represents the fundamental mode, second and third modes of vibration, respectively.

where f is the frequency of vibration in Hz, c is the velocity of the transverse wave in cm/sec, l is the length of the string in cm, T is the string's tension in dynes, and m is the string's mass per unit length in g/cm.[1]

Figure 2-17(a) shows one form of the displacement pattern that might exist for a string as the motion of the string is successively reflected from each of the ends. The points at which the string is clamped, of course, by definition can undergo no vibration; these points are called *nodes*. The points at which the maximum vibration occurs is called an *antinode*. In Figure 2-17(b) and (c) additional patterns of vibration are shown in which we can see that nodes may occur at other positions along the string in addition to the end points. These vibration patterns are characterized by the number of antinodes present being f_1, f_2, and f_3 in Figure 2-17(a), (b), and (c). Any number of antinodes may be present, but since the string is clamped at both ends the number of antinodes can never be less than one and, in general, must be an integer rather than a fractional number. Since the frequency of vibration is related to the length of the string between nodes, it follows that if there are two nodes rather than one the string is effectively one-half as long and the frequency twice as great. With three nodes the frequency is three times as great. Thus more than one frequency may be generated simultaneously with a string and all frequencies will be integral multiples (harmonics) of the

[1] In this and all succeeding equations which define the frequency of a vibrating system, the frequency is determined by two factors. First is the speed with which the disturbance moves through the material, c in this case. Second is the effective length of the system, that is, that distance the disturbance must travel before and after reflection in order that it arrives back at the same position in the original phase relation, $2l$ in this case. All equations will be written so that you can differentiate these two contributors to frequency of vibration.

frequency produced in the single antinode case (fundamental). The pattern of vibration that results in the fundamental frequency is called the fundamental or first mode; that for the second harmonic, the second mode and so on. The principles which describe the vibration of the strings may be summarized as follows: (1) For a given string and a given tension, the longer the string, the lower the frequency; (2) For a string of given length and material, the frequency varies as the square root of the tension applied, that is, the greater the tension, the higher the frequency; (3) The frequency of vibration of strings of the same length and the same tension varies inversely as the square root of the mass per unit length of the string, that is, assuming uniform density of the string, the thicker the string, the lower its frequency.

Bars

If we maintain the length of a wire and gradually increase its diameter eventually we come to the point where the added diameter has increased the stiffness of the wire so that it can no longer be considered an ideal string. At this point it is conventional to speak of the object as a bar rather than a string. The vibrational characteristics of bars differ in some important respects from those of strings. For example, in an ideal bar at least, the vibrational patterns are unaffected by the tension and influenced primarily by the stiffness. Transverse vibrations of bars may occur which are similar to the transverse vibrations in strings as discussed above, but in addition, longitudinal vibrations and torsional (twisting) vibrations can also occur in bars. Longitudinal vibrations of bars are quite often utilized in the generation of sound. However, in this chapter we will concern ourselves only with the transverse vibrations of ideal bars. A tuning fork is an example of such a sound source.

The theory of transverse vibration of bars, even when simplified, is still very complex in comparison with the theory of perfectly flexible strings. For example, in the case of strings, the disturbance travels along the string with the velocity independent of the wavelength, but in the case of bars this is not so. A bar clamped at both ends may, like a string, form one or more loops or antinodes, but the laws which regulate the frequency of the successive modes of vibration are entirely different in the two cases. The ideal bar that we will consider is assumed to be straight, uniform in crosssection and density, and not subject to tension or compression. We will also assume that the amplitude of vibration is small. We will further assume that if the bar is bent, the length of the bent bar is the same as in the unbent condition. We will consider four types of bar vibrations: (1) the bar is free at both ends; (2) the bar is clamped at both ends (we will see that the same relations obtain for both (1) and (2), (3) the bar is clamped at one end only, and (4) the bar is supported at both ends.

Bar free at both ends. With the bar free at both ends we find the frequency of vibration, f in Hz, is given by the following equation:

$$f = \frac{(4s - 1)^2}{8} \cdot \frac{\kappa}{l^2} \cdot \sqrt{\frac{E}{\rho}}$$

where s is the mode number $(1, 2, 3, \ldots, n)$, κ is the radius of gyration in cm,[2] l is the length of the bar in cm, ρ is the density of the material in g/cm³, and E is Young's elastic modulus in g/cm-sec². The frequencies of the successive symmetrical modes of vibration of the bar are proportional to $(4s - 1)^2$ or 3^2, 7^2, 11^2, 15^2, etc. The overtones, therefore, are not harmonics as in the case of the vibration of the string.

The form of the curve assumed by the bar vibrating in its fundamental or simplest mode subject to the conditions that we are describing is shown in Figure 2-18. The two nodes in this case occur at distances of 0.224l from the lengths of the bar.

Bar clamped at both ends. For a bar clamped at both ends we find the same series of vibrational frequencies as obtained for a bar free at both ends, however the arrangement of nodal positions is different.

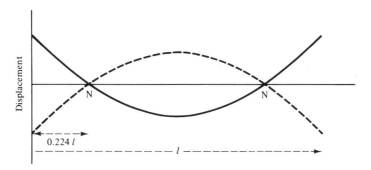

Figure 2-18   Free-free bar undergoing transverse vibration in its fundamental mode. Each node occurs at a distance 0.224l from the ends of the bar.

Bar clamped at one end only. If a bar is clamped only at one end then clearly at the clamped end no transverse displacement can occur while the other end is not similarly constrained. This, in fact, is the case and we can summarize the situation by showing the vibration pattern in Figure 2-19. Again the overtones are not harmonics of the fundamental frequency.

---

[2] κ is a function of the cross sectional form of the bar; for example, if the bar is of a circular section of radius a, then $\kappa^2 = a^2/4$. If the bar is rectangular then $\kappa^2 = T^2/12$ where T is the thickness of the bar at the point of vibration.

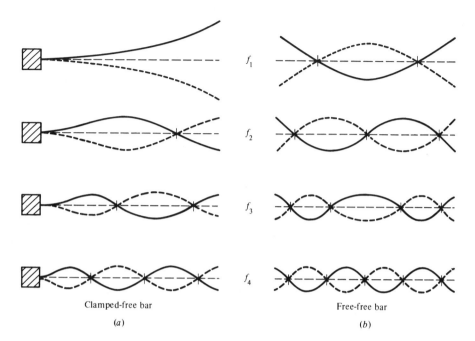

Clamped-free bar | Free-free bar

(a) | (b)

Figure 2-19 Patterns of transverse vibration in bars free at both ends (*b*) or clamped at one end and free at the other (*a*). The nodes are positioned differently in (*a*) and (*b*) and the frequencies of the overtones are also different although both cases represent a nonharmonic series.

A bar clamped at one end may be tuned to a given frequency in a number of ways. The frequency of vibration may be lowered by either increasing the mass near the free end or by reducing the cross section of the bar near the clamped end. In practice a bar may be tuned by means of a sliding collar which is clamped rigidly in the position corresponding to the required frequency. The nearer this sliding weight approaches the free end of the bar the lower will be the bar frequency of vibration.

Table 2-7(a) Characteristics of transverse vibrations of bars free at both ends (see Figure 2-19(*b*)).

No. of tones	No. of nodes	Distance of nodes from end of 1 cm bar	Relative frequency	Ratio of frequency to fundamental
1	2	0.22, 0.78	3^2	1
2	3	0.13, 0.5, 0.87	5^2	2.8
3	4	0.09, 0.36, 0.64, 0.91	7^2	5.4
4	5	0.07, 0.28, 0.5, 0.72, 0.93	9^2	8.9

Table 2-7(b) Characteristics of transverse vibrations of bars clamped at one end and free at the other end (see Figure 2-19(a)).

No. of tones	No. of nodes	Distance of nodes from end of 1 cm bar	Relative frequency	Ratio of frequency to fundamental
1	0		1.2^2	1
2	1	0.23	3^2	6.2
3	2	0.13, 0.49	5^2	17.5
4	3	0.09, 0.36, 0.64	7^2	34.4

Bar supported at both ends. If a bar is supported at both ends we have a condition in which the bar is laid across two knife edge supports but not clamped. As is the case for all bars vibrating tranversely, frequency of vibration, f, is proportional to $(\kappa/l^2)((\sqrt{E/\rho})$, but specifically in this case

$$f = \frac{\pi s^2}{2} \cdot \frac{\kappa}{l^2} \cdot \sqrt{\frac{E}{\rho}}$$

where the symbols have the same meaning as on p. 41. In this case the frequencies of the partials are proportional to the square of the partial number and the nodes, in contrast to the other bar conditions, are equidistant as in the case of a vibrating string.

Tuning fork. In its most familiar form the tuning fork consists of a U-like structure with a prong attached at the bottom of the U. One way to understand the vibrations of a tuning fork is to consider a rod free at both ends and to recall its vibrational pattern from our earlier discussion. The next step, as shown in Figure 2-20(a), is to begin to bend the straight bar, a-a, into the form of a U. It can be shown that one of the effects of such a bending is to move the nodal points more toward the center of the bar as in c-c. If a prong is added in the region at the bottom of the U which corresponds to the antinode, then, as illustrated in Figure 2-20(b), the prong will move in an up and down direction. In practice, the tuning fork is mounted on a box which serves as a sounding board and the energy of the vibrating tines is transferred through the prong to the sounding board. The efficiency of the source as a radiator is much increased by the use of the sounding board. It is important to emphasize that the same principles which applied to the vibration of a straight rod apply to the vibrations of the tuning fork.

Membranes, diaphragms, and plates

Our consideration of the vibration of strings and bars constituted a consideration of single dimension vibration. Both strings and bars, so far as our

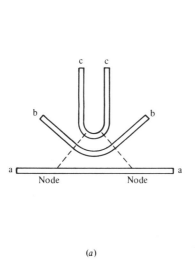
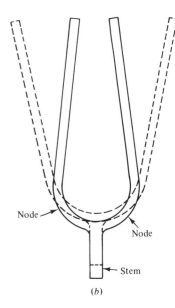

(a)   (b)

Figure 2-20 Vibrations of a tuning fork. Drawing (a) shows how the nodal points for the fundamental mode of a straight bar change as the bar is bent. Drawing (b) indicates the vibrations of the fork illustrating the placement of the stem at an antinode.

considerations are concerned, have only length. The systems included in this section are of two dimensions, they have not only length, but width as well. The importance of membranes, diaphragms, and plates arises from their very common use in acoustical systems such as earphones, special loudspeakers, or microphones. Perhaps of even greater concern to students of the speech and hearing process is the fact that these sources are commonly found in biological acoustic systems. For example, the vibrational characteristics of the vocal cords, the tympanic membrane (ear drum), and various cochlear structures all represent some combination of the features of membranes, diaphrams, and plates.

Membranes. Membranes are two-dimensional systems analogous to a string in that membranes, assumed to be perfectly flexible, uniform, and infinitesimally thick are stretched in all directions by a force which is unaffected by any transverse motion of the membrane. The detailed solution of the motion of stretched membranes is different for different shapes, rectangular, square, circular, and so forth. In most practical applications the membrane is fixed at the edge.

In a circular membrane the fundamental mode of vibration is characterized by a condition in which a single antinode is found at the middle of the membrane. The frequency of vibration, f in Hz, in this case is given by the equation

$$f = \frac{0.765}{2a} \cdot \sqrt{\frac{T}{\rho t}}$$

where a is the radius of the membrane in cm, T is the tension in dynes, ρ is the density in g/cm³, and t is the thickness of the membrane in cm. For higher modes of vibration the nodes take the form of concentric circles and the antinodes take the form of annuli located between the rings. The partials do not form a harmonic series.

Diaphragms. A diaphragm is to a membrane as a bar is to a string. That is, a diaphragm is a two-dimensional system where the stiffness (elasticity) is the dominant feature in determining the frequency of vibration and tension becomes a negligible consideration. The complete theory of a vibrating diaphragm is even more complex than that of a membrane and only approximate solutions have been obtained. The fundamental frequency of vibration, f in Hz, of a circular diaphragm clamped at the edge is estimated by the following equation

$$f = \frac{2.96}{2\pi} \cdot \frac{h}{a^2} \cdot \sqrt{\frac{E}{\rho(1 - \sigma^2)}}$$

where h is the diaphragm thickness in cm, a is the diaphragm radius in cm, E is Young's elastic modulus in g/cm-sec², ρ is diaphragm density in g/cm³, and σ is Poisson's ratio.[3] The partials are not harmonically related and the frequency of vibration is affected by the loading of the diaphragm by contact with another media such as water, or by the loading of the diaphragm by a small additional mass.

Plates. Plate is the term given to a diaphragm which is clamped at some place other than the edge, such as the middle. Their importance is perhaps marginal, but they are of historical interest at least in that bells can be considered a form of a curved plate just as a tuning fork may be considered a form of a curved bar. The vibrational patterns seen in plates are extremely complex and the mathematics which attempt to describe them is quite incomplete. In a bell as in a plate, the partials are not harmonically related.

Air columns

The simplest case of a vibrating air column within a solid enclosure is that of a parallel cylindrical pipe, such as an organ pipe, the ends of which

---

[3] Poisson's ratio is an expression of the tendency of a diaphragm to curl up sideways when it is bent lengthwise.

may be closed or open. The longitudinal vibrations of such a column of air are analogous to the corresponding vibrations in a solid bar. Usually certain assumptions are made with respect to the characteristics of the pipe, they are: (1) the diameter of the pipe is sufficiently great such that the frictional effects of the air moving within the pipe may be disregarded, (2) the diameter of the pipe is small compared to the length of the pipe and to the wavelength of the sound, (3) the walls of the pipe are rigid. In the case of an air column, the particle displacement is zero at the node and maximal at the antinode.

Pipe open at both ends. If a condensation pulse is introduced at one end of the pipe, it will be reflected from the opposite end with a reve sal of phase, that is, as a wave of rarefaction which again traverses the pipe back to the point of origin. At the origin another reflection takes place with a reversal of phase and the reflected pulse is now a condensation pulse similar to the initial pulse. Thus, the initial state of condensation is repeated after two complete traverses of the length of the pipe. This is completely analogous to the situation described on p. 38 for the vibration of strings, or on p. 40 for the vibration of bars. As was true for strings and bars, different modes of vibration can occur for air columns. The frequency, f in Hz, of these modes is given by

$$f = s \cdot \frac{1}{l} \cdot \sqrt{\frac{E}{\rho}}$$

where s is the partial number $(1, 2, 3, \ldots, n)$, l is the length of the pipe in cm, E is the elastic modulus of air in g/cm-sec^2, and ρ is the density of air in g/cm^3. The partials form a complete harmonic series, that is, as s increases, f does also in a proportional fashion.

It is important to note that the energy is radiated from the pipe at the open ends and thus damping of pipe oscillations occur. Figure 2-21(a) shows several possible modes of vibration in an open pipe. We see that in all cases of an open pipe an antinode occurs at the open end. The top drawing illustrates that for the fundamental mode of vibration a single node is located at the center of the pipe. The middle and bottom figures show the vibrational pattern of the second and third partial, respectively.

Pipe closed at one end and open at the other. In this case the initial pulse at the open end must traverse the length of the pipe four times before the cycle is repeated. This is so since the reflection of the closed end takes place without a change of phase and two reflections at the open end are necessary before the reflected pulse is restored to the initial phase. The fundamental frequency, f in cm, is therefore given when $s = 1$ in the following general relation

$$f = (2s - 1) \cdot \frac{1}{4l} \cdot \sqrt{\frac{E}{\rho}}$$

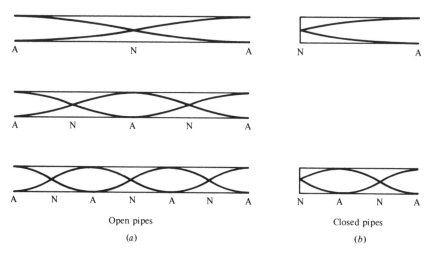

A   N   A

N   A

A   N   A   N   A

A   N   A   N   A   N   A

N   A   N   A

Open pipes

Closed pipes

(a)

(b)

Figure 2-21   Nodal patterns for the vibration of air columns.

where s is the partial number $(1, 2, 3, \ldots, n)$, l is the pipe length in cm, E is elastic modulus for air in g/cm-sec^2, and ρ is the density of air in g/cm^3. At the closed end particle displacement must be equal to zero and thus the nodal patterns are those shown in Figure 2-21(b). The top drawing shows the situation for the first partial (fundamental) and the bottom drawing shows the second partial. We can see that the effective length of the open pipe is twice that of a closed pipe of corresponding frequency. The open pipe gives a complete harmonic series while the closed pipe only gives odd harmonics of the series.

It is important to repeat that the basic characteristics of a vibrating air column are very similar to those of strings and bars in that the nodal pattern is the result of the interaction of an original disturbance and a disturbance which is reflected from the ends of the system.

ELECTRICITY

Our understanding of the basic elements of electricity is important in that laboratory generation of sound commonly makes use of electricity as the original driving source. The signal is generated by an electrical source, and controlled by electrical circuit elements. The electrical energy then drives a mechanical element such as a loudspeaker which produces sound waves.

All matter is composed of molecules which in turn are comprised of atoms. We may think of each atom as having a central nucleus around which electrons revolve. This picture of the atom is analogous to the rotation of the planets about the sun. The number of electrons in orbit in an atom varies, depending on the element; for example, hydrogen has one electron while oxygen has sixteen electrons. By convention electrons are considered as possessing a negative charge. Electrons are attracted to positively charged bodies but repelled by other electrons. Electrons can be caused to move through a conducting media, such as a metal wire, by the application of an electromotive force.

Characteristics of Electricity (Direct Current)

Charge

The negative charge on a single electron is the smallest measureable electrical unit. It represents, however, an extremely small value and for practical purposes a larger unit, the *coulomb*, has been designated. The coulomb represents the combined charge of 6.3×10^{18} electrons.

Current

Current is the rate at which electrons move in a conductor. One ampere of current is said to flow when one coulomb of charge moves past a given point in a second. This is equivalent to saying that one ampere of current flows when 6.3×10^{18} electrons move past a given point in a second. When the current flows in only one direction and does not change its value, it is called *direct current* (DC). When it changes its value or direction of flow periodically it is known as *alternating current* (AC).

Voltage

Voltage, electrical potential, or *electromotive force*, represents a capacity to do work. It causes electrons to move by imparting potential energy to them. If the electrical potential difference between two points is one volt, then in order to move one coulomb of charge from one point to the other we must expend one joule of work. As with all units of work, a joule is the product of force (acting on an object) multiplied by the distance through which that force acts. (See p. 25.) Voltage is roughly analogous to pressure in a hydraulic system.

Resistance

Some materials are composed of substances which have a large number of free electrons. That is, upon the application of an electromotive force, we can conceive of the electrons associated with atomic nuclei as leaving their orbit and moving physically from one point to another. Those materials in which this can occur are said to be good electrical conductors. By contrast, *resistance* is a measure of the opposition to electrical current flow. The unit of resistance is the ohm. One *ohm* is equal to the amount of resistance that will permit one ampere to flow when one volt is applied.

Power

If an electric current is passed through a wire, heat will be produced. When the brakes of an automobile are applied, heat is produced by the friction that occurs when the brake lining comes in contact with the brake drum. This mechanical friction, of course, is a resistance to motion as, in the same sense, is heat produced in a wire when electrical forces work against electrical resistance. The transformation of mechanical or electric energy to heat provides a common denominator with which we can define power. *Power* is the rate at which energy is expended. Thus one watt of power is equal to one joule per second.

Ohm's Law

The relationships between current, voltage, and resistance are formalized in Ohm's Law. Strictly speaking, these relations hold only for direct current and the law must be modified when considering alternating current. Ohm's Law states that current, I, is equal to the voltage applied, E, divided by the resistance, R. Figure 2-22 puts Ohm's Law in equation form and presents an illustration of its application. Power, P in watts, may be defined in terms of Ohm's Law as $P = EI$.

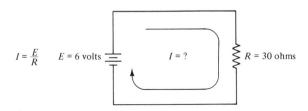

$$I = \frac{E}{R} \qquad E = 6 \text{ volts} \qquad I = ? \qquad R = 30 \text{ ohms}$$

Figure 2-22 Ohm's Law. Given a simple series circuit comprised of a DC source, E, and a resistance, R, we can find the current, I, by the equation at the left. For the values in the illustration $I = 0.2$ amperes.

Characteristics of Electricity (Alternating Current)

Inductance

When current flows through a wire a magnetic field is created. This magnetic field is a form of stored energy. We can conceive of two states: 1) no

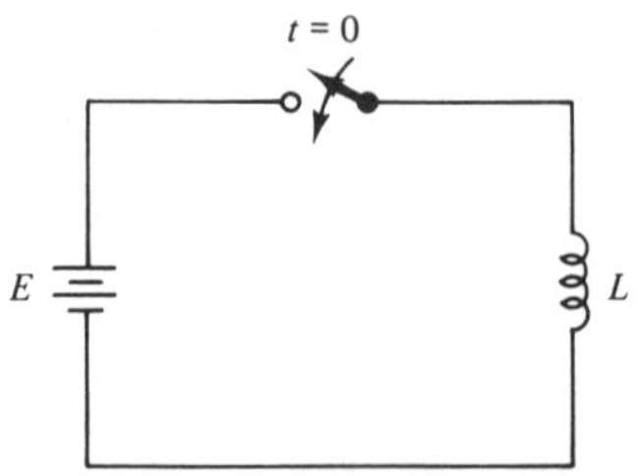

$t = 0$

Figure 2-23 Series circuit containing an inductance. The switch is closed completing the circuit, at $t = 0$. Current flow rises slowly because of the generation of a magnetic field associated with the inductance.

current flow—no magnetic field and 2) current flow—magnetic field present. The fact that energy is stored in the magnetic field can be illustrated by examining the transition between the two states. Consider the simple series circuit of Figure 2-23 consisting of a battery, switch, and a coil of wire. According to Ohm's Law, the current flow in this situation should be determined by the resistance of the wire. However, in the instant after the switch is closed to complete the circuit no current flows, but as time progresses the current rises to the value predicted by Ohm's Law. Initially, a portion of the energy being supplied by the battery is diverted to produce the magnetic field. During this time the current flow is reduced. Now let us make the other transition by opening the switch. This effectively removes the energy source (the battery) from the circuit and consequently we might expect the current flow to drop immediately to zero. Such is not the case, however, since the magnetic field was being maintained by current flow. When the current diminishes (by opening the switch) the magnetic field begins to collapse which, in turn, generates a current flow. Thus, although the switch is opened, current flow is maintained for the duration of the collapse of the magnetic field. The maintenance of this current flow across the high resistance offered by the open switch develops a high voltage which often results in an arc across the switch contacts.

If an alternating current is caused to flow in a coil of wire, each time the polarity of the current changes there will be some resistance to this change by the magnetic field that has been set up for the particular current polarity that existed previously. This resistance to current flow that we have just described is known as *inductive reactance*, X_L. This reactance is measured in ohms but, unlike electrical resistance energy, is not lost in the form of heat. Rather it is temporarily stored as energy in the magnetic field. The more rapidly the polarity changes occur in the alternating current, the greater the reactance of the coil and the less current is able to flow through the coil. This relation may be formalized by the equation

$$X_L = 2\pi f L$$

where f is frequency in Hz and L is inductance in henrys.

Capacitance

If the terminals of a battery are each connected to one member of a pair of closely spaced metal plates, current flow will initially be large. However, it will eventually cease since, according to Ohm's Law, we should expect no current flow because there is no physical connection across the plates and thus they form an infinitely high resistance. Why then was there an initial current flow? Electrons do in fact move as shown in Figure 2-24(a)

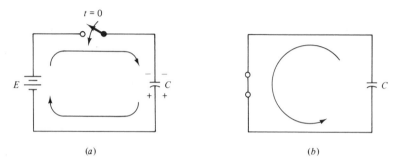

(a)   (b)

Figure 2-24 Series circuit containing capacitance. In (a) when the switch is closed at $t = 0$ current flow is initially large, but gradually ceases as a differential of electrons accumulates in the plates of the capacitor. In (b) the battery is removed and the wires from the capacitor places joined. In this case current flows until the charge on the plates is equalized.

such that an excess accumulates on the plate connected to the negative terminal while a deficit of electrons exists on the plate connected to the positive terminal. This arrangement constitutes energy storage in the form of an electrostatic field. This can be demonstrated by removing the battery and joining the wires connecting the plates as in Figure 2-24(b). At the instant the wires are joined current begins to flow and continues to do so until the number of electrons on each plate is the same, that is, until the energy storage in the electrostatic field has decayed to zero. How long the current will flow depends upon the resistance of the wires and the number of electrons stored on the plate surfaces. This ability to store energy in the form of an electric charge is known as *capacitance* and the plates that we have described are one form of a capacitor. Capacitance, C in farads, is defined by the following relation

$$C = QE$$

where Q is charge in coulombs and E is voltage in volts.

We saw that when a constant voltage was applied to the terminals of the capacitor no steady current flowed. Instead, there was brief current flow when a voltage was initially applied or removed and the plates shortened. Thus, the capacitor acts as an infinite resistance (allows no current flow) under steady state conditions. If in Figure 2-24 the battery is removed and a source of AC current substituted, the frequency of the alternation is increased as there is a greater amount of current flow. Each time the current is reversed it is as if the battery were being reconnected with opposite polarity. Since more current flows under these conditions, this implies that the effective resistance of the capacitance is decreasing. This resistance to current flow is known as *capacitive reactance* and is analogous to inductive reactance in that it represents a form of energy storage rather than energy dissipation in the form of heat. Capacitive reactance, X_C in ohms, is defined as

$$X_C = \frac{1}{2\pi} \cdot \frac{1}{fC}$$

where f is frequency in Hz and C is capacitance in farads.

Impedance

Electrical *impedance* is the total resistance to current flow and is given by the sum of the three components we have discussed: electrical resistance, inductive reactance, and capacitive reactance. In much the same fashion that displacement of a mass lags behind the applied force because of inertial effects, the current flow through an inductance lags behind the applied voltage by 90°. Thus, there is a phase difference between these two quantities. In an analogous fashion, the current flow through a capacitance leads the voltage applied by 90°, thus a phase difference also exists here. Consequently, although impedance is the sum of the quantities mentioned, they do not add in a simple fashion because of the phase differences which exist.

Resonance

Electrical *resonance* is analogous to resonance in acoustic and mechanical systems. When a voltage impulse (analogous to momentary displacement in a mechanical system) is applied to the simple series circuit of Figure 2-25(a) containing inductance, capacitance, and resistance, an oscillatory current will flow (analogous to vibratory motion). The rate of oscillation, which is called the *resonant frequency*, is approximately equal to that frequency at which the inductive reactance is equal to the capacitive reactance. The resistance in the circuit influences the resonant frequency slightly, but determines directly the duration of the oscillations (damping). The greater the resistance the shorter the time of oscillation. What is occurring in the circuit during oscillation? If the circuit is initially excited by a voltage pulse, current

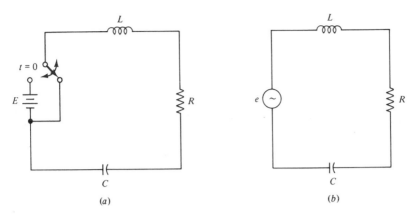

Figure 2-25 Electrical resonance in a series circuit containing resistance, inductance, and capacitance. In (a) if the switch is momentarily moved to the battery and then back to its original position, an oscillatory (AC) current will flow in the circuit. In (b) maximum current flow will occur when the frequency of e is equal to the resonance frequency of the circuit (see Figure 2-15).

is caused to flow and a magnetic field is set up by the inductance. Since the initial excitation is of short duration, after its termination the magnetic field will begin to collapse producing a current flow of its own, but of opposite polarity. This current, in turn, provides for a storage of a charge on the capacitor plate. This continues to increase until the magnetic field can provide no more current. At this point current flow in the opposite direction occurs by virtue of the charge on the capacitor. Thus, energy is alternately stored in the form of the magnetic field about the inductance and in terms of an electrostatic field on the plates of the capacitance. Such a circuit would continue to oscillate or to produce current flow of alternate polarity forever except that some resistance must inevitably exist in the wires of the circuit. Energy originally delivered to the system is gradually lost through the production of heat because of the electrical resistance, thus the amplitude of the oscillatory current flow declines eventually to zero.

If the voltage pulse in the series circuit shown in Figure 2-25(a) is replaced by an AC voltage generator as in Figure 2-25(b), we can see another manifestation of resonance. Resonance, by definition, occurs when the current flow is maximum. It will be maximum when the impedance is minimal and the impedance will be minimal when the inductive reactance is equal to the capacitive reactance. Thus if we plot current flow as a function of the frequency of the AC voltage applied, we will obtain essentially the same graph as shown in Figure 2-15. This resonant situation is again analogous to what happens in a mechanical system or in an acoustic system such as a Helmholtz resonator. The resonant frequency is that frequency at which maximum current flows or maximum displacement takes place and corresponds to the frequency of oscillation in the case of transient excitation.

Filters

Electrical filters are devices that make use of the frequency selective characteristics provided by capacitive and inductive circuit elements. A low pass filter in its simplest form is shown in Figure 2-26(a). We see that in this circuit capacitive reactance will decrease as the frequency is increased. Consequently, for high frequencies the capacitance offers a low impedance with the result that little high frequency energy appears at the output. A high pass filter is obtained by reversing the positions of the capacitance and the resistor as shown in Figure 2-26(b). In this case, at low frequencies the capacitive reactance is large and the amount of low frequency energy appear-

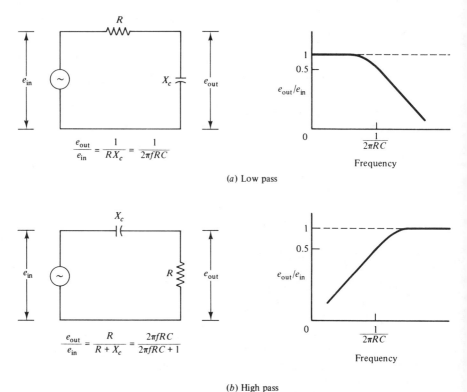

$$\frac{e_{out}}{e_{in}} = \frac{1}{RX_c} = \frac{1}{2\pi fRC}$$

(a) Low pass

$$\frac{e_{out}}{e_{in}} = \frac{R}{R + X_c} = \frac{2\pi fRC}{2\pi fRC + 1}$$

(b) High pass

Figure 2-26 Simple filters. Simple filters may be constructed using a series circuit containing resistance and either capacitance or inductance. The examples shown here use an RC combination. Below each circuit is shown the ratio of output to input voltage and to the right of each row is the frequency response. The voltage out is one-half of the input value at the position shown on the frequency axis.

ing at the output is low. A resistor and an inductor in series arrangement may also be used to achieve low and high pass effects, although their relative positions are different than in a resistance-capacitance circuit. The frequency response for each circuit is also shown in Figure 2-26. A band pass filter may be obtained by utilizing filter sections of both low pass and high pass configuration. The series resonant circuit shown in Figure 2-25(b) is the simplest example of such a circuit. We have already seen (Figure 2-15) how the voltage across the resistor changes as function of frequency. In many cases, practical filters are more complex but the principles of operation remain the same.

Filters are very useful devices in that they allow us to control the frequency composition of a stimulus and to analyze the frequency spectrum of a given signal. The acoustic or mechanical analog of these electrical filters is a very powerful concept aiding us to understand the action of the speech mechanism.

Active Network Elements

Thus far we have considered only *passive* electrical circuits. That is, no energy is supplied by these elements, their only function is energy storage or energy dissipation. While they are very useful components, the use of active or energy-supplying elements provides an increased breadth to circuit technology.

Vacuum tubes

Vacuum tubes are an example of a device which is capable of supplying energy to an electrical circuit. Vacuum tubes are so called because they are ordinarily found in the form of a sealed glass tube from which all air has been evacuated so that a vacuum exists. Typically there are several electrodes within the vacuum. One electrode is heated by externally applied current until some of the electrons break free of the electrode's metallic surface, much in the same way that steam is formed by heating water, and become available for manipulation within the vacuum tube. The simplest form of vacuum tube is the diode, so called because it has two electrodes; the cathode, which is heated and from which electrons are emitted, and a plate which is made positive with respect to the cathode by means of an external voltage. The electrons emitted from the cathode are attracted to the plate and a current exists. The importance of a diode is that the electron flow exists only in one direction—from cathode to plate, and not in the reverse direction. If more than two electrodes exist within the vacuum tube, then one or more of the electrodes can be used to control the current flow from cathode to plate. One of the very important uses of such vacuum tubes is that a very small current applied to the control electrodes is capable of controlling and regulating a very much larger electron flow from cathode to plate. This characteristic is known as amplification and is a means by which energy can be supplied to an electrical circuit.

Solid state devices

A number of solid state devices have been developed which perform functions similar to those described for vacuum tubes. They do so in a rather different way, however. Certain materials may be manufactured which contain an excess of free electrons. If voltages are applied to these materials in the proper way, electrons may be caused to flow in much the same manner as they do from cathode to plate in a vacuum tube. Thus, one can construct diodes out of solid state material as well as multielement devices similar to that which we described for vacuum tubes. One of the most common multielement solid state devices is the transistor.

ELECTROACOUSTICS

Acoustic-Electrical-Mechanical Analogs

We have already alluded to the fact that analogous effects take place in electrical, mechanical, and acoustic systems, for example, resonance effects. Our ability to understand these and other similarities between systems is aided markedly by the construction of a set of formal analogs. Such analogs make visualizing relations and actions easier when comparing an unfamiliar system with one which we know better. Figure 2-27 summarizes what is known as the impedance analogy.

Resistance

Resistance in each system is related to the dissipation of energy in the form of heat. Mechanical energy is changed into heat by motion of a mass which is opposed by mechanical friction. This is depicted in Figure 2-27 by a block sliding on a surface. Acoustic energy is changed into heat either by motion in a medium which is opposed by acoustic resistance due to medium viscosity or by the radiation of sound. Acoustic resistance in Figure 2-27 is depicted as slits through which the medium is forced to flow with consequent energy dissipation. Electrical energy is changed into heat by the passage of electric current through an electrical resistance.

Mass, inertance, and inductance

Mass is the mechanical element that opposes a change in velocity by its inertial energy. Mass is represented by a block form in Figure 2-27. Similarly,

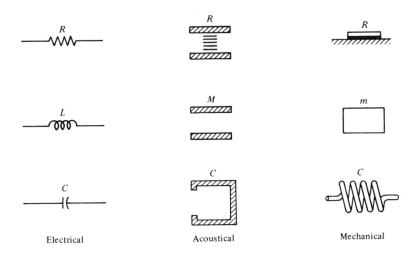

Figure 2-27 Impedance analogy relating electrical, acoustic, and mechanical systems. Electric and acoustic resistance is analogous to mechanical friction. Electric inductance, acoustic inertance and mass are analogous elements. Electrical and acoustic capacitance are analogous to mechanical compliance.

acoustic inertial energy is associated with *inertance* in an acoustic system. Inertance is the acoustic element which opposes a change in volume velocity. It is represented by a cross section of a tube in which the particles of the medium move in phase when activated by a force. *Inductance* is the electric circuit element that opposes a change in current by its electromagnetic field energy. Inductance is represented by a picture of a coil of wire.

Compliance, compressibility, capacitance

Mechanical potential energy is associated with the compression of a spring of a compliant element. *Compliance* is the mechanical element which opposes a change in the applied force and is related to the stiffness of a material. Compliance is represented by a picture of a spring. Similarly, acoustic potential energy is associated with the *compressibility* of the medium and is often referred to as acoustic capacitance. Compressibility or acoustic capacitance is the acoustic element which opposes a change in the applied pressure and is represented by a volume. Electric *capacitance* is the circuit element that opposes a change in voltage by its electrostatic field. It is represented by a diagram of a set of plates.

Several other analogies appear as we review these elemental analogies. For example, electrical current is equivalent to mechanical velocity and to acoustic volume velocity, each in its appropriate system. Further, electrical voltage is analogous to mechanical force and to acoustic pressure.

The analogies allow us to represent an acoustic system in its equivalent electrical or mechanical form. The ability to conceptually go from one system to another takes on particular importance when considering sound-generating and measuring equipment where all three systems are often involved.

Sound Measurement

There are three basic properties of sound that we are usually interested in measuring. First, we would like to know the magnitude of the sound, specifically, what is its sound pressure? Secondly, we are interested in the temporal characteristics of the sound, how long does it last and what is its waveform? Third, we are interested in the frequency characteristics of the sound, that is, its spectral characteristics.

Technology has been most highly developed in the area of electrical circuitry and for that reason almost all analysis is carried out in that mode. This requires, therefore, that the sound energy be changed into electrical energy so that these various analyses can be carried out. When one form of energy is changed into another, for example, acoustic energy into electric energy, the device that provides this transformation is known as a *transducer*, in this particular case an *acousto-electric* transducer.

Transducers

Anything that will transform acoustic energy into electric energy qualifies as an acousto-electric transducer and is commonly called a microphone. Although there are many different kinds of microphones, only a few find regular use. Commonly used microphones vary tremendously in terms of their cost, reliability, and sophistication. We will review a few of these types, commenting on their pertinent features.

Carbon. Carbon microphones find extensive use in many communication systems, primarily the telephone system. The microphone shown in Figure 2-28(*a*) consists of a small clump of carbon granules whose resistance depends upon the pressure exerted upon it. A diaphragm is connected rigidly to the carbon pack. As sound waves impinge upon the diaphragm, it is displaced varying the pressure on the carbon. If a battery is connected across the carbon pack, there will be a change in current flow as the resistance of the carbon pack changes. These changes in current flow reflect the pressure characteristics of the sound wave impinging upon the diaphragm. This AC component represents the output of the microphone. Carbon microphones are characterized by their large electrical output for a given sound pressure and their low cost. Their disadvantages are that their sensitivity tends to change with time and their frequency response is irregular, as shown in

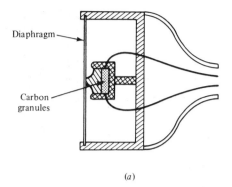

(a)

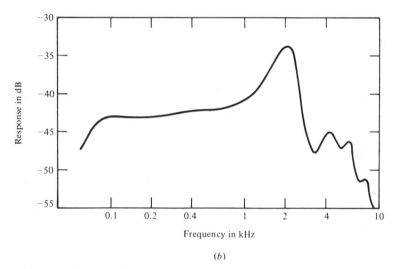

(b)

Figure 2-28 Carbon microphone. The principles of construction are shown in (a) while (b) indicates a typical pressure frequency response. The response in dB is relative to 1 volt/dyne/cm².

Figure 2-28(b). The term frequency response refers to the microphones, sensitivity at any particular frequency.

Crystal. Crystal microphones have as their transducing element a piezoelectric crystal. Such crystals generate voltage when squeezed so that their shape changes slightly. Many different types of crystals, both natural and man-made, possess this characteristic. A typical crystal microphone, shown in Figure 2-29(a), consists of a diaphragm rigidly coupled to a piezoelectric crystal. When a sound wave displaces the diaphragm the crystal is

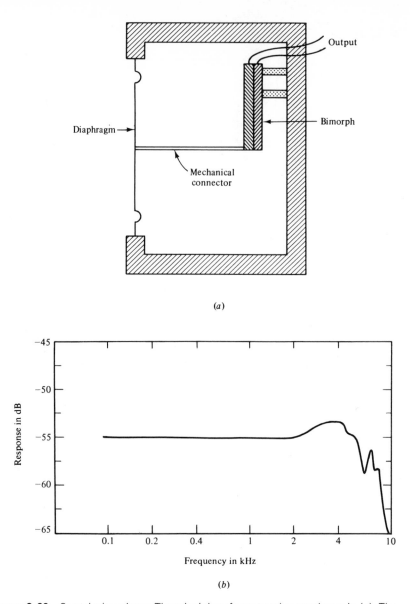

(a)

(b)

Figure 2-29 Crystal microphone. The principles of construction are shown in (a). The transducer element is a bimorph, two crystals sandwiched together. This design can give greater output voltages than a single crystal. A typical pressure frequency response is shown in (b) where the response reference is the same as Figure 2-28.

subjected to stress which generates a voltage, forming the output of the microphone. Most crystals tend to alter their piezoelectric characteristics somewhat as temperature and humidity changes. Thus, they are unsuitable for use under extreme environmental conditions. Their advantages lie in their low cost, high sensitivity, and fairly uniform frequency response.

Dynamic. The most common type of dynamic microphone is the coil type. This microphone, shown in Figure 2-30(*a*), has a small coil of wire fastened rigidly to a diaphragm. When a sound wave strikes the diaphragm it causes a movement of this small coil. The small coil is located in the field of a permanent magnet and when movement occurs a current is generated within the coil. Although the sensitivity of dynamic microphones is low

Figure 2-30   Moving coil microphone. The principles of operation are shown in (*a*). A typical pressure frequency response is shown in (*b*).

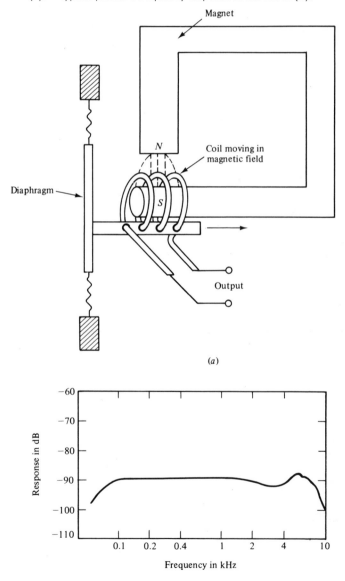

Magnet

N

Coil moving in magnetic field

Diaphragm

S

Output

(*a*)

Response in dB

−60

−70

−80

−90

−100

−110

0.1   0.2   0.4   1   2   4   10

Frequency in kHz

(*b*)

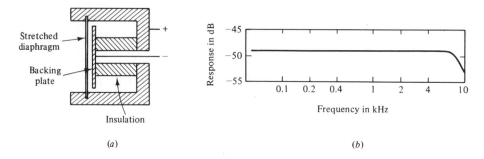

Figure 2-31 Condenser microphone. The principles of construction are shown in (*a*) and the pressure frequency response is shown in (*b*).

compared to that of carbon and crystal microphones, it possesses good stability and a good frequency response characteristic. Although more expensive than the carbon and crystal microphone, the advantages of the dynamic microphone are such that they are very widely used.

Electrostatic. The condenser microphone is a form of an electrostatic transducer. It consists of a tightly stretched metallic diaphragm which moves in response to incident sound pressure (Figure 2-31). Close to this diaphragm is a fixed metallic plate. The diaphragm and the fixed plate form an electrical capacitance, the magnitude of which varies as a function of the displacement of the diaphragm. If a DC voltage is applied to the plates of this capacitor, small variations in this DC value will occur as a result of the diaphragm movements. These small changes represent sound pressure variations and serve as the output of the microphone. The condenser microphone is used as a laboratory standard for making acoustic measurements. The advantages that have led to its adoption are its extreme reliability and the exceptionally broad range of frequencies over which its reponse is uniform. Its relatively high cost probably limits the use of the condenser microphone to the laboratory situation where precision is required.

Meters

Once the acoustic energy is in electrical form we are able to assess its sound pressure with a device called a *meter*, which can measure the voltage or current that the microphone has generated. Meters typically consist of three parts, (1) a display, (2) an amplifier, and (3) special circuitry required for the particular measurement task.

The *display function* is often carried out by a low sensitivity indicator, shown in Figure 2-32, in which the deflection of a pointer on a scale is related to the current flowing through a coil attached to the pointer. The scale is calibrated so that the deflections produced by given current flows have been noted. This type of display is known as an analog display; a second type is

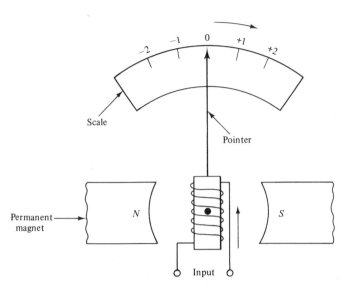

Figure 2-32 Basic analog meter movement. DC current flow in the coil will produce a magnetic field which will interact with that of the permanent magnet. The result of the interaction will be a rotation of the coil and a consequent deflection of the pointer. [*From I. J. Hirsh.* The Measurement of Hearing. (*New York: McGraw-Hill, Book Co., 1952*), *p. 42. Reprinted by permission of the author and the publisher.*]

called a digital display. In the latter case the proper numerals are illuminated by electrical means and we see no scale, only the "answer." There may be occasions when the characteristics and sensitivity of the display meter will be sufficient to make the measurement without any other aids.

Most often, and particularly in the case of measuring the electrical output of a microphone, the electrical signal is so small that the display unit itself is not sensitive enough to respond. Consequently, the signal must be made larger. This is accomplished by *amplification*. This process is discussed on p. 66. Amplification is usually implemented with vacuum tubes or transistors (see p. 55).

We have been assuming that DC current is the signal characteristic to which the meter would be responding. Sometimes this will be the case, but we may wish to measure voltage, and often we will be attempting to measure a time-varying signal such as a sinusoid. In this latter case there are different indices by which we can characterize the signal: average value, peak value, or RMS (equivalent heating) value. Special electronic circuitry, usually following the amplification, allows us a choice in the functions we wish to measure.

Cathode ray oscilloscopes

Cathode ray *oscilloscopes* are devices that display the waveform of an electrical signal. They consist of amplifiers, which turn small voltages or

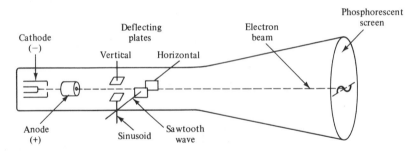

Figure 2-33 Cathode ray tube used in an oscilloscope. It is essentially a special purpose vacuum tube. Electrons emitted from the cathode are focused into a beam and accelerated by the anode, eventually falling upon the phosphorescent viewing surface. The position of the electron beam is controlled by the voltages applied to the deflection plates.

currents into larger ones, and a cathode ray tube upon which the waveform is displayed. The cathode ray tube which is shown in Figure 2-33 resembles an electrical pointer in some ways. A stream of electrons emerges from the tube's cathode. They are accelerated by positively charged electrodes and eventually impinge upon a screen which is viewed by the observer. Electrons, of course, are not visible, but the screen is coated with a substance which emits visible light when struck by electrons. Thus, whatever portion of the screen is being bombarded by electrons will glow and a point of light will be seen. The voltage to be displayed is amplified and applied to the deflection plates such that the spot of light is caused to move with an amplitude proportional to the voltage applied. An internally generated time base causes the spot to be deflected horizontally in such a way that a reproduction of the waveform is visible. It is difficult to overemphasize the importance of the cathode ray oscilloscope in the measurement of sound. This is particularly true in laboratory situations.

Spectrum analyzers

The usual *spectrum analyzer* is a device that displays voltage or its equivalent as a function of frequency. This, of course, is the usual way in which we plot spectrum. Most often this spectrum is obtained by passing the signal through a narrow band pass filter. The energy appearing at the output of this narrow filter represents the energy at the input which falls within the pass band of the filter. The analyzer has the capability of moving the spectral location of this filter. For example, the filter may initially be located so that it passes only very low frequencies but, as time progresses, the center frequency of the filter is moved upwards so that it passes frequencies of higher and higher frequency. Thus, at any particular moment in time, the output of this sweeping filter will represent the magnitude of the input signal in a particular frequency range.

Another twist to spectral analysis is to use a series of band pass filters, each located at a different, but fixed center frequency. The filters might be constructed so that the lowest filter would pass frequencies from 0 to 200 Hz, the next filter from 200 to 400 Hz, the next filter from 400 to 600 Hz, and so on. Thus, the output of each filter would represent the magnitude of the input signal for that frequency range. Thus far the analyzer sounds very much like the one described previously, except that instead of a single filter which was swept in frequency we have a number of filters which are fixed in frequency. However, there are a number of advantages in using the fixed filter analyzer. For many sound waves the spectral conditions are not constant. If it takes us a certain amount of time to sweep the single fixed filter, the spectrum of the sound may, in fact, be changing during the time the analysis is taking place. Thus, the obtained spectrum would not reflect the actual spectrum. Since in the fixed filter analyzer all filters are active simultaneously, we are able to see how the spectrum changes with time. In its original form, shown in Figure 2-34, the output of each filter went to a light and the brightness of the light depended upon the amount of energy derived from each filter. Thus, a light glowing brightly would indicate a large output in that particular filter while a light that was dim or not lighted at all would indicate little or no output. The lights were arranged in such a way that a photographic film could be passed beneath the light bank. The resulting

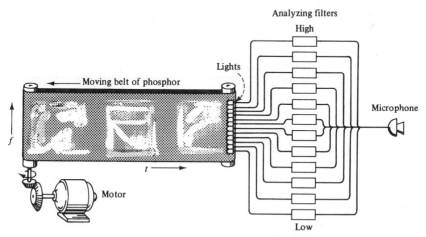

Figure 2-34 Example of a fixed frequency, contiguous, bandpass filter analyzer. The frequency, amplitude, and time characteristics of a typical speech signal are illustrated as analyzed by a sound spectrograph. [*From* Visible Speech *by R. K. Potter.* © *1947 by Litton Educational Publishing, Inc. Reprinted by permission of Van Nostrand Reinhold Company.*]

record indicates spectral intensity by the darkness of the trace, the location of the spectral energy by the position of the trace (high or low frequency), and the time at which the particular frequency-intensity conditions prevailed as shown along the horizontal dimension. This device is known as a *sound spectrograph* and finds wide application in the study of speech sounds.

Sound Production

Most sound produced for use in research in speech and hearing and for testing of hearing is produced by combinations of electrical, mechanical, and acoustic elements. The primary reason for this is that the control of the signal can be carried out much more easily and much more precisely when the signal is in electrical form rather than in acoustic form. Typically, the signal is first generated electrically, certain operations are then performed upon the signal, for example, its amplitude is changed. Finally, the signal is converted from electrical to acoustic energy by a transducer. We will discuss each of these steps in this section.

Waveform generator

A waveform generator is a device that is capable of producing a variety of periodic waveforms. The most commonly used waveform is the sine wave. Devices that produce only sine waves are often referred to as oscillators. In many cases, oscillators employ electrical resonance to produce the appropriate vibrations. As long as enough energy is supplied to a resonant circuit to compensate for its losses, the oscillations will continue.

Other commonly used periodic waveforms include square waves, triangular waves, and sawtooth waves. Nearly any conceivable waveform may be generated by an appropriate device.

Noise, although not periodic, is a very useful signal. Often the generation of noise starts with the random agitation of molecules emitted from the cathode of a vacuum tube. Electrons break free of the cathode in no particular order or with no defined interval between successive releases, thus the electron motion is not predictable, but is random. This random current flow is very small, but by appropriate techniques it may be increased and in its amplified form it finds use, eventually, as an acoustic signal.

Amplifier

The principle of amplification was described in our discussion of a vacuum tube. In this case we saw that a large current flow produced by an externally applied voltage could be controlled by a very small current flow. This process forms the basis of amplification. In the vacuum tube example, a small current flow on the control grid gives rise to a large current flow from plate to cathode. Without the process of amplification by vacuum tubes and transistors the technology of sound production, sound measurement, and sound recording would be in the horse and buggy days. Since most of our knowledge about the speech and hearing processes has been gained with the aid of acoustic technology, we owe much to the amplifier.

Electroacoustic transducers

Earlier, we discussed a number of devices that are used to transduce acoustic energy into electrical energy. All of those transducers are reversible transducers, that is, not only will they convert sound to electricity, but if electricity is fed into them they will produce a sound. Thus, in principle at least, any of the microphones we discussed may be used as sound producing devices. Unfortunately, if they are used in the same physical form in which they serve as microphones, their production of sound energy is extremely inefficient. In practice, the same principles of energy conversion are utilized, but the device is designed in such a way as to permit more efficient transduction. Although many transducer mechanisms exist, most sound production uses the dynamic principle which is the usual basis for loudspeaker and earphone designs. (Earphones are simply miniature versions of loudspeakers which are held to the listener's ears by a headband.)

The typical loudspeaker is shown in Figure 2-35. It consists of a coil of wire surrounding a permanent magnet. The coil of wire, called the voice coil, is suspended in such a way that it can move relative to the fixed permanent magnet. Attached to this coil is a large diaphragm, often of conical form, usually made of a light cardboard. The outer edge of the paper cone is suspended from a rigid structure. If an AC current is caused to flow through the voice coil, it produces a magnetic field which interacts with the field of the permanent magnet in such a way that the coil is forced to move. The movement of the coil produces a movement of the diaphragm. Because the diaphragm is relatively large, it displaces a large number of air particles and a sound wave is generated. The purpose of the large paper cone is simply to increase the efficiency of sound production by increasing the coupling between the source and the medium. The voice coil and the paper diaphragm move outward with one direction of current flow and inward with the other direction. Thus, if the waveform of the current flow was sinusoidal, the cone would execute simple harmonic motion and a sinusoidal sound wave would be produced.

The electrodynamic earphone is simply a miniature version of the loudspeaker we have just described. Earphones are widely used in the study of the hearing process because the control of the sound energy at the listener's ears is easier to achieve and the effect of other acoustic factors in the listener's

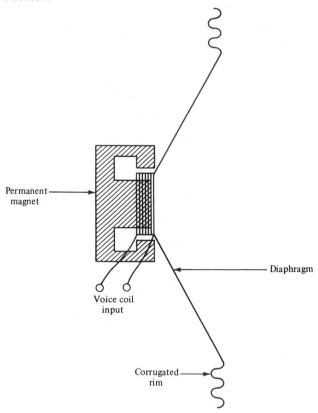

Permanent magnet

Voice coil input

Diaphragm

Corrugated rim

Figure 2-35 Electrodynamic loudspeaker. Current flow in the voice coil causes movement of the diaphragm. The large diaphragm area increases the coupling between sound source and the medium.

immediate environment are minimized. For example, a listener wearing a set of earphones can move his head freely and the sound pressure at his ears remains unchanged. This would not be the case if the sound were being produced by a loudspeaker. Additionally, if listening is being carried on in a noisy environment, the wearing of earphones reduces the effect of this noise at the listener's ears since the noise must penetrate the earphone and its cushion before reaching the listener's ears.

Sound Recording

Sound recording in speech and hearing science is a very important element in learning more about our speech and hearing mechanisms. Speech samples are recorded for future reference. Auditory stimuli are recorded for listener reaction. We will discuss several ways that sound can be recorded.

Disc recording

Elements in the system comprising the recorder consists of a microphone, an amplification circuit, and a cutting head. The cutting head is a device which transforms electrical energy into mechanical, vibratory motion and thus serves as a transducer element. As we have discussed previously, a number of elements can perform any given transducer task. Let us assume, however, that the cutting head is of the electrodynamic variety in which a current flow induces mechanical movement by means of interacting magnetic fields. The movement is produced in a device called a stylus and, in the particular cutting head we are describing, the stylus produces lateral (side to side) motion in response to the input current flow.

The recording medium is a disc made out of any of several materials. One of the requirements for the materials is that it must yield to the motions of the stylus such that grooves may be cut in its surface with relative ease. The cutting head is mounted on a carrier, the recording disc is placed on a turntable, and the cutter head lowered into the surface of the record. As the record revolves, the stylus cuts a groove through the surface. The carrier of the cutting head is designed such that as the record turns the cutting head moves laterally (typically toward the center of the disc) so as to displace each adjacent groove. A view of one of these grooves through a low power microscope reveals a series of undulations in the sides of the "valley." These, of course, are formed by the lateral vibratory movement of the stylus.

One of the advantages of disc recording is the ease with which copies may be made of the recordings. The first step in this copy process is to make a molding of the original disc such that the V-shaped valleys becomes Λ-shaped hills. This in turn serves as the master and can be used to stamp or impress its hills into other material so that the indentations produced are replicas of the original record. Many different materials are used to form copies, but one of the best in current use is a vinyl.

In order to play back a record it is necessary to reverse the recording process. The disc is placed on a revolving turntable and a device is allowed to ride in the grooves. The particular undulations of the grooves impart a motion to this device, which is also called a stylus, and the motion of the stylus then must be sensed. The mechanical motion of the stylus is transduced back into electrical energy by any of the means of transduction we have described. Typically, in disc recording this transducer is referred to as a pick-up or cartridge. Once the signal is in electrical form, it is amplified and used to drive a loudspeaker which in turn produces the sound. A summary of the sequence of recording and playing back a disc is shown in Figure 2-36.

With modern disc recording techniques, it is possible to obtain very low distortion recordings with excellent signal to noise ratio and dynamic range.

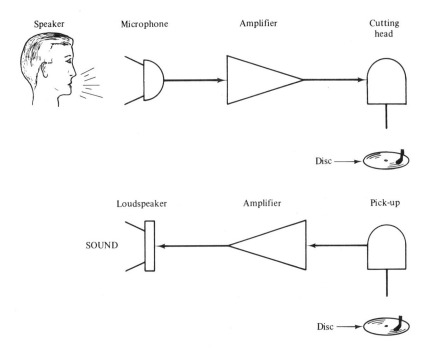

Figure 2-36   Elements of a disc recording system.

Moreover, with the recording materials that are used, it is possible to replay the same record hundreds of times with little change in the quality of the sound produced.

Optical recording

Optical recording is not as widely used as either disc or magnetic recording. However, it is used in some areas, one of them being on motion pictures.

Optical recording of sound begins in a manner similar to that of disc recording in that the sound is first transduced by microphone, electrical signals amplified by an amplifier, at which point the signal then is led to a device which controls the exposure of a photographic film. In its simplest form this is simply a small light source. Generally, the greater the instantaneous amplitude of the AC signal, the brighter the light and consequently the greater the film exposure. In some optical recording systems the same information is provided by changing the area of the film exposed to a constant intensity light.

The recording medium is photographic film which consists of a celluloid base in which is embedded a light-sensitive material. When this material is exposed to light, it changes its properties such that with subsequent chemical processing those regions of the film exposed to the light show differential light transmission as opposed to those areas that have not been exposed. One of the reasons for the relative unpopularity of optical sound recording is that photographic film is a rather expensive recording medium. This, together with the complexity of the equipment required, has limited the usefulness of this technique.

In order to play back the recorded sound a light source of constant intensity is directed onto the film. On the opposite side from the light source a photosensitive element is placed. A photosensitive element is one in which the voltage out of the element is proportional to the light falling upon it. A photographic light meter is one example of a photosensitive element. For the playback of optically recorded sound the amount of light that falls upon the photosensitive element is determined by the recorded density (opaqueness or clearness) of the film. Thus, as the film is moved in front of the light pick-up point, the light intensity varies in accordance with the original characteristics of the sound wave, and a corresponding voltage is produced. This voltage is then amplified and led to an electroacoustic transducer such as a loudspeaker.

Magnetic recording

Magnetic recording is the most widely used of the three types of recordings just discussed, and although there are a number of magnetic recording mediums, the one that we will describe is a tape with a magnetic coating.

As with the other recording techniques discussed, the first element in the recording system is a microphone. The output of the microphone is amplified and the amplified current is directed to a recording head. Recording heads are usually in the form of a letter "C" with only a very small gap. Wire is wrapped around a segment of this C through which current is caused to flow by means of the amplifier previously mentioned. The recording head and the coil of wire together form an electromagnet. That is, the current flow in the coil produces a magnetic field in the vicinity of the gap of the C. The exact characteristics of the field depend upon the nature of the current flow through the coil. Thus the electrical representation of the sound wave by means of the recording head induces a pattern of magnetic field changes which mirror those of the original sound wave.

The recording medium, as mentioned previously, consists of a thin plastic tape with a coating of magnetic material. The tape is drawn with uniform speed across the gap in the recording head and the material on the tape is magnetized. Thus, the residual magnetization in the magnetic material of the recording tape is a function of the magnetic field strength at the gap at the moment in time the tape passed over the gap.

There are certain incidental operations which occur in tape recorders that merit our attention. First, in order to improve magnetic performance, a very high frequency signal current is put on the recording head along with the audio signal. The frequency of this *bias* voltage is much too high for the ear to detect. One of the most unique features about magnetic recording is the ability to reuse the recording medium, in this case the magnetic tape. Typically, before the tape passes over the recording head it first passes over an erase head. The erase head produces a magnetic field which removes any residual magnetization related to a previously recorded audio signal. In principle any tape could be used an unlimited number of times. In practice, however, the magnetic oxide coating eventually wears off and the tape loses its magnetization potential. This state of affairs, however, is not reached until the tape has made many hundreds or perhaps thousands of passes over the recording head.

To play back this recorded material, the tape is passed over another set of heads known as play back heads. The magnetization of the tape film is sensed by a process essentially the inverse of the recording head operation. As with other play back processes, the voltage developed at the play back head is amplified and fed into a loudspeaker.

3

RESPIRATORY FUNCTION IN SPEECH

Thomas J. Hixon

INTRODUCTION

Whatever the task performed by the respiratory (breathing) apparatus, several important factors must be considered if the basic functioning of the apparatus is to be understood mechanically. Foremost among these factors are the structure of the respiratory pump, the forces applied to and by its various parts, and the movements of those parts as manifested geometrically and through volume and flow events. This chapter considers each of these factors as it relates to the adult respiratory apparatus in two important behaviors; namely, respiration for life purposes and respiration for speech purposes. Although function for life purposes is of secondary interest in this volume, it is necessary to consider such function in detail since the principles involved form a basis for understanding the mechanics of speech respiration.

The entire spectrum of speech breathing is not considered in this chapter. Interactions between the respiratory pump and larynx and upper airways are discussed in Chapters 4 and 5 where those parts and their functions are examined in detail. This is also the case for Chapter 6 where many of the concepts of this chapter and of Chapters 4 and 5 are expanded and integrated, and where the linguistic significance of respiratory function is considered.

RESPIRATION FOR LIFE PURPOSES

For life purposes, the main function of respiration is to provide oxygen to the cells of the body and to remove carbon dioxide from them. This requires movement of air to and from special gas-exchange surfaces within the body, this movement being accomplished by a remarkably engineered biological pump. This pump includes an energy source, passive elements that couple this source to the air it moves, the air itself, and the passageways through which the air is moved (Mead and Milic-Emili, 1964). Of interest in this section are the structure of this pump and a simple analysis of its behavior as a machine.

Structure of the Respiratory Apparatus

Figure 3-1 depicts a cut-away front view of the body trunk or *torso* which houses most of the important structures of the respiratory apparatus. The torso consists mainly of skeletal framework and muscular tissue and is

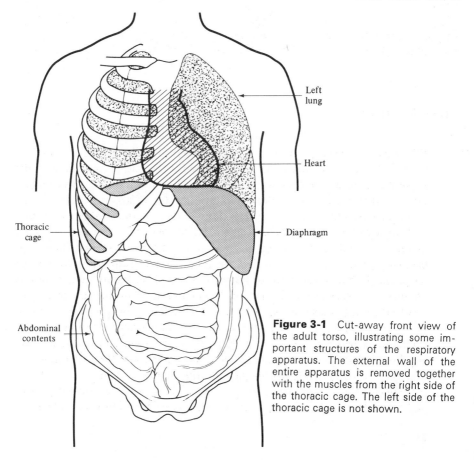

Figure 3-1 Cut-away front view of the adult torso, illustrating some important structures of the respiratory apparatus. The external wall of the entire apparatus is removed together with the muscles from the right side of the thoracic cage. The left side of the thoracic cage is not shown.

divided into upper and lower cavities by a dome-shaped partition called the *diaphragm*. The upper cavity, known as the *thorax*, or chest, is almost totally filled with the heart and various structures of the *pulmonary system* (respiratory airways and lungs), while the lower cavity, the *abdomen*, or belly, contains much of the digestive system along with various other organs and glands. Since both the thorax and abdomen participate importantly in respiratory function, it is essential that the structure of each be examined closely. Two other aspects warranting close examination here are the principle features of the pulmonary system and the unitary nature of the lungs and thorax.

Thorax

Figure 3-2 illustrates the skeletal framework of the torso, the thoracic portion of which is, perhaps, best described as a barrel-shaped cage of bone and cartilage. At the back of the torso a series of thirty-four irregularly-shaped *vertebrae* form the *vertebral column* or backbone, as it is referred to commonly. The uppermost seven vertebrae are termed *cervical* (neck); the next lower twelve, *thoracic* (chest); and the next three lower groups of five, *lumbar*, *sacral*, and *coccygeal* (collectively abdominal), respectively. The thoracic segment of the column forms only a small portion of the total cage, most of it being formed by the *ribs*, which are twelve, flat, arch-shaped bones found on each side of the body. These bones attach to thoracic vertebrae, from which they slope downward and around the sides of the thorax, giving roundness to the cage and forming its lateral walls. At the front, most of the ribs attach to bars of *costal cartilage* (rib cartilage) which in turn are connected to a long flat bone, the *sternum*, or breastbone, that serves as a front post for the thorax. Typical architecture for the thoracic cage finds the upper pairs of ribs attached to the sternum by their own costal cartilages, the lower ribs on each side sharing cartilages variously, and the lowermost two on each side "floating" without front attachments.

Completing the thoracic skeleton is the *pectoral girdle* (shoulder girdle) which is situated around the top of the barrel-shaped cage. The front of this girdle is formed by the two *clavicles* (collar bones), each of which is a bony strut running from the upper sternum over the first rib toward the side and back of the thorax. At the back, the clavicles attach to two, triangularly-shaped bony plates, the *scapulae* (shoulder blades), which complete the girdle and cover much of the upper back portion of the cage.

Both muscular and nonmuscular tissues serve to complete the vertical walls of the thorax by filling the spaces between the ribs and covering the inner and outer surfaces of the cage. The muscular tissues are especially important in respiratory function and are considered later, as is the previously mentioned diaphragm which doubles as the convex floor of the thorax and the concave roof of the abdomen.

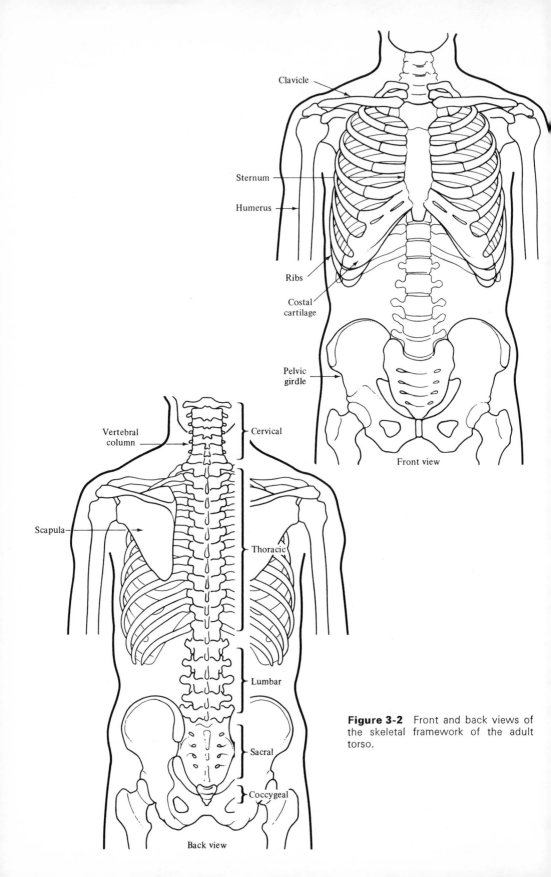

Clavicle

Sternum

Humerus

Ribs

Costal
cartilage

Pelvic
girdle

Front view

Vertebral
column

Cervical

Scapula

Thoracic

Lumbar

Sacral

Coccygeal

Figure 3-2 Front and back views of
the skeletal framework of the adult
torso.

Back view

Abdomen

The shape of the abdomen is not amenable to simple description by its skeletal structure as is the barrel-shaped cage of the thorax. The only skeleton included in the somewhat oblong-shaped abdominal cavity is the lower portion of the vertebral column at the back, and two large, irregularly-shaped *coxal bones* (hip bones) at the base. These two bones, together with the sacral and coccygeal vertebrae, form the *pelvic girdle* (bony pelvis). For the most part, the abdomen is constructed of two broad, complex sheets of connective tissue and a number of very large muscles. The two connective sheets cover the front and back walls of the abdomen and are referred to, respectively, as the *abdominal aponeurosis* and the *lumbodorsal fascia.* The muscles of concern are found on all sides of the abdomen, with those situated on the front and side walls combining with the abdominal aponeurosis to form a belly girdle that completely encloses and, in part, supports the abdominal contents. Like the muscles of the thorax, those of the abdomen are important in respiration and are discussed subsequently in this chapter.

Pulmonary system

The major features of the pulmonary system are shown in Figure 3-3. In terms of gross structure, this system is comprised of two components, the *respiratory airways* and the *lungs* (organs of respiration). The former is a highly complex and variable tract with a number of subdivisions and branches through which air can be moved to and from the lungs. The cavities of the nose, mouth, and throat (together called the *upper airways*) are included in this tract along with the *larynx* which functions as an airway valve. Since the larynx and upper airways are considered in detail in Chapters 4 and 5, discussion here is limited to the structure of the *lower airways* (the air passageways below the larynx).

Situated immediately beneath the larynx and running downward into the thorax is the *trachea* or windpipe. This is a semirigid tube composed of 16–20 C-shaped cartilages interconnected by fibrous tissue and muscle. The open ends of these cartilages face posteriorly where the tube is completed by a flexible wall shared with the *esophagus* (a muscular tube leading to the stomach). At its lower end, the trachea divides into two smaller semirigid tubes, the left and right *main-stem bronchi.* Each of these divides into *lobar bronchi*, and each of these divides, and so on through more than twenty generations. Approaching the periphery of the lung, the system finally arborizes into *terminal bronchioles, respiratory bronchioles, alveolar ducts, alveolar sacs*, and multitudes of very tiny *alveoli*, the last being the site where oxygen and carbon dioxide are exchanged during the respiratory process.

The lungs themselves are most simply described as cone-shaped structures which are of a porous, spongy texture and which possess an abundance of

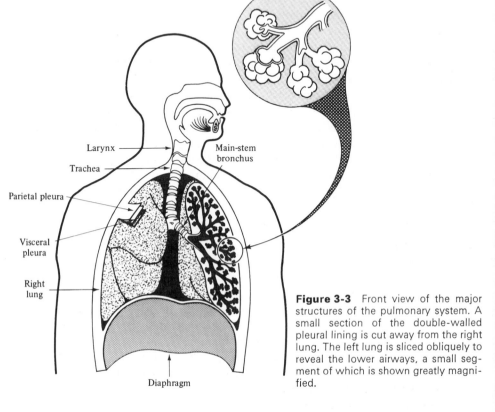

Peripheral
lower
airways

Larynx

Main-stem
bronchus

Trachea

Parietal pleura

Visceral
pleura

Right
lung

Diaphragm

Figure 3-3 Front view of the major structures of the pulmonary system. A small section of the double-walled pleural lining is cut away from the right lung. The left lung is sliced obliquely to reveal the lower airways, a small segment of which is shown greatly magnified.

resilient elastic fibers. Although a gross oversimplification of their structure, there is merit in thinking of the lungs as large air-filled elastic sacs that can change size and shape. Both lungs rest upon the top surface of the diaphragm from which they extend upward, one on each side, to almost fill the lateral chambers of the thoracic cavity. The outer surfaces of the lungs are covered with a delicate air-tight membrane called the *visceral pleura*, while a similar membrane, the *parietal pleura*, lines the inner surface of the thoracic walls and the top of the diaphragm. Together these membranes form a double-walled sac that completely encases the lungs. Both walls of this sac are covered with a thin layer of lubricating fluid which permits them to move easily upon one another, and which also serves the important function of *linking* the two pleural surfaces together in much the same manner that a film of water holds two glass plates together (Comroe, 1965).

Lungs-thorax unit

Although the lungs and thorax normally operate together as a unit, it is important to realize that their natural resting positions in the intact unit are different from their individual resting positions when the two are separated. For example, with the lungs removed from the thorax, their resting position is a collapsed state in which they contain almost no air. By contrast, the resting position of the thorax with the lungs removed is a more expanded state (greater volume). With the lungs and thorax held together as a unit by *pleural linkage*, the respiratory apparatus assumes a natural resting position between these two separate positions such that the lungs are somewhat expanded and the thorax is somewhat compressed. The springs pictured in Figure 3-4 illustrate this relationship by analogy (Comroe et al., 1962).

Figure 3-4 Spring analogy depicting the volumes (i.e., spring lengths) assumed by the lungs and the thorax when each is independent of the other and when the two are linked together by pleural linkage. The horizontal dashed lines represent lung volume levels (see Figure 3-13) appropriate to the spring lengths. [*After J. H. Comroe, Jr. et al., The Lung: Clinical Physiology and Pulmonary Function Tests. Copyright © 1962 Year Book Medical Publishers, Inc. Used by permission.*]

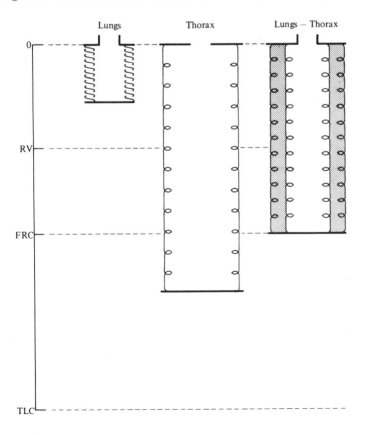

There the lungs and thorax are represented by separate springs, each in its resting position and unaffected by the other. The right side of the schema shows a different resting position for each spring when the two are held together as in pleural linkage. The net result is a stretching of the "lungs' spring" and a compression of the "thoracic spring." This coupled resting position is analogous to that designated as the *resting expiratory level* in the human respiratory apparatus. At this level the respiratory pump is in its mechanically neutral or balanced position where the force of the lungs to collapse is opposed by an equal and opposite force of the thorax (including the diaphragm and abdomen) to expand.

At this juncture it is well to distinguish three important pressures within the respiratory pump: two within the thorax and one within the abdomen. The pressure within the lungs themselves is referred to as *alveolar pressure*. That within the thorax but outside the lungs (i. e., between the two pleural walls) is designated as *pleural pressure*. Finally, the pressure within the abdomen is termed *abdominal pressure*.

Mechanics of Respiration

Assuming knowledge of respiratory structure, this section discusses the elements of normal respiration from the standpoints of dynamic performance and static properties of the respiratory pump. It is convenient to consider these elements under four headings: inspiration, expiration, the pulmonary subdivisions, and the volume-pressure relationships of the respiratory pump. The discussion under each heading is limited to respiratory function in the upright posture in normal individuals.

Inspiration

The phase of respiration where air flows into the lungs is referred to as *inspiration* or *inhalation*. Aspects of this process that warrant attention here include various aerodynamic events, the nature of thoracic enlargement, and the forces involved.

Aerodynamic events. Basic to understanding inspiration, or air movement of any type, is the principle that *air flows from regions of higher pressure to regions of lower pressure*. With the airways open and the respiratory pump in its neutral position at the resting expiratory level, the pressure within the lungs (alveolar pressure) equals that outside the body (atmospheric pressure). To accomplish inspiration, alveolar pressure must be decreased sufficiently below atmospheric that a pressure gradient will exist in favor of inward flow. This gradient is created in the human respiratory apparatus by muscular forces that increase the size of the thorax. Since, through pleural linkage,

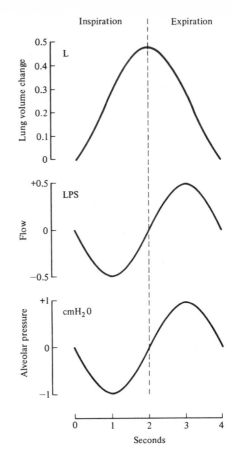

Inspiration | Expiration

Figure 3-5 Simplified illustration of lung volume (liters), flow (liters per second), and alveolar pressure (centimeters of water) changes during a quiet breathing cycle. Actually, expiration is longer than inspiration, and waves for the two phases of the breathing cycle are asymmetrical. [*From J. H. Comroe, Jr.*, Physiology of Respiration. *Copyright © 1965 Yearbook Medical Publishers, Inc. Used by permission.*]

the lungs and thorax move as a unit, any increase in thoracic volume leads to a stretching of the lungs, an expansion of alveolar air and a decrease in alveolar pressure.[1]

Figure 3-5 is a simplified illustration of selected volume, flow and pressure changes which occur during a normal breathing cycle initiated from the resting expiratory level. In that figure the relationships may be seen among (1) the amount of air within the lungs (lung volume), (2) the rate of change of lung volume (flow), and (3) the alveolar pressure. For now only the inspiratory portion of the cycle is of concern. As illustrated, there are two moments during this phase when alveolar pressure is atmospheric; at the beginning and end of inspiration (zero and two seconds on the horizontal

---

[1] Air molecules within the lungs provide pressure (force per unit area) by colliding with one another and with the structures of the lungs. When the volume of air within the lungs is expanded, the molecules are less crowded, so they are involved in fewer collisions and the pressure is lower. Conversely, when the volume is decreased, collisions are more frequent and the pressure is greater. Specifically, volume and pressure are inversely related, providing temperature remains constant and providing the respiratory airways are closed to the outside. Under such circumstances, doubling the volume halves the pressure and halving the volume doubles the pressure.

axis). Since no pressure gradient exists at these two moments, flow is also zero. During inspiration alveolar pressure drops below atmospheric magnitude (to -1 cm H_2O), the extent of its drop and the shape of the pressure curve depending, for the most part, upon the rapidity and extent of lung enlargement and the degree to which the respiratory airways are open. Since flow is proportional to the pressure difference between the lungs and atmosphere, changes in flow follow those in alveolar pressure. The specific relationship between flow and pressure depends, of course, upon the type of flow being generated.[2] As can be seen in Figure 3-5, the most rapid negative (inspiratory) flow during the cycle is about -0.5 liter per second and occurs when alveolar pressure is lowest (i. e., when the pressure difference between the lungs and atmosphere is greatest). Throughout inspiration, the volume of air within the lungs is continuously increasing, until by the end of a normal inspiration, the lung volume is about 0.5 liter greater than it was at the resting expiratory level.

Changes in thoracic volume. Aware that thoracic enlargement leads to inspiratory flow, it is relevant to examine the nature of changes in thoracic volume during inspiration. This is done most simply by considering the three dimensions in which the size of the thorax increases; these being vertical, anteroposterior, and transverse. Vertical enlargement is easiest to explain in that it results primarily from lowering the base of the thorax (diaphragm) as shown schematically in Figure 3-6. The anteroposterior and transverse increases, illustrated in Figure 3-7, are the result of somewhat more complex thoracic changes involving movements of the ribs and sternum. Recall that the ribs attach to the vertebral column posteriorly, from which they slope downward and forward toward the front of the thoracic cage. Upon elevation, the ribs go through two types of movement, one likened to the raising of a "pump handle," the other likened to the raising of a "bucket handle." In the pump-handle movement the front ends of the ribs move upward and forward along with the sternum, the result being an enlargement in the anteroposterior diameter of the thorax. The action described as "bucket handle" amounts to an outward *eversion* (rotation) of each rib around an imaginary line joining its two ends. This action results in a widening of the thorax transversely, the extent of increase being greater in the lower than upper thorax because the lower ribs swing through arcs of larger imaginary circles (Siebens, 1966).

---

[2] The two flows most commonly recognized are laminar and turbulent. Laminar flow is smooth or streamline with its driving pressure being directly related to flow. Turbulent flow, on the other hand, is erratic in both direction and magnitude, its driving pressure being proportional to the square of flow. Turbulence can occur at high flows in smooth straight tubes, or at low flows in tubes containing irregularities such as the partial closure of the respiratory airways by the larynx. Both laminar and turbulent flow may exist in different portions of the respiratory airways at the same time. During normal respiration, flow is mostly laminar, while at higher than usual flows it becomes predominantly turbulent. For additional information read Comroe (1965) and Rouse and Howe (1953).

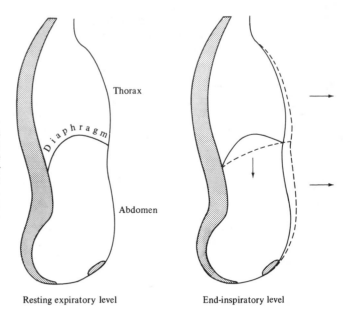

Figure 3-6 Resting and end-inspiratory positions of various respiratory structures during quiet breathing. Vertical increase in the thorax is caused mainly by footward displacement of the diaphragm, which in turn increases abdominal pressure and drives the abdominal wall outward.

Thorax

Abdomen

Resting expiratory level   End-inspiratory level

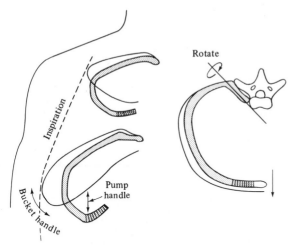

Rotate

Inspiration

Bucket handle

Pump handle

Figure 3-7 Front and top views of ribs, illustrating the "pump handle" and "bucket handle" motions responsible for anteroposterior and transverse diameter changes in the thorax. [*After R. Cherniack and L. Cherniack,* Respiration in Health and Disease *(Phila., Penna.: W. B. Saunders Company, 1961).*]

Forces of inspiration. The muscular energy expended during inspiration serves to overcome (1) resistance to air flow through the respiratory airways, (2) resistance to the deformation of respiratory tissues, and (3) elastic recoil of the lungs-thorax unit (Mead and Martin, 1968). More than a dozen muscles may be involved in providing this energy at one time or another during inspiration. Their individual mechanical contributions depend upon various factors, the most important including (1) other muscles that are active simultaneously, (2) the amount of air within the lungs, and (3) the forcefulness of the respiratory maneuver (Campbell, 1958). The structure and function of the most important inspiratory muscles are considered here, this discussion being divided to consider separately the forces of quiet inspiration and those of forced inspiration. It should be borne in mind that the descriptions offered for individual muscle behaviors are based on the assumption that only the muscle under consideration is active, a convenient, but in most instances, an unrealistic assumption. Also, where controversy surrounds the function of certain muscles, the descriptions given are based on what is judged to be the most compelling experimental evidence. All of the statements that follow concerning the consequences of individual muscle activities assume that the muscles are shortening during contraction.

Quiet inspiration. Resting individuals take air into their lungs a dozen or more times a minute. This inward flow of air, called *quiet inspiration*, usually goes unnoticed, despite the fact that *active* muscular contraction is needed to enlarge the thorax. Two muscles, the diaphragm and the external intercostals,

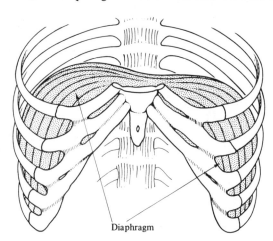

Diaphragm

Figure 3-8 Muscles of quiet inspiration.

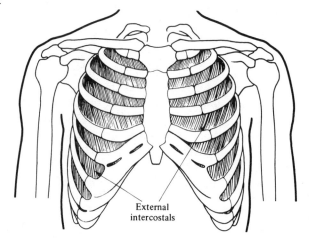

External intercostals

are most responsible for thoracic enlargement under these circumstances and as such are classified as the muscles of quiet inspiration. Figure 3-8 depicts their structure and shows their location within the body.

The *diaphragm* is a dome-shaped structure of muscle and tendon which bears resemblance to an inverted bowl. Its centermost part consists of a thin, flat, *central tendon*, while the remainder is formed by a rim of muscle which radiates downward from the edges of the tendon. The bottom of this muscular rim attaches around the internal circumference of the lower portion of the thorax; these attachments include the bottom of the sternum, the lower ribs and their cartilages, and the first three or four lumbar vertebrae. When the muscular rim contracts, the diaphragm is pulled downward and slightly forward, thus increasing the thoracic cavity in a vertical direction. Contraction of the diaphragm also increases the circumference of the thorax through elevation of the lower ribs. The combined action of lowering the base of the thorax and expanding its circumference is sufficient to account for most of the change in thoracic volume during quiet inspiration. In association with this volume change, the component of diaphragmatic activity which is resolved into footward displacement of the structure, causes an increase in abdominal pressure and a driving outward of the abdominal wall (see Figure 3-6).

The *external intercostal* muscles are eleven relatively thin layers of muscular tissue which completely fill the rib interspaces. Each runs between the lower edge of one rib and the upper edge of the rib immediately below, the individual fibers running forward and downward. Although structurally inaccurate, it is useful to think of the external intercostals, from a mechanical viewpoint, as a large sheet of muscle linking other ribs to the fixated first rib, the cervical vertebrae, and the base of the skull (Draper et al., 1959). When the external intercostals shorten during contraction, each elevates the rib below, thus increasing the anteroposterior and transverse dimensions of the thorax. Also, they tense the tissue-filled rib interspaces, preventing them from being sucked inward during inspiration.[3]

As mentioned above, most of the change in thoracic volume during quiet breathing is accounted for by diaphragmatic activity. It should be understood, however, that there exists a substantial capability for independence of motion between the thoracic cage and the diaphragm-abdomen unit (Konno and Mead, 1967). Witness to this is the ability to inspire mainly with either the thoracic muscles or the diaphragm. A further example is the ability to produce paradoxical movements of the thorax and diaphragm-abdomen during breathing. The main point to be made is that it is possible to move air both in and out of the lungs through a wide variety of relative displacements of the thoracic cage and diaphragm-abdomen.

[3] The intercartilaginous (between the costal cartilages) segment of the *internal intercostal* muscles is so arranged that the internal intercostals also exert inspiratory force on the thoracic cage (Taylor, 1960). Their main function is expiratory, however, and they are discussed as such in the section on expiratory forces.

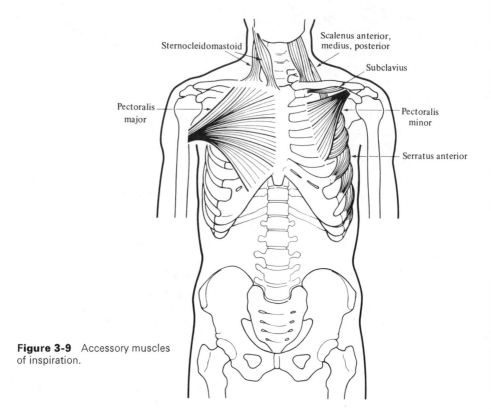

Figure 3-9 Accessory muscles
of inspiration.

Forced inspiration. Inspiration of a more vigorous nature than that of the resting individual is called *forced inspiration*. Innumerable gradations of forced inspiration may occur in terms of both the volume of air inspired and the effort exerted during the inspiratory maneuver. During these more vigorous intakes of air, *accessory muscles* are employed to help the diaphragm and external intercostals increase thoracic volume. These muscles, shown in Figures 3-9 and 3-10, warrant individual consideration.

The *sternocleidomastoid* is a relatively large muscle located on the side of the neck, its fibers originating from the bony skull behind the ear and passing downward in two divisions. One division inserts into the top surface of the clavicle while the other attaches to the top portion of the front of the sternum. With the head held in a fixed position, contraction of the sterno-cleidomastoid raises the sternum, and because of their attachments thereto, the ribs are elevated.

The *scalenus muscle group* includes three muscles found on the side of the neck: the *scalenus anterior*, *medius*, and *posterior*. The anterior originates as four tiny muscular tabs from the third through sixth cervical vertebrae.

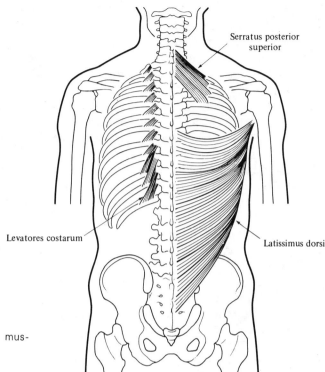

Figure 3-10 Accessory muscles of inspiration.

These tabs converge into a relatively thick muscle bundle which runs downward and laterally to insert along the inner border of the top surface of the first rib. The medius arises as tiny tabs from the lower six cervical vertebrae. Fibers descend along the side of the vertebral column and, like the anterior segment, merge into a single bundle, this one inserting along the upper border of the first rib just behind the scalenus anterior. The final member of the group, the posterior, is located behind the medius. The fibers of the posterior muscle arise from the lower two or three cervical vertebrae as muscular tabs which converge as they pass downward and laterally to attach to the outer surface of the second rib. Upon contraction of the scalenus group, the first two ribs are elevated.

The *subclavius* is a relatively small, narrow muscle originating on the undersurface of the clavicle and running slightly downward and toward the midline where it attaches to the junction of the first rib and its cartilage. Contraction of the subclavius brings about an elevation of the first rib, providing the clavicle is braced.

The *pectoralis major* is a large, fan-shaped muscle found on the upper front wall of the thorax. It arises from the *humerus* (the major bone of the upper arm) and fans out widely across the thorax, having a complex insertion which includes the front surfaces of the upper costal cartilages, the sternum, and the inner half of the clavicle. When the upper arm is held in a fixed position, contraction of the pectoralis major draws the sternum and ribs upward.

The *pectoralis minor* is a relatively large, thin muscle situated underneath the pectoralis major. It originates from the front surface of the scapula and radiates downward toward the midline where its fibers insert into the outer surfaces of the second through fifth ribs near their cartilages. If the scapula is anchored, the pull of the pectoralis minor will lift ribs two through five.

The *serratus anterior* is a large thin muscle located on the side wall of the thorax. It arises from the front surface of the scapula and passes forward around the side of the thoracic cage, where it diverges into a number of thin, finger-like muscular tabs. These insert into the outer surfaces of the upper eight or nine ribs. If the scapula is secured in position, action of the serratus anterior will raise the upper ribs.

The *levatores costarum* (rib raisers) are twelve small muscles located on the back of the thoracic cage. These originate from the seventh cervical and upper eleven thoracic vertebrae with each muscle extending downward and slightly outward to the back surface of the rib immediately below the vertebra of origin. In the lower thorax some muscle fibers also extend to the second rib below. When the levatores costarum contract, they raise the ribs.

The *serratus posterior superior* muscle is located on the upper back portion of the thorax. It is a flat, thin muscle originating from the back of the vertebral column; points of origin include the seventh cervical and the first three or four thoracic vertebrae. Fibers of the serratus posterior superior slant downward across the back of the thorax to insert as muscular tabs into the second through fifth ribs. This muscle serves to elevate the ribs to which it attaches.

The *latissimus dorsi* is a large muscle located on the back of the body, its fibers originating from the humerus and fanning out to run downward across the back of the lower thorax. This muscle has a complex insertion into the lower portion of the vertebral column and lower ribs. Attachments include the lower six thoracic, the lumbar, and the sacral vertebrae, as well as the posterior surfaces of the lower three or four ribs. When the humerus is braced, contraction of the fibers inserted into the lower ribs will elevate them.

Expiration

Air flow from the lungs is termed *expiration* or *exhalation*. As with inspiration, features of expiration that warrant consideration here are the aerodynamic behavior of the respiratory pump and the forces applied to and by its various parts.

Aerodynamic events. Remember that alveolar pressure is equal to atmospheric at the end of inspiration. Air will flow out of the lungs if alveolar pressure is made to exceed that of the atmosphere by an amount sufficient to overcome resistance, that is, if a pressure gradient is established in favor of outward flow. In the human respiratory pump this is accomplished at times by nonmuscular forces, and at other times by both muscular and nonmuscular forces, which reduce the size of the lungs-thorax unit, thereby compressing the alveolar air and raising its pressure above atmospheric.

Consideration has already been given to volume, flow, and pressure changes associated with the inspiratory phase of the quiet breathing cycle. In the right half of Figure 3-5, those same aerodynamic events are illustrated for a *quiet expiration.* There alveolar pressure is seen to be atmospheric at both the beginning and end of expiration (two and four seconds on the abscissa), rising to $+1$ cm H_2O in between. As pressure fluctuates, flow increases from zero to approximately $+0.5$ liter per second and then decreases to zero, the maximum flow coinciding with maximum alveolar pressure. The shapes of the pressure and flow curves during quiet expiration are determined mainly by the recoil forces of the lungs and thorax (including the diaphragm and abdomen), and the resistance to flow through the airways. The 0.5 liter or so of air taken into the lungs during inspiration is expelled as expiration proceeds, until the normal volume at the resting expiratory level is attained.

Forces of expiration. As with inspiration, the forces exerted during expiration serve to move air and nonelastic tissues and to overcome the elastic recoil of the lungs-thorax unit. Two types of expiration, passive and active, are employed in meeting the various demands for expelling air from the lungs. In the case of the latter, the mechanical contributions of the muscles involved are dependent upon the same factors as previously discussed for the inspiratory muscles.

Passive expiration. Expiration above the resting expiratory level is usually *passive.* As such it is accomplished not by muscular effort, but by nonmuscular forces which return the lungs and thorax to their usual volumes at the resting expiratory level. During *quiet* inspiration, potential energy is created by the contraction of inspiratory muscles and stored in the stretched elastic fabric (tissues) of the lungs. When the inspiratory muscles are relaxed, the external force (muscular effort) distending the lungs no longer exists. Consequently, the stored energy is released and the lungs recoil toward a smaller volume—like a stretched spring recoils when released. Being linked to the thorax, the recoiling lungs pull inward on the thoracic walls and upward on the diaphragm. This action causes the thoracic cavity to decrease in size along the dimensions in which it expanded during inspiration; namely, vertically, anteroposteriorly, and transversely. The total force of lung recoil at any instant depends only in part upon the recoil force of the actual elastic fabric of the lungs. Other factors contribute, the most important of which is a very special surface film found within the lungs. This film coats the inside of each of the tiny alveoli, forming a liquid-air interface (boundary) whose surface tension causes it to recoil like a tiny bubble. The combined recoil force of the 300 million or so alveolar surfaces is responsible for as much or more of the total lung recoil as the actual elastic fabric of the lungs. This is clearly demonstrated by the fact that it requires less than half the pressure to fully inflate a lung when fluid-filled than when air-filled (Radford, 1964). The basis for this difference is that in the fluid-filled lung the normal liquid-air interface of each alveolus is replaced by a liquid-liquid interface whose surface tension is negligible (Comroe, 1965).

Unlike quiet inspiration, deep inspiration[4] involves the storage of potential expiratory energy within the elastic tissues of lungs *and* thorax (including the diaphragm and abdominal structures). Therefore, following deep inspiration *both* the lungs and thorax recoil toward smaller volumes with the sum of their recoil forces determining the total force of passive expiration. It is important to realize that the thorax contributes to the development of positive passive expiratory forces *only* at relatively high lung volumes (above 55% of the vital capacity) where it is expanded beyond its own resting position, and therefore, tends to recoil to a smaller size. Otherwise, and as is the case in quiet expiration, the forces of the thorax and lungs are in opposition with the lungs attempting to reduce their size and the thorax attempting to increase its size, i. e., the two springs are working against one another.

Lest it be misunderstood from previous discussion, it is important to note that the inspiratory muscles do not cease their activity the instant flow changes direction between inspiration and passive expiration (Agostoni, 1964). They actually continue their activity into the early part of expiration (beyond the two second point in Figure 3-5) with the force they exert gradually decreasing and acting as a releasing brake against the lung recoil forces just described. Thus, while the term passive expiration characterizes most expirations above the resting expiratory level, such expirations are only truly passive (i. e., involve no muscular effort) after the inspiratory muscles have ceased their activity.

Active expiration. Although most expirations are passive, countless degrees of *active* expiration are possible in which muscular forces are employed to reduce the volumes of the lungs and thorax. The term "active expiration" has two meanings as it is used in this chapter: one relative to the use of muscular effort above the resting expiratory level and the other for expirations below that level. Above the resting level, active expiration is accomplished by using expiratory muscles to decrease the size of the thorax with greater force than the decrease caused by passive (nonmuscular) forces alone.

---

[4] Deep inspiration in this context is defined as any inspiration where the thorax is expanded beyond its own resting position (lungs removed). In the spring analogy of Figure 3-4, deep inspiration would involve a stretching of the thoracic spring to a length greater than that shown for the normal resting position of the thorax alone.

By analogy, this amounts to a forcing of the stretched lungs-thorax spring unit back to its resting position rather than permitting it to return there of its own accord. In the respiratory pump this action results in a more rapid than usual reduction in lung volume and a substantial increase in both alveolar pressure and flow. As for expirations below the resting level, the term "active expiration" always applies. This is because any decrease in thoracic volume from the resting level, like any increase from that level, requires the use of muscular force, regardless of the depth or forcefulness with which the expiration occurs.

It should be apparent by this juncture that while expirations above the resting level can be either passive or active, those below the resting level must be active. Knowing this, it is relevant to examine the muscles responsible for active reduction of thoracic size under the conditions just described. Each of the muscles of concern has one or both of two important mechanical functions: (1) it lowers the ribs and/or sternum to decrease the antero-posterior and transverse dimensions of the thorax, and (2) it raises the abdominal pressure and forces the diaphragm upward, thus decreasing the vertical dimension of the thorax. Figures 3-11 and 3-12 show the expiratory muscles, each of which warrants consideration with reference to its structure and function.

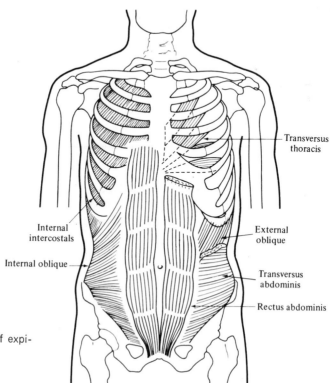

Figure 3-11   Muscles of expiration.

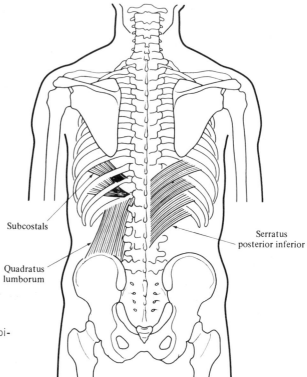

Figure 3-12 Muscles of expiration.

Subcostals

Serratus posterior inferior

Quadratus lumborum

The *internal intercostals* are eleven thin muscles situated within the rib interspaces underneath the external intercostals. They extend from around the sides of the thorax to the sternum but do not fill the interspaces at the back of the thoracic cage. The fibers of the internal intercostals run upward and forward from the upper border of one rib to the lower border of the rib immediately above, their course being at approximately right angles to the fibers of the external intercostals. From a mechanical viewpoint it is useful to think of the internal intercostals as a sheet of muscle linking the ribs to the pelvic girdle through a number of other muscles, principally those of the abdomen. Upon contraction, the internal intercostals pull the ribs downward and stiffen the rib interspaces.

The *transversus thoracis* is a thin, fan-shaped muscle found on the inside, front wall of the thorax. It originates at the midline on the inner surface of the lower sternum and the fourth or fifth through seventh costal cartilages. From this broad origin it fans out across the thorax and divides into a number of muscular tabs which insert variously into the inner surface of the costal cartilages and bony ends of ribs two through six. The upper fibers run nearly vertically, while the intermediate and lower fibers run obliquely and horizontally, respectively. When the transversus thoracis contracts, it exerts a downward pull on the ribs to which it attaches.

The *subcostal* muscles are located on the inside back wall of the thorax. These vary considerably in number from person to person, being most often located and best developed in the lower portion of the rib cage. The subcostals originate close to the vertebral column on the inner surfaces of ribs, from which their fibers extend upward and laterally, inserting into the inner surface of the rib immediately above the rib of origin, or skipping a rib or two in their course and inserting into higher ribs. Upon contraction, the subcostals act to depress the ribs.

The *serratus posterior inferior* muscle is located on the lower back portion of the thorax. This thin, flat muscle originates from the lower two thoracic and upper two or three lumbar vertebrae. Its fibers slant upward across the back of the thorax diverging into four flat muscular tabs which insert into the lower borders of the last four ribs on the back of the cage. When the serratus posterior inferior contracts, it pulls down on the lower ribs.

The *quadratus lumborum* is a flat sheet of muscle located on the back wall of the abdominal cavity. It arises from the top of the coxal bone and its fibers run upward and slightly toward the midline, diverging into several muscular tabs. These insert into the first four lumbar vertebrae and the lower border of the inner half of the lowest rib. Contraction of the quadratus lumborum depresses the lowest rib.

The *latissimus dorsi* was discussed earlier in this chapter as a muscle of inspiration. While the fibers attached to the lower three or four ribs are capable of raising them during inspiration, contraction of the muscle as a whole compresses the lower portion of the thoracic cage. Therefore, it is not contradictory to view the latissimus dorsi as a muscle of both inspiration and expiration.

The next four muscles are usually regarded as the most important muscles of active expiration. They are referred to collectively as the abdominal muscles, and include the rectus abdominis, external oblique, internal oblique, and transversus abdominis.

The *rectus abdominis* is a long, ribbon-like muscle found on the front of the abdominal cavity. It originates from the upper front edge of the coxal bone and runs upward, parallel to the midline, to insert into the fifth, sixth, and seventh costal cartilages and lower sternum. The rectus abdominis is encased in a fibrous sheath or sleeve which is formed by the complex abdominal aponeurosis. Together with the rectus, this sheath forms a front post for the abdomen which can be viewed as a continuation of the sternal post of the thoracic cage. When the rectus abdominis contracts, it draws the lower ribs and sternum downward and forces the abdominal contents inward.

The *external oblique* is a very broad, flat muscle which is situated on the side and front portions of the lower thorax and abdomen. This muscle arises as a number of tabs from the outer surface of the lower eight ribs and its fibers run downward across the abdomen at various angles. Fibers toward the back of the body descend nearly vertically to insert into the upper surface of the top portion of the coxal bone, while others run obliquely downward and toward the front of the abdomen to attach to the abdominal aponeurosis near the midline. When it contracts, the external oblique draws the lower ribs downward and displaces the contents of the abdomen inward, thus raising the abdominal pressure.

The *internal oblique* is a large, flat muscle located on the side and front walls of the abdominal cavity. It lies under the external oblique and has a rather extensive origin which includes much of the upper surface of the coxal bone and the lumbodorsal fascia. The fibers of the internal oblique fan out across the abdomen to insert into the abdominal aponeurosis and the costal cartilages of the lower three or four ribs. Upon contraction, this muscle drives the abdominal wall inward and draws the lower ribs downward.

The *transversus abdominis* is a flat, broad muscle located on the front and side of the abdomen under the internal oblique. It has a complex origin which includes the upper surface of the coxal bone, the lumbodorsal fascia, and the inner surfaces of the costal cartilages of ribs seven through twelve. The fibers of the transversus abdominis run horizontally around the abdomen where, at the front, they attach to the abdominal aponeurosis. When the transversus abdominis contracts, it displaces the abdominal wall inward, thereby elevating. abdominal pressure.

Pulmonary subdivisions

The pulmonary system is capable of holding various amounts of air. This air can be measured with a number of different simple devices, some of which trace out a permanent record of air volume changes called a *spirogram*. Figure 3-13 shows an example of such a tracing and illustrates in principle the various *lung volumes* and *capacities* (Pappenheimer et al., 1950).

Lung volumes. The primary lung volumes are four in number and mutually exclusive (i. e., they do not overlap).

The *tidal volume* (TV) is the amount of air inspired or expired during a respiratory cycle. Under usual conditions, its magnitude is dictated by the oxygen needs of the body. In the resting individual it is termed *quiet tidal breathing* and its magnitude may be determined from a single respiratory cycle or from the average volume of a series of quiet breaths.

The *inspiratory reserve volume* (IRV) is the maximum amount of air that can be taken into the lungs and airways from the *end-inspiratory level* (i. e., the peak of each tidal volume cycle).

The *expiratory reserve volume* (ERV) is the greatest volume of air that can be expired from the resting expiratory level.

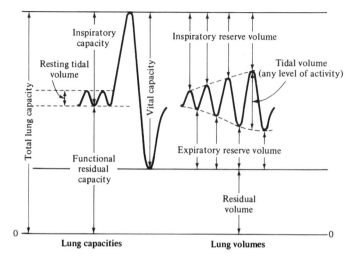

Figure 3-13 Spirogram illustration of lung volumes and lung capacities. [*After J. Pappenheimer et al., "Standardization of definitions and symbols in respiratory physiology,"* Fed. Proc., *9 (1950), 602-5.*]

The *residual volume* (RV) is the amount of air that remains in the lungs and airways at the end of a maximum expiration. Of the four primary lung volumes the RV is the only one that cannot be measured directly, since no matter how forceful the expiration, the pulmonary system cannot be emptied. It is possible, however, to indirectly estimate the residual volume through the use of special respiratory tests (Mead and Milic-Emili, 1964).

Lung Capacities. Like the primary lung volumes, the lung capacities are also four in number. In the case of each capacity, it includes two or more of the lung volumes just discussed.

The *inspiratory capacity* (IC) is the maximum volume of air that can be inspired from the resting expiratory level. This capacity is the sum of the tidal volume and the inspiratory reserve volume.

The *vital capacity* (VC) is the greatest amount of air that can be expelled from the lungs and airways after a maximum inspiration. It encompasses all of the primary lung volumes except the residual volume.

The *functional residual capacity* (FRC) is the volume of air contained within the lungs and airways at the resting expiratory level. It includes the expiratory reserve and residual volumes.

The *total lung capacity* (TLC) is the volume of air contained within the lungs and airways at the end of a maximum inspiration. This capacity includes all four of the primary lung volumes.

To give some indication of the relative magnitudes of the various pulmonary subdivisions, sample values for all the lung volumes and capacities are presented in Table 3-1. The data shown are for a healthy, young, adult male, breathing at sea level in a standing position. It should be appreciated that these values vary with many factors, including posture, age, height, weight, sex, and altitude (Comroe et al., 1962).

Table 3-1   Values (in liters) for the various pulmonar subdivisions of a healthy, young, adult male, breathing at sea level in a standing position.

Lung volume or capacity	Magnitude (L)
Tidal Volume	0.5
Inspiratory Reserve Volume	2.5
Expiratory Reserve Volume	2.0
Residual Volume	2.0
Inspiratory Capacity	3.0
Vital Capacity	5.0
Functional Residual Capacity	4.0
Total Lung Capacity	7.0

Volume-pressure relationships

Much of the discussion to this point can be integrated into a single graph, a knowledge of which serves as an important basis for understanding the discussions on speech respiration to follow. Such a graph, known as a volume-pressure diagram (Rahn et al., 1946; Campbell, 1958, 1968), is of analytical value in relating the nonmuscular and muscular forces of respiration to each

Figure 3-14   Lung volume-alveolar pressure relations during relaxation, maximum expiration and maximum inspiration, with a spirogram showing lung volume subdivisions. [*After E. Agostoni and J. Mead, "Statics of the Respiratory System," in W. Fenn and H. Rahn (eds)., Handbook of Physiology (Washington, D.C.: Amer. Physiol. Soc., 1964).*]

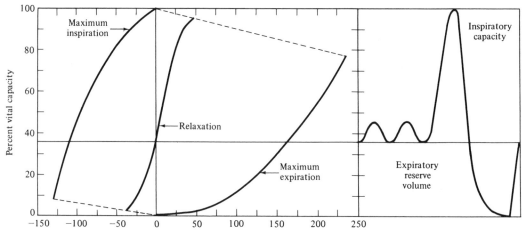

other, to the alveolar pressure, and to the various levels of the lung volume. One form of the volume-pressure diagram is illustrated in Figure 3-14 along with a spirogram of the pulmonary subdivisions for reference. There the amount of air within the lungs (expressed as percent of the vital capacity) is displayed on the vertical axis, with alveolar pressure on the horizontal axis. Points to the right of zero (atmospheric pressure) represent pressures greater than atmospheric; those to the left are subatmospheric. The three curves shown represent the volume-pressure relations during (1) relaxation, (2) maximum expiration, and (3) maximum inspiration.

Relaxation pressure. The pressure produced entirely by nonmuscular forces of the respiratory mechanism is termed the *relaxation pressure*. This pressure, developed in the lungs and airways when the respiratory muscles are relaxed, varies in magnitude depending upon how much the lungs are inflated or deflated from the resting expiratory level. At lung volumes above the resting position, relaxation results in passive expiration through generation of a positive pressure (above atmospheric). This pressure decreases as the lungs are deflated from the total lung capacity to the resting expiratory level. Relaxation at lung volumes below the resting level results in subatmospheric alveolar pressure, with the magnitude of this pressure increasing (i. e., becoming less subatmospheric) as the lungs inflate from the residual volume to the resting expiratory level.[5] In the midvolume range, relaxation pressure changes nearly in direct proportion to volume, while at the extremes of lung volume, pressure changes more abruptly. The basis for the differences at the volume extremes is the relative stiffness of the lungs and thorax, the lungs being stiffer at high lung volumes and the thorax being stiffer at low volumes.[6]

Departures from relaxation pressure can be achieved at any lung volume through the use of muscular effort (Mead et al., 1968). Pressures less than the relaxation pressure (i. e., to the left of the curve) require that a "net" *inspiratory* muscle effort be added to the relaxation pressure. Those pressures which exceed the relaxation pressure (i. e., those to the right of the curve) require that a "net" *expiratory* muscle effort be added to the relaxation pressure. It is important to specify "net" in such descriptions since although pressures less than relaxation can be produced solely through inspiratory effort and

[5] Up to now inspiration has been considered as an active process. Following expiration below the resting expiratory level, however, inspiration may be passive. This can be demonstrated by the simple experiment of expiring to the residual volume and then relaxing. Upon relaxation, the respiratory pump recoils back to its resting level without the aid of muscular effort. For an analogy, consider the action of a compressed spring when it is released.

[6] Although beyond the scope of this chapter, it should be mentioned that the relaxation pressure for the total respiratory apparatus can be analyzed into several components. Most commonly partitioned are the pressure caused by recoil of the lungs and the pressure due to recoil of the thorax (including the diaphragm and abdomen). For a detailed account of the various components, see Agostoni and Mead (1964), and Konno and Mead (1968).

pressures more than relaxation can be produced solely through expiratory effort, it is possible to depart from the relaxation pressure curve with both inspiratory and expiratory forces operating simultaneously but with one or the other being in preponderance. Furthermore, it is possible to stay on the relaxation pressure curve during muscular effort (i. e., to produce a pressure equal to the relaxation pressure at any lung volume) by exerting inspiratory and expiratory forces which are equal and thus cancelling. It follows that pressure equal to the relaxation pressure at a given lung volume cannot be used as evidence for a lack of muscular effort.

Maximum pressures. The curves labelled *maximum expiration* and *maximum inspiration* in Figure 3-14 show, respectively, the greatest positive and negative pressures that can be developed through the use of muscular effort. As such, these curves define the limits within which respiratory function must occur, or to which it is possible to depart from the relaxation pressure at each lung volume. As with relaxation pressure, pressures developed during maximum efforts depend upon lung volume. The maximum expiratory pressure, for example, decreases as the lungs deflate from the total lung capacity to the residual volume. Maximum inspiratory pressure, on the other hand, increases (i. e., becomes less subatmospheric) as the lungs are inflated from the residual volume to the total lung capacity. Maximum expiratory pressures are greater at higher lung volumes because the relaxation pressure is greater and because the expiratory muscles are stretched to more optimum lengths for generating tensions (Siebens, 1966). Along similar lines, greater negative pressures can be produced at lower volumes since the respiratory pump recoils toward a larger volume with greater force, and because the inspiratory muscles are operating under more favorable length-tension conditions.

RESPIRATION FOR SPEECH PURPOSES

Knowing the elements of normal respiration, attention is now directed toward respiratory function in speech. This calls for discussion of the task facing the respiratory pump as well as examination of how that task is accomplished by the body machinery.

Role of the Respiratory Pump in Speech

The ease with which breathing occurs in speech gives little hint as to the important role the respiratory pump plays in man's ability to communicate orally. Viewed broadly, that role is to provide the driving forces necessary for the generation of sounds, those forces being supplied in the form of pressures and flows which act upon and interact with various structures within the head and neck. To be more specific, the respiratory pump participates in speech by displacing structures, creating pressures behind valves, and generating flows through constrictions within the larynx and upper airways. These activities, in association with intricate and rapid maneuvers of other parts of the speech apparatus, create the disturbances of air that constitute speech at the acoustical level. Since respiratory forces provide the basic energy source for all speech and voice production in the English language, the events of speech respiration are of fundamental importance in any account of oral communication. Within the broad spectrum of physiological function in speech, the respiratory pump is involved in the regulation of such important parameters as speech and voice intensity (loudness), vocal fundamental frequency (pitch), linguistic stress (emphasis), and the division of speech into various units (syllables, words, phrases, etc.). Each of these involvements is considered in this volume, some in this chapter and others in Chapters 4, 5, and 6.

Mechanics of Speech Respiration

Most accounts of speech breathing portray it as a simple and relatively featureless behavior of the speech apparatus, albeit a behavior of primary importance. Actually, there is great complexity in the events of respiration during speech, complexity that equals and in many respects surpasses that of events in other parts of the speaking machinery. This section considers the more important mechanical aspects of respiratory function in speech and relates these to the general problem which speech imposes upon the respiratory pump. First considered are the demands of steady utterances, then the demands of conversational speech.

Demands of steady utterances

The simplest mechanical problem facing the respiratory pump in speech is that where the average pressure, flow, and resistance of the upper airways are relatively constant throughout the utterance. Speech activities meeting these criteria are the focus of this section, their being a useful starting point for the study of speech breathing physiology. The discussion offered here deals with the aerodynamic events associated with such utterances as well as the forces provided by the respiratory pump.

Aerodynamic events. Figure 3-15 illustrates in simplified form the nature of volume, flow, and pressure events associated with a prolonged utterance produced throughout most of the vital capacity. The speech activity in this

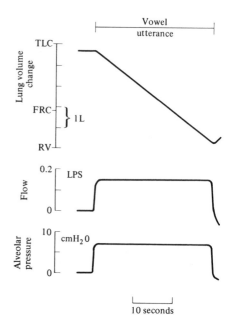

Figure 3-15 Lung volume change (liters), flow (liters per second) and alveolar pressure (centimeters of water) during an isolated vowel utterance produced throughout most of the vital capacity.

instance consists of an isolated sustained vowel produced at constant normal loudness and pitch levels. However, the data are representative of *average values*[7] for a variety of utterances consisting mainly of equally stressed syllables as when repeating a single syllable, counting, reciting the alphabet, etc. (Draper et al., 1959; Bouhuys et al., 1966). The top tracing in Figure 3-15 shows lung volume decreasing at a constant rate during the speech activity, from near the total lung capacity to near the residual volume. Flow and alveolar pressure show abrupt increases at the onset of speech activity, maintenance at constant values during the utterance, and abrupt decreases at the end of speech. Since both pressure and flow are constant during the utterance, it follows that the average resistance offered by the larynx and upper airways is also constant since, by definition, resistance is the ratio of pressure to flow (resistance = pressure/flow).

[7] The recordings shown are simplified in several ways. For example, they do not portray rapid variations associated with vocal fold vibration or the heartbeat. Although they represent the average values for a variety of utterances, the particular example shown is for a prolonged vowel and therefore gives no indication of the nature of rapid changes in pressure, flow, and volume that occur during syllable utterances. In effect, the tracings of Figure 3-15 have high frequency information (rapidly changing events) "filtered off" them. It is assumed that the alveolar pressure recording approximates that which would be obtained just below the larynx (i. e., subglottal or tracheal pressure). Actually, alveolar and subglottal pressures differ by a small amount during speech because of a resistive pressure loss between the alveoli and the larynx, this loss increasing slightly with decreasing lung volume (Bouhuys et al., 1966).

Respiratory forces. Both muscular and nonmuscular forces are involved in the regulation of respiratory behavior for utterances like that illustrated in Figure 3-15. The general problem of combining such forces to achieve a desired alveolar pressure is the concern of the next four sections which consider, respectively, the total force provided, the activity of specific muscles involved in providing this total force, the special role played by hydraulic events within the abdomen, and the effect of changing body posture within a gravity field.

Muscular pressures. Recall that the relaxation pressure curve portrays the nonmuscular forces of respiration, with the magnitude of the pressure developed during relaxation depending upon how much air is contained within the lungs. It is useful to think of the relaxation pressure as a spring-like background force that is expiratory at lung volumes above the resting expiratory level and inspiratory at lung volumes below that level. Recall further that departures from relaxation pressure can be achieved at any lung volume through the use of muscular effort, with (1) pressures less than the relaxation pressure resulting from "net" or solely inspiratory efforts, (2) pressures greater than the relaxation pressure resulting from "net" or solely expiratory efforts, and (3) pressures equal to the relaxation pressure indicating either no muscular effort (i. e., muscular relaxation) or equal and simultaneous inspiratory and expiratory efforts. By viewing the relaxation pressure and departures from it in these terms, it is possible to use the volume-pressure diagram to graphically determine the sign and magnitude of muscular force that must be added to the spring-like background force to achieve the alveolar pressure required for any utterance (Hixon et al., 1968b; Mead et al., 1968). The main point to keep in mind for any such analysis is that *the amount of muscular pressure required at a given instant during speech depends upon the alveolar pressure needed and the relaxation pressure available at the prevailing lung volume.*

Figure 3-16 presents an example of the application of the type of analysis just described. The alveolar pressure from the normal loudness utterance of Figure 3-15 is replotted in the upper half of the figure (this time against lung volume) together with the relaxation volume-pressure characteristic of the respiratory apparatus (illustrated earlier in Figure 3-14). Note that the needed alveolar pressure of 7 cm H_2O is less than the relaxation pressure during the early part of the utterance (throughout the high lung volumes), equal to it at one point (where the curves intersect), and greater than it during the latter part of the utterance (throughout the low lung volumes). Since the difference between the alveolar pressure and relaxation pressure represents the muscular pressure, the horizontal distance (i. e., the hatched area) between the speech curve and the relaxation pressure curve indicates the muscular pressure that must be added to the relaxation pressure to achieve the alveolar pressure needed at each lung volume for speech. For convenience this pressure differ-

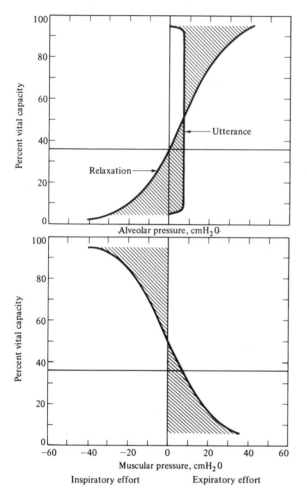

Figure 3-16 Upper: Lung volume-alveolar pressure relations during relaxation and during an isolated vowel utterance of normal loudness produced throughout most of the vital capacity. [*Relaxation curve after E. Agostoni and J. Mead, "Statics of the Respiratory System," in W. Fenn and H. Rahn (eds.),* Handbook of Physiology (*Washington, D.C.: Amer. Physiol. Soc., 1964*).] Hatched area between the curves shows the muscular pressure required for the utterance. Lower: Lung volume-muscular pressure relations replotted from data of the upper graph. Negative values represent net inspiratory forces and positive values represent net expiratory forces.

ence is plotted in the lower half of Figure 3-16. The horizontal axis depicts muscular pressure, with negative and positive values representing net inspiratory and net expiratory forces, respectively. Examination of the muscular pressure graph reveals that at high lung volumes a net inspiratory force is added to the relaxation pressure, the magnitude of this force decreasing as speech proceeds and air leaves the lungs. Near 50% of the vital capacity the net force is zero, while below that level a positive muscular pressure is required in increasing amounts as lung volume continues to decrease. For this particular utterance, then, where a constant alveolar pressure of 7 cm H_2O is required, the sign of the muscular pressure provided at high lung volumes is opposite to that of alveolar pressure and flow. In other words, a situation exists where inspiratory effort is exerted during an expiratory task, namely, speech production. This is not unlike the situation discussed earlier where during quiet breathing the activity of the inspiratory muscles persists into expiration. In the present situation, inspiratory effort is employed at high lung volumes in order to counteract the full force of the spring-like recoil of the respiratory pump, a recoil that would provide more pressure than needed were the relaxation pressure not opposed to some extent at high lung volumes (Bouhuys et al., 1966). The negative muscular work done in opposing the excessive relaxation pressure in this circumstance may be thought of as a "braking" or "checking" action against the spring-like background force. In contrast to high lung volumes, at intermediate lung volumes (between about 50% and 35% of the vital capacity) the relaxation pressure is insufficient to meet the demands of the utterance. It is necessary, therefore, to supplement the background force through the contribution of a positive muscular pressure. This means that within the intermediate range of lung volumes the relaxation and muscular pressures are of the same sign for this utterance. Such is not the case below the resting level since the muscular pressure added must overcome the inspiratory recoil of the pump and, beyond that, provide sufficient pressure to meet the demands of the utterance. It should be noted that for this seemingly simple utterance of sustaining a vowel, the muscular pressure needed is initially opposite in sign to the recoil pressure of the pump, then in the same sign as that of the pump, and finally again opposite in sign to the pump but with the sign of both the muscular pressure and recoil pressure being opposite to their respective signs at high lung volumes.

Some may find it useful at this juncture to consider the muscular pressure problem in analogous terms such as apply to the simple mechanical system shown in Figure 3-17. There in place of the respiratory apparatus is a hand bellows which, in functional analogy to the human respiratory pump, has (1) a mechanism (hand power) to pull its handles apart, corresponding to negative muscular pressure or inspiratory effort, (2) a countermechanism (again hand power) to push its handles together, corresponding to positive muscular pressure or expiratory effort, and (3) a spring between the handles corresponding to the relaxation pressure provided by the lungs-thorax unit, which will exert varying degrees of inspiratory or expiratory force on the handles depending on how far the spring is stretched or compressed from its resting length. Although the system of Figure 3-17 has general application to all aspects of the muscular pressure problem, two examples of its functional equivalence should serve sufficiently to illustrate the usefulness of reasoning by analogy. For a first example, consider the functional analogy of the mechanical system to the "checking" action of the human pump. Suppose the handles of the bellows were maximally widespread (i. e., the total lung capacity of the bellows) and then released. If the pressure created within the bellows chamber by the recoiling spring exceeded that desired,

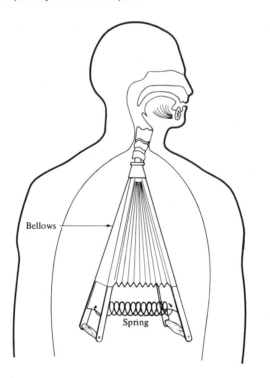

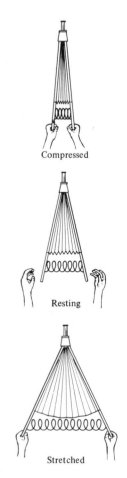

Figure 3-17   Bellows-spring analogy for the respiratory pump. Equivalents are : (1) hand forces to pull the handles apart, representing inspiratory effort, (2) hand forces to push the handles together, representing expiratory effort, and (3) a spring between the handles, representing the background force of the lungs-thorax unit. Smaller models on the right depict various functional situations.

this pressure could be reduced to a specified level by the simple opposing maneuver of pulling with appropriate force on the handles of the system. As a second example, consider the application of the analog to a situation where a positive muscular pressure is needed as would be the case if it were a requirement that a steady chamber pressure be maintained below resting spring length (i. e., the resting expiratory level). In such a circumstance it would be necessary to compress the system by pushing on the handles of the bellows with an appropriately increasing force that would overcome the inspiratory recoil of the spring and add an amount of pressure equal to the desired chamber pressure.

Since alveolar pressure demands differ for different utterances, speech activities requiring pressures other than the 7 cm H_2O considered in Figure 3-16 require different muscular pressures at each lung volume. This is illustrated in Figure 3-18 where the alveolar and muscular pressures for a soft and very loud utterance are contrasted with a normal-loudness utterance. It is clear in Figure 3-18 that an even greater negative muscular pressure must be used to counteract the relaxation pressure at high lung volumes for the soft than for the normal-loudness utterance. In addition, this counteraction must continue to a lower lung volume for the softer of the two utterances. In terms of the preceding analogy, these events would require that the recoil of the stretched lungs-thorax spring be opposed more and to shorter spring lengths to achieve a lower chamber pressure for the less demanding pressure maneuver. Continuing with the soft-normal contrast, less positive muscular pressure needs to be added to the relaxation pressure at low lung volumes for the soft than for the normal loudness condition, a situation that by analogy requires less forceful pushing on the bellows handles for the condition requiring lower pressure. Where the alveolar pressure demand is great, such as for the very loud utterance depicted in Figure 3-18, a positive

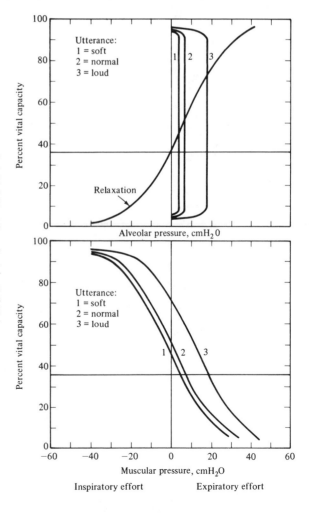

Figure 3-18 Upper: Lung volume-alveolar pressure relations during relaxation and during three isolated vowel utterances of different loudnesses produced throughout most of the vital capacity. [*Relaxation curve after E. Agostoni and J. Mead, "Statics of the Respiratory System," in W. Fenn and H. Rahn (eds.),* Handbook of Physiology *(Washington, D.C.: Amer. Physiol. Soc., 1964).*] Lower: Lung volume-muscular pressure relations replotted from data of the upper graph. Negative values represent net inspiratory forces and positive values indicate net expiratory forces.

muscular pressure is required throughout most of the vital capacity. This is because the relaxation pressure does not exceed the needed alveolar pressure over most of the lung volume range. A compression of the bellows system would be required at nearly every spring position were this task subjected to analog treatment.

By this point it should be obvious that with knowledge of the relaxation pressure characteristic, the alveolar pressure developed during speech, and the lung volume at which speech is produced, it is possible to specify the muscular pressure that is required at every instant. Thus the respiratory pump accomplishes the task which speech imposes upon it by adding, at each instant, a muscular pressure that is precisely equal to the difference between the alveolar pressure desired and the relaxation pressure available. The important implication of this statement is that *each alveolar pressure produced in speech demands a different muscular pressure at each lung volume.*

Electromyographic activity. Informed of the magnitude and sign of the total muscular pressure applied during speech, it is relevant to examine the specific muscles involved in the active regulation of this pressure. This requires consideration of the time course of muscle activity and how that activity relates to the mechanical properties of the respiratory pump as well as the demands placed upon it. Beginning with an utterance of normal loudness, Figure 3-19 presents an account of several of the more important muscles involved. The upper part of that figure is a duplication of the lower half of Figure 3-16, while the lower part of the figure is a diagrammatic representation of the temporal activity[8] of six muscles which play a part in generating the muscular pressures depicted in the upper graph (Draper et al., 1959; Ladefoged, 1967). Of the muscles considered, previous description has characterized the diaphragm and external intercostals as inspiratory, the internal intercostals, external oblique and rectus abdominis as expiratory, and the latissiumus dorsi as potentially inspiratory or expiratory. During a deep inspiration, such as that preceding speech initiated near the total lung capacity, the diaphragm, external intercostals and accessory muscles are

[8] This activity is determined through study of the voltage variations associated with muscle activity. The technique used is termed *electromyography* and involves the sensing of electrical activity of muscles through metal electrodes placed on the body surface over muscles or inserted directly into muscles through the skin. Electrical changes occur when a muscle is active under three circumstances: (1) miometric contraction in which it shortens, (2) isometric contraction in which its length does not change, and (3) pliometric contraction in which it lengthens under the influence of other forces acting on it (Agostoni, 1964). There is no way to unequivocally differentiate among these three types of activity in the respiratory muscles during speech. Inferences must be made about the type of activity on the basis of the mechanical behaviors of various parts of the respiratory pump and on the pressure changes associated with their actions. Figure 3-19 amounts to a binary statement of the activity of each muscle considered. It indicates only when a muscle is, or is not, active electrically and says nothing about the tensions created by the different muscles at different times.

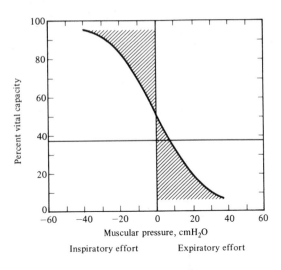

Figure 3-19   Upper: Lung volume-muscular pressure relations during an isolated vowel utterance of normal loudness produced throughout most of the vital capacity (see Figure 3-16). Negative values represent net inspiratory forces and positive values represent net expiratory forces. Lower: Diagrammatic representation of the temporal activity of six muscles involved in generating the muscular pressures depicted in the upper graph. [*Lower graph is after M. Draper, P. Ladefoged, and D. Whitteridge, "Respiratory muscles in speech."* J. Speech Hearing Research, 2 (*1959*), *16–27.*]

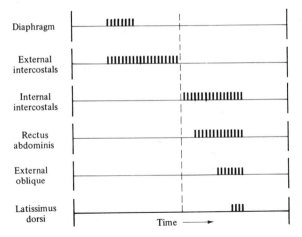

active. As shown in Figure 3-19, the diaphragm and external intercostals remain active as speech begins despite the fact that expiration is occurring. This observation is consistent with the negative muscular pressure requirement shown in the upper part of the figure. There is reason to believe that other inspiratory muscles may participate in this counteraction behavior (Eblen, 1963), however, insufficient research has been done to determine this unequivocally. In any event, the activity of the chief muscle of inspiration, the diaphragm, is seen to cease early in the utterance despite the fact that the relaxation pressure exceeds the needed alveolar pressure (i. e., the muscular pressure is negative). The activity of the external intercostal muscles proceeds well into the utterance and, although not determinable from Figure 3-19, it diminishes gradually until the muscular pressure demand is zero. This, recall, is the instant when the available relaxation pressure is equal to the alveolar pressure demanded for the utterance. For the utterance to continue below the lung volume corresponding to the instant of zero muscular pressure it is necessary that a positive muscular pressure be added to the relaxation forces of the pump. This pressure is provided initially by the internal intercostal muscles which are activated the moment a positive muscular pressure is needed and which increase their level of activity as the lung volume reduces further. As the pump passes through the resting expiratory level and is faced with the problem of overcoming its inspiratory recoil, abdominal muscles (i. e., the external oblique and rectus abdominis) are brought into play to supplement the contribution of the internal intercostals. Finally, at the lower extreme of the lung volume (near RV) the latissimus dorsi becomes active. Assuming its activity to be expiratory, then at least four muscles are implicated as expiratory participants in speech near the end of the utterance where the negative recoil of the respiratory apparatus is maximum. There is reason to suspect that other expiratory muscles may be involved in respiratory regulation at low lung volumes (Hixon et al., 1968a), however, as with the inspiratory muscles at high lung volumes, experimental information is incomplete.

It is important to mention that the account just offered is not entirely universal among speakers or to repeated utterances by the same individual. Although it represents the usual pattern of activity for normal speakers who do not use their diaphragms, it is possible to consciously depart from this pattern. While many combinations of muscle activity could achieve the same end result (i. e., the desired alveolar pressure), certain combinations are undoubtedly more efficient than others from the viewpoint of function of the body machinery. With regard to this point, it is interesting to note and tempting to ascribe significance to the fact that there is no antagonistic muscle activity (i. e., no simultaneous inspiratory and expiratory activity) at any point throughout the utterance depicted in Figure 3-19. If the activities of the muscles portrayed are representative of other muscles with similar functions, then the muscular pressure values shown are related solely to inspiratory activity at high lung volumes and solely to expiratory activity at low lung volumes. This again is not meant to imply that the muscles function in this fashion under all circumstances. Indeed, there is evidence (Draper et al., 1959) that some individuals occasionally use inspiratory and expiratory muscles simultaneously during speech.

Since each alveolar pressure produced in speech demands a different muscular pressure at each lung volume, it would be expected that muscular

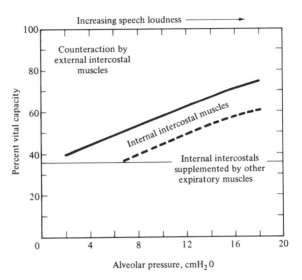

Figure 3-20 Graphic portrayal illustrating which muscles or groups of muscles are active at different lung volumes and alveolar pressures (or loudnesses) during speech where the diaphragm is inactive. [*After M. Draper, P. Ladefoged, and D. Whitteridge, "Respiratory muscles in speech," J. Speech Hearing Research, 2 (1959), 16–27.*]

activity would likewise be different for different alveolar pressures at different lung volumes. This is evident in Figure 3-20 which graphically portrays the dependence of muscular activity upon alveolar pressure and lung volume. From Figure 3-20 predictions can be made as to which muscles or groups of muscles will be active at different lung volumes and alveolar pressures during speech where the diaphragm is inactive (Draper et al., 1959; Ladefoged, 1967). The vertical axis in that figure represents lung volume, the horizontal dimension represents alveolar pressure.[9] Assuming a relatively steady alveolar pressure with decreasing lung volume, the pattern of muscular activity when speaking at a given average alveolar pressure can be determined by following any vertical line downward. For example, when speaking from near the total lung capacity with an alveolar pressure of 10 cm H_2O the external intercostal muscles cease their activity at about 58% of the vital capacity, the internal intercostals take over from there to approximately the 44% level and thereafter the internals are supplemented by other expiratory muscles. The significant point to be made in conjunction with Figure 3-20 is that speech using relatively high alveolar pressures involves less "checking" on the part of the external intercostals and earlier and greater activity of the internal inter-

[9] Figure 3-20 is redrawn from the work of Draper et al. (1959). Their study was based on esophageal pressure measurements which were assumed to be the equivalent of tracheal or alveolar pressures. Esophageal and alveolar pressures actually differ by an amount equal to the volume-dependent recoil pressure developed by the stretched lungs (Bouhuys et al., 1966; Ladefoged, 1967, 1968). Unfortunately, lung recoil data were not obtained for the subjects studied by Draper et al. (1959); hence, the original version of Figure 3-20 cannot be adjusted with great precision. A good approximation to the truth has been provided in Figure 3-20, however, by correcting the original pressure data on the basis of predicted static recoil pressures for the lungs of healthy normal subjects (Agostoni and Mead, 1964).

costals and other expiratory muscles than speech requiring low alveolar pressures. Furthermore, the determinants of the activities of specific muscles are largely those discussed earlier in the muscular pressure problem; namely, the alveolar pressure required and the recoil force contributed by the lungs-thorax unit.

Abdominal hydraulics. Despite the diaphragm's status as the most important muscle of inspiration, it has been noted above that this structure ceases its electrical activity at high lung volumes in most speakers, although there is a continuing need for negative muscular pressures for certain types of utterances. The generation of such pressures without recourse to the diaphragm is made possible in the upright posture because of the influence of gravity on the abdominal contents (Bouhuys et al., 1966). From a mechanical viewpoint, the abdomen may be likened to a liquid-filled container (see Figure 3-21) in which its top (the diaphgram) and part of its lateral wall (the abdominal wall) are distensible (Agostoni and Mead, 1964). The weight of the abdominal contents is supported in part by the wall of the abdomen and in part by pleural pressure. The latter manifests itself as an upward force pulling on the relaxed diaphragm, this pull being transmitted to the ab-

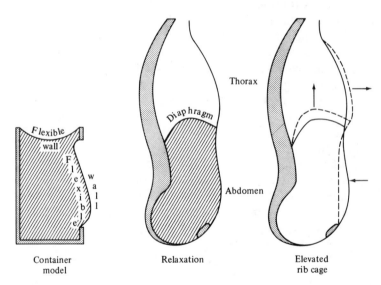

| Container model | Relaxation | Elevated rib cage |

Figure 3-21 Container model of the diaphragm-abdomen system, together with illustrations of the resting and elevated rib cage positions of various respiratory structures. During relaxation the abdominal contents are supported against gravity by the wall of the abdomen and by lung recoil acting to elevate the diaphragm. Elevation of the rib cage through muscular effort causes it to expand, the diaphragm to be sucked upward, and the abdominal wall to be sucked inward. [*After E. Agostoni and J. Mead, "Statics of the Respiratory System," in W. Fenn and H. Rahn (eds.),* Handbook of Physiology (*Washington, D.C.: Amer. Physiol. Soc., 1964*).]

dominal contents to support it in a manner somewhat analogous to the support of a water column by suction in a drinking straw. Through various respiratory maneuvers the relative support of the abdominal contents can be shifted in favor of either the abdominal wall or the negative pleural pressure, support in favor of the latter being of foremost importance to the generation of negative muscular pressure at high lung volumes during speech. As shown previously, a low alveolar pressure demand at high lung volume finds the external intercostal muscles active even in the absence of diaphragmatic activity. These, and possibly other inspiratory muscles acting on the walls of the thorax, elevate the rib cage and expand it to a size greater than it would assume during relaxation at the same lung volume (Konno and Mead, 1967; Hixon et al., 1970). An elevated rib cage in combination with a relaxed abdominal wall and a relaxed diaphragm causes most of the support of the abdominal contents to be shifted to the pleural pressure (Mead et al., 1968). During such a maneuver the relaxed diaphragm is sucked upward, the abdominal pressure becomes more negative than its value during relaxation at the same lung volume, and the abdominal wall is sucked inward. With a pressure more negative than usual acting on the abdominal side of the diaphragm, a downward pull is placed on the structure, this pull balancing that of the negative pleural pressure. The significant aspect of abdominal hydraulics in this circumstance is that the weight of the abdominal contents provides a mechanism against which the rib cage muscles can decrease pleural pressure. Were it not for the hydraulic properties of the abdomen in the upright posture, the rib cage muscles would be relatively ineffective in lowering pleural pressure without active contraction of the diaphragm. The next section examines a circumstance where the abdomen does not exert this important influence.

Effects of posture. Departures from the upright posture have marked effects on the behaviors and interactions of various respiratory parts, these effects being related mainly to the influence of gravity. As an illustration of the complexity of events involved, the more important contrasts of function in the upright and supine (i. e., lying on the back) postures are considered here. In the upright posture, gravity acts in an expiratory direction on the rib cage and in an inspiratory direction on the abdomen (see Figure 3-22). The effect is mainly on the abdomen, being greater at low than high lung volumes because the height of the abdomen is greater and its wall less stiff in the former situation (Agostoni and Mead, 1964). As discussed in the previous section, the abdominal contents are supported against gravity by the abdominal wall and the upward lifting force of the negative pleural pressure. In shifting from the upright to supine posture, a new mechanical situation exists wherein the gravitational effect is expiratory on both the rib cage and abdomen. Compared to the upright posture there is less gravitational effect with changes in lung volume in the supine posture because the height of the

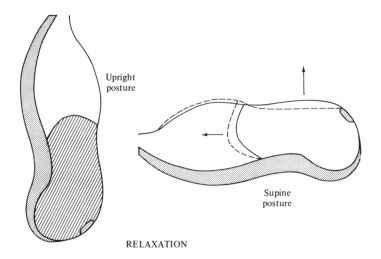

Upright
posture

Supine
posture

RELAXATION

Figure 3-22 Resting positions of various respiratory structures during relaxation in the upright and supine postures. Gravity acts in the expiratory direction on the rib cage and in the inspiratory direction on the abdomen in the upright posture. In the supine position, gravity acts in the expiratory direction on both the rib cage and abdomen. The diaphragm is displaced headward in the supine posture and the forces of the abdomen which act to distend the diaphragm are balanced by the diaphragm's own elastic force. [*After E. Agostoni and J. Mead, "Statics of the Respiratory System," in W. Fenn and H. Rahn* (*eds.*), Handbook of Physiology (*Washington, D.C.: Amer. Physiol. Soc., 1964*).]

abdomen is less (Agostoni and Mead, 1964). A significant feature of shifting to the supine posture is that pleural pressure no longer has a major role in supporting the abdominal contents. With gravity acting on the relaxed abdomen, the diaphragm is displaced into the rib cage until the forces acting to distend it are balanced by its own elastic force. As a consequence of this headward displacement of the diaphragm, the resting expiratory level of the pump changes from its upright value of approximately 35% of the vital capacity to a supine value of about 20%. An important outcome of this total set of events is a change in the relaxation volume-pressure characteristic of the mechanism. Figure 3-23 shows the relaxation pressure curves for both the upright and supine postures. The two curves differ in slope and shape with the supine curve being displaced to the right (i. e., the spring-like background force is greater at corresponding lung volumes in the supine than upright posture). The lower half of Figure 3-23 shows the muscular pressures needed for the production of the normal loudness utterance depicted in the upper part of the figure. A greater negative muscular pressure is required throughout the high lung volumes for the supine than upright posture, this negativity continuing to a lower lung volume in the supine than upright position. At low lung volumes, less positive muscular pressure is needed in the supine than upright posture for the same utterance. On first consideration it seems a simple problem of adding somewhat different muscular pressures to the relaxation pressure at each lung volume for the two postures. However, the pump is operating under very different mechanical conditions, a principal difference being the function of the diaphragm in the two positions. While abdominal hydraulics enable a footward pull to be placed on the relaxed diaphragm in the upright posture, they do not enable such a circumstance to exist in the supine posture (Hixon et al., 1970). Consequently, conditions requiring a negative muscular pressure at high lung volumes in the supine posture require that the diaphragm be active. In effect this activity is needed to overcome the influence of gravity on the abdominal contents, an influence which causes the diaphragm to be displaced headward.

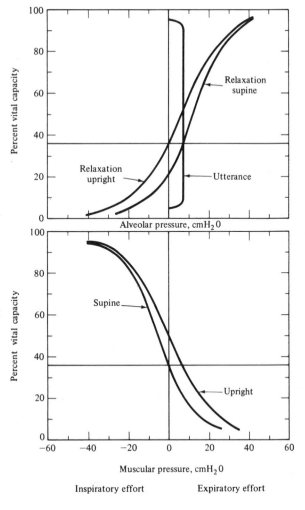

Figure 3-23   Upper: Lung volume-alveolar pressure relations during relaxation in the upright and supine postures and during an isolated vowel utterance of normal loudness produced throughout most of the vital capacity. [*Relaxation curves after E. Agostoni and J. Mead, "Statics of the Respiratory System," in W. Fenn and H. Rahn (eds.),* Handbook of Physiology, *(Washington, D.C.: Amer. Physiol. Soc., 1964)*.] Lower: Lung volume-muscular pressure relations replotted from data of the upper graph. Negative values represent net inspiratory forces and positive values represent net expiratory forces.

While only two postures have been considered here, it should be realized that every postural change requires a different solution to the mechanical problem of providing a given alveolar pressure. Indeed, the complexity of respiratory function in speech becomes staggering when consideration is given to the innumerable postures in which the body is oriented and reoriented with respect to gravity. In this regard it should be noted that while the influence of gravity is manifested in other parts of the speech mechanism with postural change, the functional adjustments that must be made by the respiratory pump far exceed those required in other parts of the speaking machinery.

Demands of conversational speech

The mechanical problem facing the respiratory pump in conversational speech is far more complex than that imposed by steady utterances. This section deals with some important features of that problem by considering selected aspects of three general topics: aerodynamic events, forces provided by the respiratory pump, and neurophysiological mechanisms which govern in part the actions of the respiratory machinery. Unless otherwise indicated, discussion of each topic is limited to function in the upright posture.

Aerodynamic events. For the speech activities discussed thus far the task of the respiratory pump is that of providing steady average pressures, flows, and resistances during single expirations throughout most of the vital capacity. Conversational speech is not characterized by aerodynamic events of this nature (except for brief durations), nor is it often produced on expirations encompassing a great deal of the vital capacity. As for the pressures, flows, and resistances, they are in nearly constant states of change during conversational speech, these changes often being rapid and of substantial magnitude. The specific nature of such changes depends upon a host of factors that can be categorized broadly into the following: (1) where within the total speech apparatus the aerodynamic events are examined (e. g., alveolar pressure, nasal flow, laryngeal resistance, etc.), (2) what phonetic factors are involved (e. g., specific sounds produced, serial ordering of sounds, etc.), and (3) what prosodic features are operating (e. g., variations in speaking rate, vocal pitch, stress, etc.). While the entire topic of aerodynamic events is within the province of speech breathing mechanics, the specific details of pressure, flow, and resistance changes have been judged to be more appropriately considered in this book within the broader context of speech physiology (Chapter 6) and following discussion of the dynamics of laryngeal (Chapter 4) and articulatory (Chapter 5) valving mechanisms. This leaves as the major area for discussion here the lung volume variations in conversational speech.

Lung volume changes. In breathing for life purposes, approximately 0.5 l of air is exchanged during each quiet tidal breath. By definition, breathing of this type occurs between the resting expiratory level and the tidal end-inspiratory position, the range between these covering approximately 10% of the vital capacity. While it is possible to consciously restrict speech to this limited range of lung volumes or to produce it within nearly any segment of the vital capacity, there are roughly defined lung volume limits within which certain types of utterances typically occur (Hixon et al., 1970). For example, as is illustrated in Figure 3-24, in the upright posture most conversational speech of normal loudness is produced within the midrange through volumes encompassing approximately 60 to 35% of the vital capacity. Deeper breaths are taken for speech of this nature than during normal quiet tidal breathing. Indeed, seldom are running speech phrases on new breaths initiated from lung volumes at or below the quiet end-inspiratory level. Of the many factors influencing the depth of inspiration during conversational utterances, the most important is the alveolar pressure demanded for the

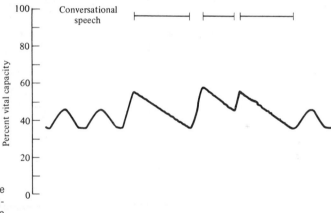

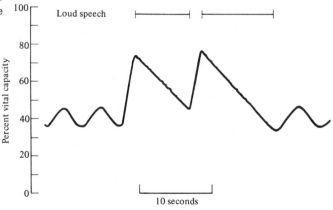

Figure 3-24 Lung volume changes characteristic of conversational and loud speech in the upright posture. Utterance is during the bracketed time segments shown above each of the tracings.

ensuing utterance. Witness to this pressure influence is very loud speech which demands high alveolar pressures and is usually initiated from higher lung volumes (e. g., 80–60% VC) than speech of normal loudness. As a further example, very soft speech, which demands low alveolar pressures, is frequently initiated at lower lung volumes than normal speech, however, still from volumes generally above the tidal end-inspiratory level. In the upright posture, breathing phrases are usually terminated slightly above or at the resting expiratory level (around 40–35% VC) during conversational utterances of normal loudness, with occasional phrases encroaching modestly upon the expiratory reserve volume. These latter instances most often result from the speaker's desire to complete a continuing utterance without inspiratory interruption to the communication process. Soft speech finds expiratory phrases ending near the same lung volumes as normal speech, while loud utterances are frequently terminated at lung volumes above the resting expiratory level, sometimes appreciably above.

The lung volumes used for conversational speech in other postures differ from those in the upright position (Hixon et al., 1970). In the supine posture, for example, volume events occur at lower levels of the vital capacity than in the upright position. Remember that in shifting from the upright to supine posture, the resting level of the respiratory pump decreases from approximately 35% VC to about 20% VC. As with the upright position, the supine speaker uses lung volumes above his resting expiratory level (20% VC) with his inspirations in preparation for speech involving deeper breaths than for quiet breathing. For speech of normal loudness most events occur between 45 and 20% VC in the supine position, with soft speech being initiated from somewhat lower lung volumes and loud speech being initiated from higher levels (e. g., 60 to 50% VC). As with the upright posture, relatively few expirations during speech in the supine posture extend below the resting level of the respiratory pump. In further similarity to the upright position, the supine speaker's loud speech phrases are more likely to end at higher lung volumes than normally loud or soft speech.

Mechanical factors are in part responsible for the use of the midvolume range of the vital capacity for speech, and for the utterance of most speech above the resting expiratory level. Use of the midvolume range is more desirable than use of either the upper or lower end of the vital capacity, since at these extremes the respiratory mechanism is stiffer and, therefore, mechanically more costly to control with muscular forces. By restricting utterances to lung volumes above the resting expiratory level, the speaker can take advantage of the positive recoil force of the respiratory mechanism to help drive his speech mechanism. Speech above the resting level is desirable also for the fact that no muscular energy needs to be expended against inspiratory recoil forces as would be the case for speech produced at volumes below the resting level.

The relative partitioning of volume change between the rib cage and abdomen-diaphragm during speech depends upon various factors, including the regulatory idiosyncrasies of the speaker, the loudness of speech, and the phonetic and prosodic content of the utterances (Hixon et al., 1970). Some speakers use predominantly rib cage motion to displace volume during speech while others use predominantly abdominal motion. The reasons for the choice of one motion over the other by a given speaker are uncertain, however, speakers are highly consistent with respect to how their rib cage and abdomen interact with changes in lung volume during speech.

Of final interest here are the temporal aspects of lung volume changes in conversational speech. It has been noted that the quiet breathing cycle is repeated twelve or more times a minute and involves expirations that are slightly longer than inspirations. For speech, the frequency of breathing typically decreases and the relative durations of the inspiratory and expiratory phases change considerably (see Figure 3-24). The inspiratory phase of the cycle, for example, is usually more abrupt than in quiet breathing since the speaker inspires rapidly during speech in order to minimize interruption to the speaking situation. The expiratory phase, on the other hand, is typically lengthened for speech since air leaves the lungs more slowly because of the high resistances in the upper airways. The result is an expiratory phase that is many times longer than the expiratory phase of quiet breathing and many times longer than the inspirations associated with either speech or quiet breathing. It is difficult to characterize the temporal aspects of volume events during speech in any quantifiable manner. Perhaps the most useful summary statement on temporal aspects is that while life respiration is highly regular in rate and rhythm, a hallmark of the volume events of conversational speech is the irregularity of the breathing cycle.

Respiratory forces. As with steady utterances, both muscular and non-muscular forces are involved in the regulation of the respiratory pump for conversational speech. These are considered in the next two subsections.

Muscular pressures. The muscular pressure problem in conversational speech can be viewed in the same terms and subjected to the same type of graphical volume-pressure solution as the problem for steady utterances. Recall that the muscular pressure required at a given instant during speech depends upon the alveolar pressure demanded and the relaxation pressure available. As noted previously, the lung volumes used in conversational speech are for the most part in the midrange of the vital capacity (i. e., about 60 to 35% VC). Referring to the volume-pressure diagram of Figure 3-14, it can be seen that the relaxation pressure available within those lung volume limits ranges between 10 and 0 cm H_2O. If 7 cm H_2O is taken as the average alveolar pressure required for normal loudness conversational speech, the relaxation pressure throughout most of the midrange of volumes is less than that demanded of the respiratory pump. Accordingly, a positive muscular pressure must be added to the relaxation pressure. This muscular pressure must be gradually increased so as to compensate for the decreasing recoil force of the respiratory pump with reducing lung volume. This aspect of the muscular pressure problem for conversational speech is solved in a manner identical to that discussed earlier for sustained utterances. In the present instance, however, positive muscular pressures are generally involved since the range of lung volumes characteristically used by normal speakers involves relatively low relaxation pressures. Remember that negative muscular pressures are demanded only when the alveolar pressures needed are more than the pressure available through the combined recoil force of the lungs and thorax (including the diaphragm and abdomen). Another feature which distinguishes the muscular pressure problem in conversational speech from that in sustained utterances is that during conversational speech there are frequent demands for rapid changes in muscular pressure. These may be viewed as "pulsatile" variations in muscular pressure which are provided in addition to the usual background level of alveolar pressure for steady utterances. The specific nature of these pulsatile variations is discussed in Chapter 6, where it is shown how they are of great linguistic significance as, for example, in stress (emphasis) contrasts. It is sufficient here to point out that these abrupt changes in muscular pressure are of brief duration (about 75–150 msec) and involve magnitudes of change in the neighborhood of 1–3 cm H_2O during normal loudness speech in the midvolume range (Netsell, 1969).

The bellows-spring analogy considered earlier for sustained utterances can be extended to apply to conversational speech. Figure 3-25 shows how the problem may be conceptualized as involving the parallel (i. e., simultaneous) solution of two problems. The left side of Figure 3-25 illustrates that component of the solution which provides a relatively constant alveolar pressure in the face of a continuously changing elastic recoil. There, with the wrists of the operator locked, movements of the arms provide the *gradual* changes in muscular pressure needed for utterance. These changes result from forcing the handles of the bellows toward one another to augment the spring-like background force within the range of lung volumes of interest here. This component of the muscular pressure solution may be designated as the "volume solution" since changing lung volume dictates that a changing muscular pressure adjustment be made. The right side of Figure 3-25 combines this volume solution with the second component which may be designated as the "pulsatile solution." There, in addition to the volume solution accomplished by gradual inward movement of the arms, brief and rapid changes in muscular pressure (i.e., pulsatile changes) are accomplished, in analogy, by simultaneous rapid movements of the hands as performed through unlocked wrists. Thus, the problem imposed upon the respiratory

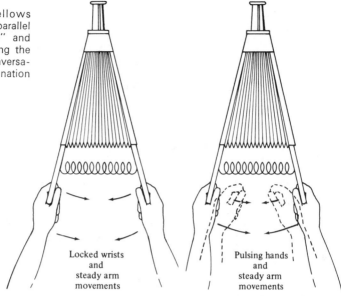

Volume solution   Pulsatile solution

Figure 3-25 Spring-bellows analogies portraying the parallel solution of the "volume" and "pulsatile" problems facing the respiratory pump in conversational speech. For explanation see text.

Locked wrists and steady arm movements

Pulsing hands and steady arm movements

pump in conversational speech is solved, in analogy, by taking into account the slowly needed muscular pressure adjustments with arm movements and the more rapid variations with sudden and small movements of the hands. Although the nature of muscular pressure changes in running speech is relatively well understood, the muscular events within the respiratory apparatus which govern these changes are not well defined. The following section reviews the essential features of what is known about the specific muscular events.

Electromyographic activity. With positive muscular pressures being demanded during conversational speech, it follows that expiratory muscles are implicated in the mechanical events of such utterances. Examination of Figures 3-19 and 3-20 reveals that the muscles most important to the maintenance of a relatively steady alveolar pressure within the midvolume range are the internal intercostals. As discussed in the previous section, the "volume solution" for sustained utterances and conversational speech is conceptually identical. Accordingly, the important aspect to be discussed in this section is the manner in which the so-called "pulsatile" pressure changes are accomplished within the midvolume range. A great deal of controversy surrounds the activity of muscles in supplying these "pulsatile" variations (Stetson, 1951; Ladefoged et al., 1958; Draper et al., 1959; Hoshiko, 1960; Hardy, 1967; Ladefoged, 1967). Although there is general agreement that thoracic muscles are the chief regulators of muscular pressure changes under these circumstances, it is not agreed as to which specific muscles or groups of muscles are involved nor what their specific involvements are. Most experimental study has been centered on the intercostal muscles. The preponderance of available evidence suggests that the internal intercostal muscles are one of the principal generators for pulsatile variations of typical magnitude. These small and fast acting muscular generators appear to provide bursts of electrical activity in association with their discrete and brief contractions when the conditions of utterance call for rapid and small pressure variations of respiratory origin. Assuming that these bursts cause displacements of the thorax, the available evidence suggests that the muscles of greatest importance to everyday speech are the internal intercostals. They are so positioned and of such a size that they can importantly influence rib cage volume and introduce rapid and small variations in the driving pressure supplied to the larynx and upper airways. There is further evidence (Ladefoged et al., 1958) to suggest that very large pulsatile changes, such as those associated with very emphatic utterances, involve activity of the abdominal muscles. Such information, in conjunction with existing knowledge about respiratory mechanics, makes it seem reasonable to speculate that pulsatile variations of substantial magnitude may involve expiratory muscles in addition to the internal intercostals and abdominals.

It should be noted that the above discussion pertains to the regulation of pulsatile pressure variations within the midrange of the vital capacity. Out of this range, and especially at higher lung volumes, the muscular forces governing alveolar pressure may operate in quite another manner (Ladefoged et al., 1958; Hardy, 1970). At least part of the capability for developing pulsatile variations at high lung volumes seems related to the ability to rapidly and momentarily decrease the counteracting muscular forces which may be used to oppose the recoil of the lungs and thorax at very high lung volumes. The external intercostal muscles have been implicated in this type of activity (Ladefoged et al., 1958) by the fact that they can briefly decrease their counteracting force and permit the spring-like background force of the respiratory mechanism to exert rapid increases in pressure. Such a mechanism can be considered with reference to the bellows analogy: If the handles of the spring-bellows system were initially widespread and the arms of the operator used in opposition to the strong recoil provided by the spring at large chamber volumes, then very rapid releases of the wrists of the operator would bear functional analogy to rapid and brief decrements in external intercostal activity within the chest. Under these circumstances, the driving forces to the bellows are provided by the spring, with the spring being able to exert these brief increases in pressure only during intermittent relaxation of the hand-wrist component.

Neurophysiological mechanisms. Although discussion up to this juncture has been dominated by consideration of consciously controlled muscular events within the torso, there is evidence that load compensating reflexes within the intercostal muscles also are operative during speech (Sears and

Newsom Davis, 1968). Such reflexes are in response to mechanical valving (i. e., articulatory gestures) within the larynx and upper airways, valving, which by its action, causes very rapid loading and unloading of the respiratory pump. Variations in load cause transient changes in pressure and flow which in turn result in small but rapid changes in lung volume. Such volume changes are in addition to those produced by the conscious driving of the respiratory muscles. When the pump is loaded during conversational speech, such as is the case when the larynx closes abruptly, transient pressure build-ups are reflected back to the torso and a small volume increase results. Conversely, when the pump is unloaded during conversational speech, such as is the case when the larynx opens abruptly and air escapes rapidly from the lungs, a slight reduction in lung volume occurs. In the face of these rapid volume changes, the gamma-loop system[10] functions at the spinal level as a servo-mechanism that performs an automatic length stabilization of the intercostal muscles to compensate for the transient loading changes through which the muscles must work. The gamma-loop system has the capability to serve in this function by virtue of its sensitivities to length and rate of change in length of intercostal muscles (Matthews, 1964). To the extent that intercostal adjustments relate to overall respiratory function, these sensitivities represent displacement equivalents of volume and flow, respectively (Agostoni and Fenn, 1960). As transient length changes occur in the muscles of the torso, intercostal spindle receptors are deformed by these changes and the gamma-loop makes reflexive stabilization adjustments of which the speaker is totally unaware (Matthews, 1964). The responses are such that when loading on contracting inspiratory or expiratory intercostal muscles is made to increase, there is an associated increase in their respective electrical activities; conversely, when loading on them is decreased, there is a decrease in their electrical activities (Sears and Newsom Davis, 1968). In addition to positive experimental evidence that reflex responses are elicited by artificially imposed load variations during spontaneous breathing (Newsom Davis et al., 1966) and during utterance (Sears and Newsom Davis, 1968), two other observations about speech breathing seem to accord well with the general nature of the reflex stabilization. Outward displacements of the torso wall, for example, have been shown (Cooker, 1963) to be symmetrically associated with laryngeal and upper airways valving during speech. These displacements follow transient pressure changes related to loading of the respiratory pump and, as

---

[10] Following Smith (1969) and Abbs (1971), the gamma-loop system is defined at a segmental level and includes (1) the gamma efferent fibers, (2) the spindle fiber controlled by the efferent fibers, and (3) the synaptic connections made by the spindle afferent fibers with alpha motorneuron. See Campbell (1964), and Ruch et al. (1965) for more detailed discussions. An excellent account of muscle spindle anatomy and physiology is provided in the motion picture film entitled "The Muscle Spindle" by Dr. Ian A. Boyd, Institute of Physiology, University of Glasgow. This film is available through John Wiley and Sons Film Library.

such, they may be viewed as reflections of articulatory events within the head and neck. If outward displacements are assumed to indicate volume increases (Hixon, 1970b), and thus variations in intercostal muscle length, then it seems reasonable to suppose that the gamma-loop system responds to these variations by stabilizing the demanded length changes of the muscles. For another example, multiple bursts of electrical activity have been recorded from intercostal muscles during utterance segments where respiratory loading could account for the electrical activity as well, if not better, than could specific voluntary commands to muscle generators (Ladefoged, 1968).

Finally, the operation of the gamma motor system during speech may be far more complex than has been suggested by the above description of function at a gamma-loop reflex level alone. There appears to be good evidence for gamma system activity at supraspinal levels and for involvement of the gamma system in both the initiation and control of voluntary movement (Campbell, 1964, 1968; Sears, 1966; Abbs, 1971). Study of the gamma system has shown it to have specific cortical representation very similar to that for the alpha motorneuron system and for its activity to precede that of alpha motorneurons during spontaneous movements (Mortimer and Akert, 1961). One of the possible functional linkages between the gamma and alpha systems that has been suggested is a parallel driving of the intrafusal and extrafusal muscle systems. Given this arrangement it may be conceptualized that the alpha system provides the coarse action of the respiratory muscles and the gamma system provides fine adjustments in the muscles (Granit, 1955; Campbell, 1968). For speech, which is a learned motor skill, the rapid variations in respiratory load may become predictable through repeated performance and therefore anticipated and compensated for by appropriately regulated activities of both gamma and alpha motor systems (Sears and Newsom Davis, 1968). In view of what is becoming known about the neurophysiology of respiration, there may soon be valid physiological bases for choosing among possible explanations of speech breathing data and for determining their implications for theoretical models of speech breathing mechanics (Ladefoged, 1968) and the clinical management of patients (Hixon, 1970a).

REFERENCES

Abbs, J. 1971. The influence of the gamma motor system on jaw movement during speech. Ph.D. Thesis. Univ. Wisconsin.

Agostoni, E. 1964. Action of respiratory muscles, pp. 377–86. *In* W. Fenn and H. Rahn (eds.) *Handbook of Physiology, Respiration 1, Sect. 3.* Washington, D.C.: Amer. Physiol. Soc.

AGOSTONI, E. and FENN, W. 1960. Velocity of muscle shortening as a limiting factor in respiratory air flow. *J. of Appl. Physiol.* 15: 349–53.

AGOSTONI, E. and MEAD, J. 1964. Statics of the respiratory system, pp. 387–409. *In* W. Fenn and H. Rahn (eds.) *Handbook of Physiology, Respiration 1, Sect. 3.* Washington, D.C.: Amer. Physiol. Soc.

BOUHUYS, A., PROCTOR, D., and MEAD, J. 1966. Kinetic aspects of singing. *J. Appl. Physiol.* 21: 483–96.

CAMPBELL, E. 1958. *The Respiratory Muscles and the Mechanics of Breathing.* Chicago, Ill.: Year Book Medical Publishers, Inc.

CAMPBELL, E. 1964. Motor pathways, pp. 535–43. *In* W. Fenn and H. Rahn (eds.) *Handbook of Physiology, Respiration 1, Sect. 3.* Washington, D.C.: Amer. Physiol. Soc.

CAMPBELL, E. 1968. The respiratory muscles. *In* A. Bouhuys (ed.) *Sound Production in Man. Annals of the N.Y. Acad. Sci.* 155: 135–40.

CHERNIACK, R. and CHERNIACK, L. 1961. *Respiration in Health and Disease.* Phila., Penna.: W. B. Saunders Co.

COMROE, J. H., Jr. 1965. *Physiology of Respiration.* Chicago, Ill.: Year Book Medical Publishers, Inc.

COMROE, J. H., Jr., FORSTER, R. II, DuBOIS, A., BRISCOE, W., CARLSEN, E. 1962. *The Lung: Clinical Physiology and Pulmonary Function Tests.* (2nd ed.) Chicago, Ill.: Year Book Medical Publishers, Inc.

COOKER, H. 1963. Time relationships of chest wall movements and intraoral pressures during speech. Ph.D. Thesis. Univ. Iowa.

DRAPER, M., LADEFOGED, P. and WHITTERIDGE, D. 1959. Respiratory muscles in speech. *J. Speech Hearing Research* 2: 16–27.

EBLEN, R. 1963. Limitations of the use of surface electromyography in studies of speech breathing. *J. Speech Hearing Research* 6: 3–18.

GRANIT, R. 1955. *Receptors and Sensory Perception.* New Haven, Conn.: Yale University Press.

HARDY, J. 1967. Electromyographic evidence of syllable pulses in respiratory muscles. Paper presented to the Convention of the Amer. Speech and Hearing Assoc., Chicago, Ill.

HARDY, J. 1970. Discrete contractions of respiratory musculatures associated with |CV| syllable trains. Paper presented to the Convention of the Amer. Speech and Hearing Assoc., New York, N.Y.

HIXON, T. 1970. Clinical implications of recent advances in speech breathing mechanics. Paper presented to the Convention of the Amer. Speech and Hearing Assoc., New York, N.Y.

HIXON, T. 1970. Respiratory mechanics during speech production. Paper presented to the Meeting of the Amer. Assoc. for the Advancement of Science, Chicago, Ill.

HIXON, T., MEAD, J., and GOLDMAN, M. 1970. Separate volume changes of the rib cage and abdomen during speech. Paper presented to the Convention of the Amer. Speech and Hearing Assoc., New York, N.Y.

HIXON, T., MINIFIE, F., PEYROT, A., and SIEBENS, A. 1968. Mechanical behavior of the diaphragm during speech. Paper presented to the Fall Meeting of the Acoustical Society of America, Cleveland, Ohio.

HIXON, T., SIEBENS, A., and EWANOWSKI, S. 1968. Respiratory mechanics during speech production. Paper presented to the Spring Meeting of the Acoustical Society of America, Ottawa, Canada.

HOSHIKO, M. 1960. Sequence of action of breathing muscles during speech. *J. Speech Hearing Research* 3: 291–96.

KONNO, K. and MEAD, J. 1967. Measurement of the separate volume changes of rib cage and abdomen during breathing. *J. Appl. Physiol.* 22: 407–22.

KONNO, K. and MEAD, J. 1968. Static volume-pressure characteristics of the rib cage and abdomen. *J. Appl. Physiol.* 24: 544–48.

LADEFOGED, P. 1967. *Three Areas of Experimental Phonetics.* London, England: Oxford Univ. Press.

LADEFOGED, P. 1968. Linguistic aspects of respiratory phenomena. *In* A. Bouhuys (ed.) *Sound Production in Man. Annals N.Y. Acad. Sci.* 155: 141–51.

LADEFOGED, P., DRAPER, M. and WHITTERIDGE, D. 1958. Syllables and stress. *Miscellania Phonetica* 3: 1–15.

MATTHEWS, P. 1964. Muscle spindles and their motor control. *Physiol. Rev.* 44: 219–88.

MEAD, J., BOUHUYS, A., and PROCTOR, D. 1968. Mechanisms generating subglottic pressure. *In* A. Bouhuys (ed.) *Sound Production in Man. Annals N.Y. Acad. Sci.* 155: 177–81.

MEAD, J. and MARTIN, H. 1968. Principles of respiratory mechanics. *J. Amer. Physical Therapy Assoc.* 48: 478–94.

MEAD, J. and MILIC-EMILI, J. 1964. Theory and methodology in respiratory mechanics with glossary of symbols, pp. 363–76. *In* W. Fenn and H. Rahn (eds.) *Handbook of Physiology, Respiration 1, Sect. 3.* Washington, D.C.: Amer. Physiol. Soc.

MORTIMER, E. and AKERT, K. 1961. Cortical control and representation of fusimotor neurons. *Amer. J. Phys. Med.* 48: 228–48.

NETSELL, R. 1969. A perceptual-acoustic-physiological study of syllable stress. Ph.D. Thesis. Univ. Iowa.

NEWSOM DAVIS, J., SEARS, T., STAFF, D., and TAYLOR, A. 1966. The effects of airway obstruction on the electrical activity of intercostal muscles in conscious man. *J. Physiol.* (London) 185: 19P.

PAPPENHEIMER, J., COMROE, J. H., JR., COURNAND, A., FERGUSON, J., FILLEY, G., FOWLER, W., GRAY, J., HELMHOLZ, H., JR., OTIS, A., RAHN, H., and RILEY, R. 1950. Standardization of definitions and symbols in respiratory physiology. *Fed. Proc.* 9: 602–15.

RADFORD, E., JR. 1964. Static mechanical properties of mammalian lungs, pp. 429–49. *In* W. Fenn and H. Rahn (eds.) *Handbook of Physiology, Respiration 1, Sect. 3.* Washington, D.C.: Amer. Physiol. Soc.

RAHN, H., OTIS, A., CHADWICK, L., and FENN, W. 1946. The pressure-volume diagram of the thorax and lung. *Amer. J. Physiol.* 146: 161–78.

ROUSE, H. and HOWE, J. 1953. *Basic Mechanics of Fluids.* New York: John Wiley & Sons, Inc.

RUCH, T., PATTON, H., WOODBURY, J., and TOWE, A. 1965. *Neurophysiology* (2nd ed.) Philadelphia, Penna.: W. B. Saunders Co.

SEARS, T. 1966. The respiratory motorneuron: integration at spinal segmental level, pp. 33–47. *In* J. Howell and E. Campbell (eds.) *Breathlessness.* Oxford, England: Blackwell Scientific Publications.

SEARS, T. and NEWSOM DAVIS, J. 1968. The control of respiratory muscles during voluntary breathing. *In* A. Bouhuys (ed.) *Sound Production in Man. Annals N.Y. Acad. Sci.* 155: 183–90.

SIEBENS, A. 1966. The mechanics of breathing. *In* C. Best and N. Taylor (eds.) *The Physical Basis of Medical Practice.* (8th ed.) Baltimore. Md.: The Williams & Wilkens Co.

SMITH, J. 1969. Fusimotor neuron block and voluntary arm movement in man. Ph.D. Thesis. Univ. Wisconsin.

STETSON, R. H. 1951. *Motor Phonetics.* Amsterdam: North-Holland Publishing Co.

TAYLOR, A. 1960. The contribution of the intercostal muscles to the effort of respiration in man. *J. Physiol.* 151: 390–402.

4

PHONATION

David J. Broad

INTRODUCTION

Speech is a type of communication that depends on the transmission of sound waves through air. In order for such waves to exist, of course, a speaker must generate them by some action of his speech mechanism. One of the main anatomical locations for sound production in speech is the *larynx*, which is attached to the upper end of the trachea in the anterior part of the neck, as shown in Figure 4-1. The larynx acts as a valve that opens for the passage of air and closes when food or other foreign bodies enter the throat. The necessity for this arrangement arises from the fact that both food on its way to the stomach and air on its way to the lungs traverse the same passageway through the *oropharynx* and *laryngopharynx*. The primary biological function of the larynx is the protection of the lower airways from foreign bodies. It can also help regulate airflow into and out of the lungs. By closing completely and locking air in the lungs, the larynx helps stabilize the thorax for bodily exertions such as lifting weights or defecation. Air flowing through the larynx can make various sounds that give rise to its function as a speech organ.

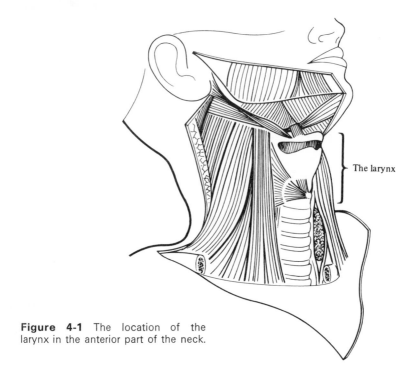

The larynx

Figure 4-1 The location of the larynx in the anterior part of the neck.

The sounds produced by the larynx include voice and whisper, and the general term *phonation* refers to any type of laryngeal sound production in speech. This chapter describes the physical mechanisms of phonation. These include the acoustics of sound generation in the larynx and the adjustments of the larynx that control the type of sound produced. An understanding of the anatomical structure of the larynx is obviously basic to an understanding of its function. We will begin by introducing the minimum anatomical concepts that are needed to explain the most elementary aspects of phonation. This will permit a discussion of several aspects of phonation at a fairly early stage in the chapter and will provide a context for the later introduction of the remaining anatomical concepts necessary for a more comprehensive understanding of phonation.

THE CARTILAGINOUS FRAMEWORK FOR PHONATION

The larynx consists of soft tissues that are supported by a system of semirigid cartilages. These cartilages form a skeleton for the larynx that provides a convenient reference for defining the anatomy of the laryngeal ligaments, membranes, and muscles. The cartilages are connected by joints that allow the cartilages to move in relation to one another. Motions of the laryngeal cartilages are essential to the physiological function of the larynx since they permit it to assume a variety of different configurations that, among other things, open and close the larynx and determine the kind of sound that it produces.

The Major Laryngeal Cartilages

The *cricoid* cartilage is a ring-shaped structure connected to the top of the trachea, as shown in Figure 4-2. Its center hole is the upward continuation of the tracheal passageway and in this sense the cricoid may be thought of as the uppermost tracheal ring. The cricoid differs from the horseshoe-shaped tracheal rings, however, in that it is a complete ring closed at the back where a massive *lamina* or plate extends vertically. Anteriorly, the cartilage becomes thinner to form the less massive cricoid *arch*. The *cricotracheal ligament* connects the cricoid cartilage to the trachea.

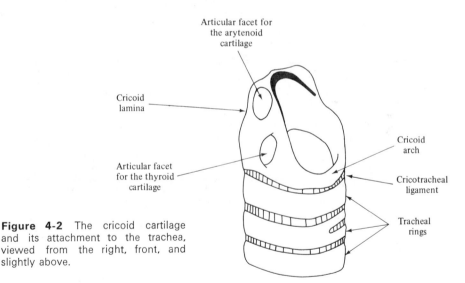

Articular facet for the arytenoid cartilage

Cricoid lamina

Articular facet for the thyroid cartilage

Cricoid arch

Cricotracheal ligament

Tracheal rings

Figure 4-2 The cricoid cartilage and its attachment to the trachea, viewed from the right, front, and slightly above.

A pair of *facets* (articular surfaces) on the lower lateral surfaces of the cricoid cartilage are where the *thyroid* cartilage connects to the cricoid, as shown in Figure 4-3. The thyroid cartilage is formed by two relatively flat plates, the thyroid *laminae*, which come together in the front to form the thyroid *angle*. Anteriorly, the upper borders of the thyroid laminae slope sharply downward to form a V-shaped space just above the thyroid angle;

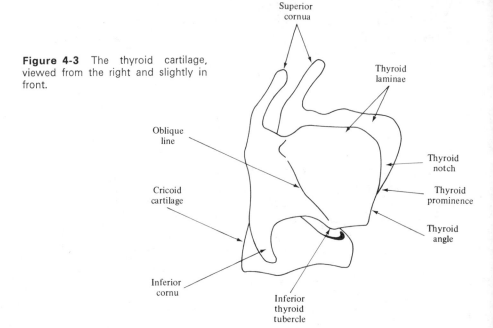

Figure 4-3 The thyroid cartilage, viewed from the right and slightly in front.

this space is called the thyroid *notch*. In the male larynx the upper part of the thyroid angle projects forward and is called the thyroid *prominence* or "Adam's apple." The *oblique line* is a ridge that runs diagonally down the surface of the thyroid lamina to end in the *inferior thyroid tubercle*.

There is a significant difference between the thyroid cartilages of adult males and females, as illustrated in Figure 4-4. In females the angle between the two laminae is approximately 120° and the thyroid prominence does not project very far forward. In males, on the other hand, the angle is a smaller one of approximately 90° and the thyroid prominence projects fairly far forward. Thus, in males, the thyroid cartilage is more elongated in the front-back direction than it is in females. This can be observed informally by noting that males tend to have more prominent Adam's apples than females.

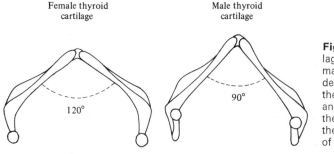

Figure 4-4 The thyroid cartilages of a female (left) and a male (right) seen from above to demonstrate the differences in the angles between the laminae and in the forward projections of the thyroid angles. The fronts of the cartilages are toward the top of the figure.

Two pairs of horns or *cornua* extend upward and downward from the back of the thyroid cartilage. The shorter downward projecting pair are the *inferior cornua* and the longer upward projecting pair are the *superior cornua*. The inferior cornua have smooth facets on their inner surfaces where the thyroid cartilage connects to the cricoid at the *cricothyroid* joints. The cricothyroid joints permit the cricoid and thyroid cartilages to rotate around a horizontal axis passing through the two joints.

The cricoid cartilage has a second pair of facets on the rim of the lamina that are for the *cricoarytenoid* joints which connect the cricoid to the *arytenoid* cartilages. There are two arytenoid cartilages, one left and one right, that rest on the articular facets of the cricoid cartilage. An arytenoid cartilage is shown in Figure 4-5. The stubby knob at the side and bottom of the cartilage is the *muscular process* where three different laryngeal muscles attach. The underside of the muscular process is a concave facet that fits the convex articular facet of the cricoid. Since the muscular process is convex on top and concave on the bottom, it has, somewhat, the overall shape of a cupped hand. Forward from the muscular process the arytenoid tapers and curves into a forward projecting point, the *vocal process*. Upward from a base formed by the muscular process and the vocal process the arytenoid projects in a thinning and backward-curving arch to terminate in the *apex* at the top. The posterior surface of the arytenoid is concave.

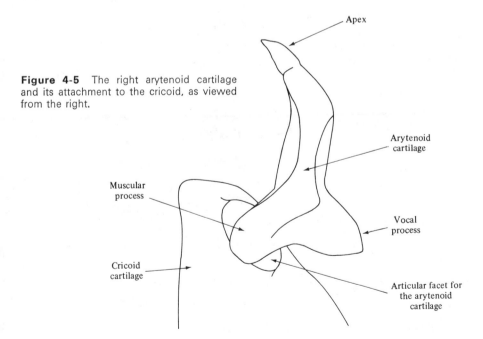

Figure 4-5 The right arytenoid cartilage and its attachment to the cricoid, as viewed from the right.

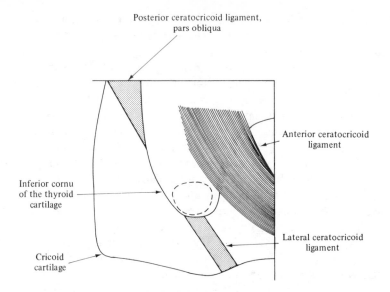

Posterior ceratocricoid ligament,
pars obliqua

Anterior ceratocricoid
ligament

Inferior cornu
of the thyroid
cartilage

Lateral ceratocricoid
ligament

Cricoid
cartilage

Figure 4-6   The cricothyroid joint and the ceratocricoid ligaments. In the upper part of the figure the ligaments are viewed from the right; in the lower part of the figure they are viewed from behind.

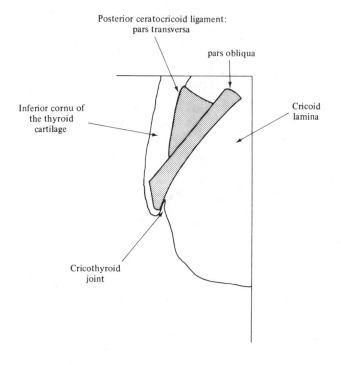

Posterior ceratocricoid ligament:
pars transversa

pars obliqua

Inferior cornu of
the thyroid
cartilage

Cricoid
lamina

Cricothyroid
joint

The Laryngeal Joints

The cricoid, thyroid, and arytenoid cartilages form the main semirigid framework of the larynx. They support the softer tissues and it is through motions in the cricothyroid and cricoarytenoid joints that the soft tissues are maneuvered into the positions for the different modes of phonation. These very important motions can be understood rather simply by considering the shapes and positions of the joints. Since the joints are where the cartilages contact each other mechanically, it is apparent that the cartilages can move only in ways that the joints permit. Just as the knee joint permits certain motions in the leg and prevents others, the laryngeal joints limit and define the mechanical adjustments in the larynx.

The thyroid and cricoid cartilages are in contact at the two cricothyroid joints. The inner surface of the inferior cornu of the thyroid cartilage is a smooth facet that contacts the corresponding facet on the cricoid cartilage. The joint is held together by the *ceratocricoid* ligaments, as shown in Figure 4-6. There are three ceratocricoid ligaments: anterior, posterior, and lateral. According to Mayet and Mündnich (1958) the posterior ceratocricoid ligament is often observed to have two parts: a cranially and medially directed *pars obliqua* and a short horizontally directed *pars transversa*. These ligaments limit the relative motions of the cricoid and thyroid cartilages. Mayet and Mündnich found that the cricothyroid joints behave in the following manner: The primary motion is a rotation of the two cartilages with respect to one another about a horizontal axis that passes through the two joints. This motion is illustrated in Figure 4-7. When the cricoid arch

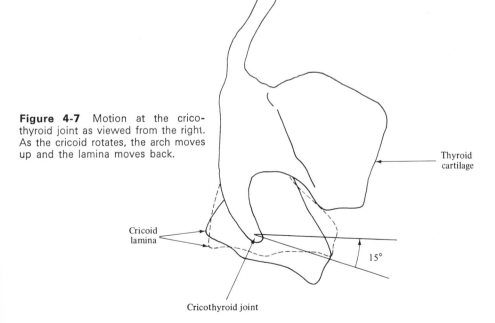

Figure 4-7 Motion at the crico-thyroid joint as viewed from the right. As the cricoid rotates, the arch moves up and the lamina moves back.

Thyroid cartilage

Cricoid lamina

15°

Cricothyroid joint

is rotated upward toward the thyroid angle, the upper rim of the cricoid lamina is simultaneously rotated backward. This motion also carries the arytenoid cartilages backward. As rotation in the cricothyroid joints is continued, the ceratocricoid ligaments are stretched slightly and they oppose further rotation. The ligaments are fairly strong and not very distensible; they limit the rotary motion to a maximum of about 15°. When the cricothyroid joints are in their equilibrium position, the ceratocricoid ligaments are slightly lax and may permit some very limited translatory movement between the cartilages. This freedom of movement rapidly disappears as the ligaments are tensed by rotation, however, and it is the rotary movement in the joints that dominates the relative motions of the cricoid and thyroid.

The arytenoid cartilages are coupled with the cricoid cartilage through the cricoarytenoid joints. The motions permitted by the cricoarytenoid joints are determined by the geometry of the articular surfaces of the cartilages. The excellent account of these joints given by Sonesson (1959) has been confirmed by von Leden and Moore (1961). A schematic transverse crosssection through the cricoarytenoid joints is shown in Figure 4-8. The articular facet of the cricoid is shaped like a convex section of a circular cylinder. The articular surface of the arytenoid, on the other hand, is shaped like a concave section of a circular cylinder that fits closely to the corresponding surface of the cricoid. The posterior cricoarytenoid ligament aids in holding the two cartilages tightly together and helps limit the motions in the joints to movements that maintain the contact between the two surfaces. The two types of motion possible under this condition are illustrated in Figure 4-9. First, the arytenoid can slide along the articular surface of the cricoid parallel to the cylinder axis.

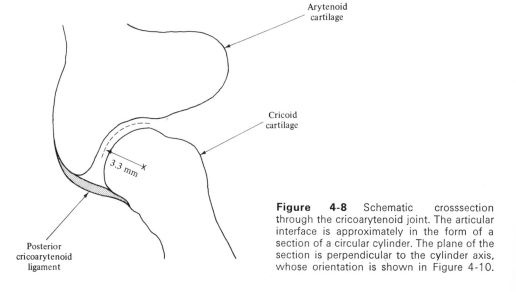

Arytenoid
cartilage

Cricoid
cartilage

3.3 mm

Posterior
cricoarytenoid
ligament

Figure 4-8 Schematic crosssection through the cricoarytenoid joint. The articular interface is approximately in the form of a section of a circular cylinder. The plane of the section is perpendicular to the cylinder axis, whose orientation is shown in Figure 4-10.

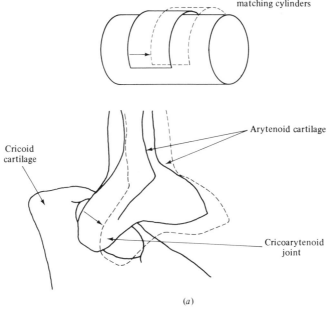

Paraxial (gliding) motion of two matching cylinders

Arytenoid cartilage

Cricoid cartilage

Cricoarytenoid joint

(*a*)

Figure 4-9 The motions of the cricoarytenoid joint. Upper: In the gliding motion the arytenoid slides parallel to the joint axis, analogously to the paraxial motion of two matching cylinders shown above. The cartilages are viewed from the right side. Lower: In the rocking motion the arytenoid rotates about the joint axis, analogously to the rotary motion of two matching cylinders illustrated below. The maximum rotary motion is about 30°. The arytenoid is viewed along the joint axis from the same direction as in Figure 4-8.

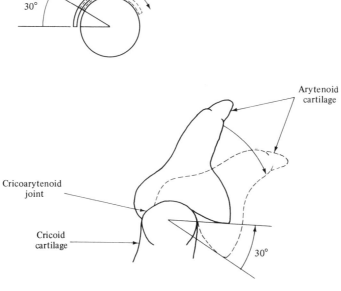

Rotary (rocking) motion of two matching cylinders

30°

Arytenoid cartilage

Cricoarytenoid joint

Cricoid cartilage

30°

(*b*)

This is the *gliding* motion of the arytenoid (Figure 4-9(*a*)). The constraints of the joints limit the extent of the gliding motion to a maximum of about 2 millimeters. Second, the arytenoid can slide over the articular surface of the cricoid in a direction perpendicular to the cylinder axis. This is the *rocking* motion of the arytenoid (Figure 4-9(*b*)). The rocking motion is actually a rotation of the arytenoid cartilage around the axis of the joints. The rocking motion has a range of approximately 30° and is the major component of the motions of the arytenoid cartilage. In particular, the rocking motion can carry the arytenoid toward and away from the mid-sagittal plane. Movement of a structure toward the mid-sagittal plane is called *adduction* and movement away from this plane is called *abduction*.

The axis of the cricoarytenoid joints is directed obliquely to the major body planes. As shown in Figure 4-10, the axis is directed downward, forward, and outward. This means that when the arytenoid is adducted in a rocking motion the vocal process not only comes toward the midline but it also rotates somewhat downward. Conversely, when the arytenoid is abducted the vocal process is rotated upward as well as outward.

Many of the functions of the larynx can be understood in terms of the motions that have just been described. Basically, there are three motions that are important to remember: the mutual rotation between the cricoid and thyroid cartilages determined by the cricothyroid joints and the gliding and rocking motions of the arytenoid cartilages.

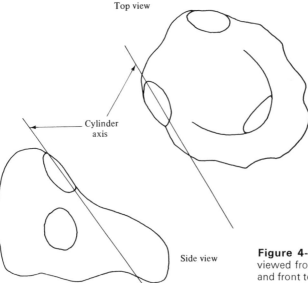

Top view

Cylinder axis

Side view

Cricoid cartilage

Figure 4-10 The cricoid cartilage viewed from the side and from the top and front to show the orientation of the axis of the cricoarytenoid joint. The axis is directed outward, forward, and downward.

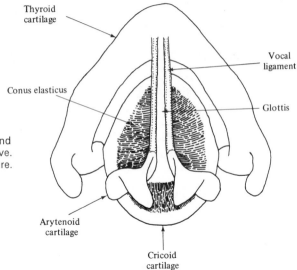

Figure 4-11 The conus elasticus and vocal ligament as seen from above. The front is toward the top of the figure.

THE CONUS ELASTICUS AND THE VOCAL LIGAMENTS

As shown in Figure 4-11, the respiratory passageway is continued upward from the circular opening of the cricoid cartilage by a membranous boundary that converges into a slit-like opening. This membrane is the *conus elasticus* which arises in a full circle from the top of the cricoid cartilage. At its top the conus elasticus ends in a thick, tough edge called the *vocal ligament*. The vocal ligament attaches in back to the vocal process of the arytenoid cartilage and in front to the inner surface of the thyroid angle. The thick anterior part of the conus elasticus is the *median cricothyroid ligament*. This ligament attaches to the inferior rim of the thyroid angle. Figure 4-12 is a frontal crosssection through the larynx showing the conus elasticus and its related

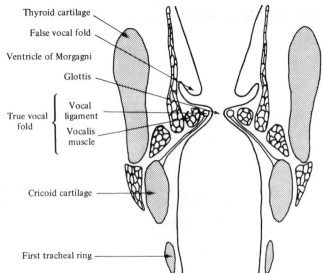

Figure 4-12 A frontal cross-section through the larynx showing the conus elasticus and vocal ligament.

structures. The conus elasticus consists of a yellow, elastic connective tissue. Attached to its inner surface is a layer of mucous membrane that is continuous with the mucosal lining of the trachea. At the level of the vocal ligament the mucous membrane is folded around the ligament to enclose the *true vocal fold*. The upper end of the trachea is thus funneled through the slit-shaped opening bordered by the true vocal folds. This opening is the *glottis*. The border of the glottis has two parts. Anteriorly, the true vocal folds are the *membranous* border of the glottis. Posteriorly, the arytenoid cartilages form the *cartilaginous* border of the glottis.

The glottal opening is regulated mostly by motions in the arytenoid cartilages. During respiration the arytenoids are abducted and the glottis is relatively wide. During inspiration the arytenoids are somewhat more widely abducted than during expiration. When a foreign body enters the throat, the larynx closes in a reflex action in which the arytenoids are rapidly adducted to close the glottis, thus preventing the foreign body from entering the lower airways. This protective function is carried out mainly by other parts of the larynx that lie above the true vocal folds, though the closure of the glottis is an integral part of this function (Pressman and Kelemen, 1970). The opening of the passageway to air by abduction of the arytenoids and its closing to things other than air by adduction of the arytenoids is part of the primary biological function of the larynx. The abductory and adductory adjustments of the vocal folds also enter into speech production.

LARYNGEAL SOUND PRODUCTION

The airflow that is nozzled through the glottis produces sound, and different basic modes of sound production result from two distinct types of glottal valving action, voicing and whispering. Most other modes of laryngeal sound production can be understood in terms of these two fundamental mechanisms.

Voicing

Voicing is perhaps the most important type of phonation since it serves as a primary source of acoustic energy in speech. The presence or absence of voicing in speech sounds is a phonetic signal and it is mainly by changes in the voice source that changes in the perceptual pitch and loudness of speech utterances are made. Singing depends on a fine control of the laryngeal voice source. In ordinary speech this fine control is used to signal different levels of emphasis and emotional qualities, as well as the ordinary meanings that

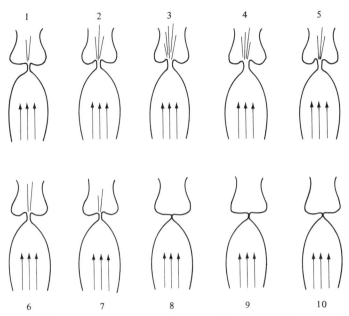

Figure 4-13 Series of frontal crosssections of the vocal folds showing the phases of the normal vibratory cycle during voicing. The sections are schematized from Figure 4-12. The arrows represent the force of the subglottal pressure; air flows through the glottis in sections 1 through 7. [*After H. Hollien, R. Coleman, and P. Moore,"Stroboscopic laminagraphy of the larynx during phonation,"* Acta Oto-Laryngol., 65 (1968), 209–15, Fig. 9.]

are attached to different stress and intonation patterns. During voicing the arytenoid cartilages are adducted to constrict the glottis. When a subglottal air pressure is applied, the vocal folds are moved cyclically toward and away from the midline to open and close the glottis and to permit the emission of a quasi-periodic train of air puffs. These air puffs are the acoustic source of voicing. One cycle of vocal fold movement in voicing is shown in Figure 4-13, which is a sequence of frontal sections of the larynx based on the stroboscopic laminagraphic observations by Hollien, et al. (1968). Section 1 shows the glottis partially open permitting some airflow. The vocal folds move away from each other in the succeeding sections to attain a maximum opening in section 4. Then the folds move back together to attain glottal closure as shown in sections 8, 9, and 10. The cycle then repeats starting with section 1.

The way that sound results from the intermittent flow of air through the glottis is actually relatively simple. Since sound is a type of vibratory air movement, any mechanism that produces a vibration in the air will be a sound source. In the case of voicing, the source of the vibration is the rapid interruption of the air movement through the glottis. Each puff excites the adjacent air in the vocal tract and the sequence of puffs forms the recurrent acoustic excitation that we hear as voicing.

The opening and closing of the vocal folds involves a relatively rapid back and forth movement in the form of a complex vibration. The complexity of vocal fold vibration arises largely from the fact that the vocal folds do not move as rigid units. Rather, different parts of the folds vibrate in different, but related ways. As shown in Figure 4-13, when the vocal folds start opening from complete closure, the folds move apart first at the bottom of their contact. The opening is continued as the line of contact moves upward until the folds are finally separated at the topmost contact. The bottom parts of the folds thus have a head start on the upper parts and this lead is maintained throughout the vibratory cycle. Thus the lower portions of the true vocal folds are the first to reach their maximum excursion and they are the first to recontact each other at the end of the closing phase of the vibratory cycle. As a consequence, the closure is made from the bottom up, with the upper parts of the folds being the last to achieve closure. Also, during the opening phase the folds are blown upward as they are blown apart.

Vocal fold vibration results from a dynamic alternation of forces that open and close the glottis. Since the forces arise from the aerodynamic, muscular, and elastic forces in the larynx, their description is called the *aerodynamic-myoelastic* theory of voice production (van den Berg, 1958). Although the theory is somewhat complicated, we might mention some of the major physical forces that it takes into account.

Figure 4-14 shows a simplified mechanical model of the glottis proposed by Ishizaka and Matsudaira (1968, 1972). Assuming that the two folds act with bilateral symmetry, the model is simplified without loss of physical applicability by lumping the two folds into the single equivalent fold on the left. To account for vertical phase differences, the fold is represented by two masses m_1 and m_2 which can move independently of one another. Horizontal displacements x_1 and x_2 of m_1 and m_2 determine the horizontal areas A_1 and A_2 of the lower and upper parts of the glottis according to the simple relations $A_1 = 2l_g x_1$ and $A_2 = 2l_g x_2$, where l_g is the length of the glottis. The factor 2 arises from the bilateral symmetry of the larynx. The average particle velocities of airflow through A_1 and A_2 are denoted by U_1 and U_2 respectively. The stiffnesses represented by the springs s_1 and s_2 are the result of the *longitudinal tension* of the vocal fold. If the masses m_1 and m_2 are displaced distances $x_1 - x_0$ and $x_2 - x_0$ from their rest displacements x_0, then the springs will exert forces equal to $s_1(x_1 - x_0)$ and $s_2(x_2 - x_0)$ to restore the masses to the equilibrium position x_0. The stiffness s_3 is the *mechanical coupling stiffness* between the upper and lower parts of the vocal fold. The coupling stiffness resists deformation of the vocal fold in the sense that the force it develops is proportional to the difference between the displacements

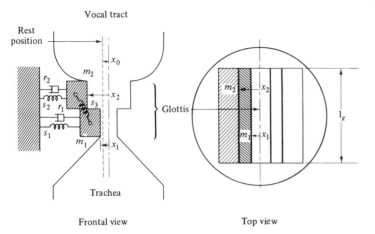

Figure 4-14   A two-degree-of-freedom mechanical model of the larynx. At the left the model is seen in a frontal crosssection; at the right it is seen from above. The displacements of m_1 and m_2 are x_1 and x_2, respectively. The glottal length is l_g, so that the glottal areas are $A_1 = 2l_g x_1$ and $A_2 = 2l_g x_2$ for the respective lower and upper sections. [*After K. Ishizaka and M. Matsudaira,* SCRL Monograph No. 8, (*Santa Barbara: Speech Communications Research Laboratory, 1972*).]

of m_1 and m_2 and acts to pull them back together. The dashpots r_1 and r_2 in Figure 4-14 represent *resistances* which arise from dissipative forces, such as the viscous forces in the tissues, and which act to decrease the velocities of the two masses.

The *aerodynamic* forces acting on the vocal folds are the intraglottal air pressures. These pressures are governed approximately by *Bernoulli's law* which is a simplified statement of the conservation of energy:

$$P + \tfrac{1}{2}\rho U^2 = \text{constant}$$

where P is the air pressure, ρ is the air density, and U is the air velocity. Hence when the air velocity increases, this is compensated by a decrease in air pressure, and vice versa. Just below the vocal folds the air pressure is approximately the same as the subglottal pressure. At the upper outlet of the glottis, the air pressure is somewhat less than atmospheric pressure, since at this point the sum of the kinetic energy of the air (due to its velocity) and its potential energy (due to its pressure) must approximately equal the static potential energy due to atmospheric pressure. Thus in traversing the glottis, the air pressure drops continuously from the subglottic pressure to less than atmospheric pressure. Ishizaka and Matsudaira have shown that, due to the different aerodynamic considerations that apply at the inlet and the outlet of the glottis, the effective air pressures that act on the masses m_1 and m_2

behave in quite different ways. To illustrate this, we will consider a special case.

For a given value of the subglottal pressure suppose that there is some value of the upper and lower glottal areas $A_1 = A_2 = A$ such that, if no other mechanisms were present, the air pressures acting on m_1 and m_2 would exactly balance the tension forces from s_1 and s_2. This configuration of static equilibrium is called the *operating* point of the mechanical model. If we now introduce a small perturbation ΔA_2 in the upper area, then the changes in the air velocities U_1 and U_2 will be approximately

$$\Delta U_1/U_1 = \Delta A_2/A_2 \qquad \Delta U_2/U_2 = 0$$

Hence, when the upper mass moves, the air velocity in the upper part of the glottis stays about the same and so, by the Bernoulli principle, does the air pressure acting on m_2. On the other hand, the air velocity through the lower glottis *increases* when A_2 increases, and consequently the air pressure acting on m_1 *decreases*. Ishizaka has called this phenomenon an *aerodynamic coupling force* between m_1 and m_2 since it is a change in the air pressure acting on m_1 that is due to a change in the displacement of m_2. Also, since the pressure on m_1 drops as A_2 increases, the aerodynamic coupling force due to an *increase* in A_2 will act to decrease A_1; hence its action is opposite to that of the mechanical coupling stiffness s_3 and behaves as a *negative coupling stiffness*. Ishizaka's analysis shows, in fact, that vocal fold vibration can occur only if the effect of this negative stiffness due to the aerodynamic coupling force is *greater* than that of the mechanical coupling stiffness.

Similarly, we can assume a small change ΔA_1 in the displacement of m_1 from the operating point. Now the air velocities change approximately by

$$\Delta U_1/U_1 = -\Delta A_1/A_1 \qquad \Delta U_2/U_2 = 0$$

Again, only the velocity in the lower glottis is significantly affected, but this time the air velocity *decreases* as A_1 increases or, in terms of pressure, the air pressure acting on m_1 increases as A_1 increases. Thus the change in air pressure due to ΔA_1 acts in the same direction as ΔA_1, i. e., it acts to enhance the initially assumed perturbation. Hence the aerodynamic effect of ΔA_1 is opposite to that of the stiffness s_1 and consequently, this effect also can be viewed as negative stiffness.

The aerodynamic forces just mentioned act to enhance any displacement of m_1 away from the operating point either in inward or outward directions. Such an equilibrium is called *unstable*. Ultimately, the excursion of the vocal fold away from unstable equilibrium is limited in the inward direction by glottal closure and in the outward direction by the fact that s_1 and s_2 increase nonlinearly with wide displacements. Sustained oscillation of the folds results from a dynamic interchange between the mechanical and aerodynamic forces acting on the folds and the momentum of the masses m_1 and m_2. Full explication of the vibration requires not only a consideration of how large the forces concerned are, but also a consideration of when they act, i. e., a consideration of the relative phases of the forces, displacements, and velocities of m_1 and m_2. Since the aerodynamic forces on m_2 change only slightly in relation to those on m_1, the main source of motion for m_2 is its mechanical coupling to m_1 through the stiffness s_3. In this sense, m_2 is "dragged along" by m_1 and this is why the upper part of the vocal fold lags behind the lower part in the vibratory cycle.

In his physiological investigations, Hiroto (1966) had noted the evident mechanical importance of the vertical phase differences in the vocal fold vibration. His suggested *mucoviscoelastic aerodynamic* theory for the phenomenon is an anticipation of the physical mechanism just described, especially in its emphasis on the participation of the mucous membrane as a mechanical element more or less loosely coupled to the vocal ligament. If the membrane were rigidly coupled to the ligament, it is obvious that no vertical phase differences could exist, and, more seriously in view of the necessary condition that the aerodynamic coupling force exceed the mechanical coupling force, the vocal fold vibration could not take place at all.

It is most important to understand clearly the way that vibration of the vocal folds produces voice in the larynx. Ordinarily, a vibrating object, such as a tuning fork, produces sound by transmitting its motion directly to the surrounding air. Vocal fold vibration produces sound in quite a different way. Direct transmission of the vibration of the vocal folds to the adjacent air is not acoustically significant in voicing. Rather, the primary acoustic effect of the vibrating folds is the rapid valving of the airflow through the glottis and it is this modulated airstream that is the true acoustic source of voicing.

The laryngeal voice source can produce sounds with a large range of intensities, frequencies, and qualities. In sections below we will explore the behavior and control of the voice source in more detail.

Whispering

If the vocal folds are separated somewhat so that the glottis is a relatively narrow slit, then air flowing from the lungs will be funneled by the conus elasticus into a converging and rapidly moving stream. If the air emitted from the glottis is moving fast enough, the emergent flow becomes turbulent; it becomes random and irregular and contains a large number of small circulating eddies. The turbulent air motion is an acoustic source of the noisy sound that we recognize as whispering. As with voicing, the production of sound in whispering is the result, then, of a particular kind of air movement through the glottis. In the case of voicing the sound results from the regular pulsation of airflow, while in whispering it results from the turbulence of a rapid airflow. Turbulent airflow occurs at other places in the vocal tract to produce fricative sounds such as [f]. Various shapes of the glottal opening have been observed for whispering. The usual "whispering position" involves a relatively wide opening between the arytenoid cartilages and a relatively narrow opening between the true vocal folds, and most of the turbulent airflow is presumably channeled between the arytenoids.

Breathy Voicing

The vocal folds can be adducted from the whispering adjustment to form yet a more narrow glottal slit. In this adjustment the glottal airflow can be turbulent and produce noise as in the whispering adjustment. The glottis is also narrow enough for vocal fold vibration to occur. As the vocal folds vibrate without actually closing, the airstream is modulated rapidly between smaller and greater flow. As in the case of pure voicing, this rapid and approximately periodic variation in the airflow is a quasi-periodic source of sound. The production of both turbulent noise and a periodic tone at the same time is called *breathy voicing*. Sometimes speakers will substitute breathy voicing for voicing in speech, either as a personal speech habit or because the individual larynx may not be able to make a complete glottal closure. Breathy voicing can be considered to include the continuum of phonation types that lies between the extremes of pure voicing and pure whispering. This corresponds to the continuum of narrow glottal openings that lies between the non-opening for pure voicing and the more open constrictions that produce pure whispering. In this sense the so-called normal voice may often employ breathy voicing a substantial proportion of the time.

The voicing component of breathy voicing is acoustically similar to ordinary voicing in that it is a more or less periodic sound source. The voicing in breathy voicing is, however, acoustically different from pure voicing in that the higher harmonics tend to be weaker than those of pure voicing. The origin of this difference is the absence of a complete glottal closure in breathy voicing. When the airstream is shut off sharply by the closures in regular voicing, a sharper tone results that is relatively rich in higher harmonics. When there is no closure, however, the rapid changes in the air movement through the glottis are smoother and the higher harmonics are greatly reduced in intensity. Perceptually the breathy voice can be described as "softer" or "less rich" than non-breathy voicing.

PHONETIC ASPECTS OF PHONATION

So far we have considered the most elementary physical aspects of phonation. With this basic foundation we can mention the ways that laryngeal sound production enters into speech. The larynx participates in speech sound formation in three different and somewhat overlapping ways: First, any speech sound can be classified according to its associated laryngeal action such as voiced, voiceless, whispered, etc. For example, a phonetic difference between [z] and [s] is that [z] is voiced and [s] is voiceless. Second, changes in the intensity and fundamental frequency of voicing are used to produce different levels of syllable stress and different intonation patterns in utterances. This is a *prosodic* function of the larynx. Third, the true vocal folds can be used to form the speech sounds known as *glottal articulations*.

Laryngeal Actions

The laryngeal actions are phonetic categories for classifying speech sounds according to the type of sound that is made in the larynx (Peterson and Shoup, 1966). The laryngeal actions include voicing, breathy voicing, and whispering. In phonetic practice it has been found necessary to include some additional types of voicing in the set of laryngeal actions. The term "voiced" is reserved for the type of voice production that is very nearly periodic or "smooth."

In voiced sounds the durations of successive fundamental periods do not differ greatly from one another. Depending on the laryngeal adjustment or on the physical condition of the vocal folds, however, a kind of sound can be produced that is similar to voicing except that the durations of successive periods vary widely from one period to the next. This can occur in two different ways. Most commonly, the successive fundamental periods may be alternately short and long. In this case, the alternate periods resemble each other more than the successive periods do. Less commonly, the voice source may exhibit more or less random variation in the durations and forms of successive periods. In either case, when the sound has widely varying fundamental periods we have the condition termed *laryngealization*. Laryngealization can occur in hoarse voice; it can also occur normally at the ends of declarative utterances in which the fundamental frequency of the voice drops rapidly. Laryngealization can occur normally in other circumstances as well.

Pulsation (Peterson and Shoup, 1966) or *vocal fry* (Wendahl et al., 1963) is another laryngeal action that resembles voicing except that in pulsation the fundamental frequency is quite low (20–90 Hz) and the durations of

Table 4-1 The laryngeal actions and their associated sound wave types and degrees of glottal opening.

Laryngeal action	Glottal opening	Sound type
voiceless	wide	no sound
whispered	narrow	random noise
breathy voicing	very narrow	random noise plus quasi-periodic pulses
voicing	closed	quasi-periodic pulses
laryngealization	closed	recurrent nonperiodic pulses
pulsation	closed	quasi-periodic pulses of very low frequency

the separate glottal air puffs tend to be quite short in relation to the time that the glottis is closed.

The laryngeal actions that involve sound production are voicing, laryngealization, pulsation, breathy voicing, and whispering. To be phonetically complete, a further case must be taken into account: This is the condition in which the vocal folds are so widely separated that no phonetically significant sound is produced. This is the voiceless laryngeal action. Consonants such as [p], [t], [k], [f], [θ] [s], and [ʃ] are produced with voiceless laryngeal action. The laryngeal actions mentioned here are listed in Table 4-1 along with their glottal configurations and types of sound produced. Some of the terminology is rather unfortunate since the same term "voicing" can be used

Figure 4-15 Acoustic waveforms and corresponding phonetic symbols of the vowel [a] produced by a normal male speaker using various laryngeal actions.

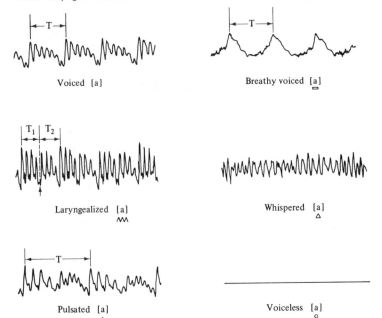

Voiced [a]

Breathy voiced [a]

Laryngealized [a]

Whispered [a]

Pulsated [a]

Voiceless [a]

both in the broad sense for any production of sound by sequences of glottal air puffs and in the narrow sense for the case in which the sequence is relatively regular. In the later sections of this chapter we will, for the most part, be discussing voicing in the more narrow sense.

Figure 4-15 shows the acoustic waveforms of the vowel [a] produced with various laryngeal actions. For the voiceless production the waveform has approximately zero energy. In the voiced [a] the regular spacing of the fundamental periods can be noted. By contrast, the laryngealized vowel has successive periods that are quite different. The distinguishing characteristic of the pulsated vowel is its relatively long fundamental period. Random noise can be seen in the whispered and breathy vowels; in the breathy voicing a periodic component can be seen that is absent in the whispered vowel. The regular-appearing oscillations in the whispered vowel are due to the resonant response of the supraglottal vocal tract to the random noise excitation; they are not related to any periodic behavior of the glottis. With each waveform a corresponding phonetic symbol is given.

Prosody Formation

During voicing the sound produced in the larynx can change in its intensity, fundamental frequency, and quality. These changes are important in speech since they are used to produce emphasis and intonation patterns. The physical attributes of speech that signal such linguistic quantities as stress and intonation are called *prosodic parameters*. Acoustically, the prosodic parameters include the fundamental frequency of the voice, the intensity of the voice, and the durations of the individual speech sounds. The fundamental frequency is determined physiologically by the vocal fold vibration rate and the voice intensity depends in part upon the intensity of the laryngeal voice source. Phonetic segment duration is determined physiologically, for the most part, by the rates of movement of the supraglottal articulators. Hence the larynx is not the only physiological locus for prosody formation, as we shall see in Chapter 6. Its key role in determining fundamental frequency and intensity implies, however, that the laryngeal voice source carries a major functional load in forming the prosodic patterns of utterances.

In English, syllable stress is an essential component of word formation and dictionaries of English include stress marks in their word pronunciations. For example, in a word such as "inspiration" the four syllables have three levels of stress: the third syllable has the major stress, the first syllable has a strong but somewhat lesser degree of stress, and the second and fourth syllables are weakly stressed. If the major stress were placed on a different syllable the pronunciation would sound strange to a native speaker of English. Stress differences are in part made in the larynx, though other variables such as vowel duration and vowel quality significantly contribute to syllable stress. Stressed vowels tend to have higher fundamental frequencies, greater durations, and higher acoustic intensities than their unstressed counterparts. The significant differences in the intensity and fundamental frequency of the voice in stressed syllables are largely due to changes in the intensity and fundamental frequency of the laryngeal voice source.

Similarly, in a question such as "We are going?" the interrogative can be signaled by a rising intonation at the end. The intonation pattern is almost entirely determined by the fundamental frequency of the laryngeal voice source. As we shall see, this behavior is determined both by the larynx itself and by subglottal respiratory actions. Various intonation patterns in English are used to signal questions, statements, and commands, along with the almost unlimited variety of fine nuances of meaning that convey information about the speaker's attitude toward what is being said. A fine control of the fundamental frequency of the glottal voice source is essential for producing utterances with normal and variously communicative intonation patterns.

The exact behavior of the larynx in the formation of prosodic patterns is not clearly known at present. This is largely due to the fact that the larynx is very difficult to observe during speech. Nevertheless, we do know some things about the ways in which changes in the adjustment of the larynx bring about changes in the intensity and fundamental frequency of the voice. We know, for example, several different possible ways that the fundamental frequency of the voice can be changed. This actually creates a problem in studying the prosodies since when we observe a change in the fundamental frequency there is no easy way of telling which of the several possible mechanisms have actually been used to bring it about. Later in this chapter we will discuss the different mechanisms that exist for controlling fundamental frequency, while Chapter 6 will tell us about how they participate in prosody formation. For the present it is most important to be aware that the laryngeal voice source is the primary physiological locus for producing prosodic variations in utterances and that the formation of prosodic patterns is essential to the normal production of speech.

Glottal Articulations

The third phonetic aspect of laryngeal function in speech is the use of the larynx to articulate speech sounds. The true vocal folds can act as a pair of articulators to produce the glottal articulations, which include the glottal stop and the glottal fricatives.

The glottal stop, which is symbolized phonetically [ʔ], often occurs in some English dialects as the second consonant in such words as "bottle" or "button." Also a glottal stop often precedes a vowel that is at the beginning of an utterance. To produce the glottal stop the arytenoid cartilages are completely adducted to close the glottis, so that an expiratory air pressure can be built up in the trachea. This air pressure can then be released by abducting the arytenoids. The sudden release of the blocked air results in an impulse-like or popping sound at the glottis. Phonetically the glottal stop is similar to other stops, such as [p], [t], or [k], in that it involves a closure of the vocal tract that permits the build-up of an air pressure that can be released to produce an acoustic burst. It is different from the other stops in that the closure is made at the glottis.

The second type of glottal articulation is the glottal fricative which is symbolized by [h] if it is voiceless or by [ɦ] if it is voiced. As with other fricative sounds, glottal fricatives involve degrees of opening that permit airflow. Aside from their being produced at the glottis, the [h] and [ɦ] differ from other fricatives in that they inherently involve a dynamic change in the articulatory constriction. The [h] is produced by a rapid adductory shift of the arytenoids which changes the glottis from the wide opening for voiceless laryngeal action to the narrower opening for whispered laryngeal action. Similarly, the [ɦ] is produced by a dynamic shift from the very narrow opening for breathy voicing to a complete adduction for voicing. The [h] occurs normally in words such as "home" or "have." The [ɦ] may sometimes occur in English between vowels in words such as "Ohio" or "aha." The rapid movements of the arytenoids during these sounds can be seen clearly in motion pictures of the larynx.

RESPIRATORY DETERMINANTS OF VOICE

The air pressure in the trachea below the vocal folds is the subglottal pressure. As we learned in Chapter 3, subglottal pressure originates from respiratory actions of the thoracic and abdominal muscles and recoil forces that change the volume of the lungs. Changes in the subglottal pressure change the sound that is produced in the larynx, and it is primarily through changes in the subglottal pressure that sublaryngeal respiratory actions influence the voice.

Increasing the subglottal pressure increases the intensity of the sound produced. A number of experimental studies (van den Berg, 1956; Ladefoged and McKinney, 1963; Isshiki, 1964; Cavagna and Margaria, 1965) have shown that the acoustic intensity of voicing is approximately proportional to the third or fourth power of the subglottal pressure. This means that if the subglottal pressure is doubled, the intensity of the voice is multiplied by a factor of between 8 and 16. This can be stated somewhat differently by using the decibel measure of sound intensity described in Chapter 2. We find that every doubling of the subglottal pressure adds 9 to 12 decibels to the intensity of the voice. Hence the voice intensity is quite sensitive to changes in the subglottal pressure. Small changes in the sublaryngeal respiratory actions can evidently have substantial effects on the sound produced in the larynx.

In addition to its effect on voice intensity, the subglottal pressure also affects the fundamental frequency of the voice source. Increasing the subglottal pressure tends to raise the fundamental frequency. This effect is acoustically significant, though in speech it is perhaps not as great an influence on fundamental frequency as the internal adjustment of the larynx is. The experimental evidence on the magnitude of fundamental frequency variations resulting from subglottal pressure changes is not yet clear. The effect can, however, be demonstrated informally by having someone sing a steady note and giving him an unexpected push in the abdomen. There will be a momentary rise in the subglottal pressure and a dramatic change in the voice can be heard. The change may be heard largely as an increase in loudness, but some rise in the pitch may also be noted.

The quality of the sound produced in the larynx is also influenced by changes in the subglottal pressure. For example, shouting is accomplished largely by raising the subglottal pressure. In addition to its greater intensity, shouting is qualitatively different from regular voicing. This can be demonstrated simply by playing back, at equal intensities, tape recordings of shouting and of normal voicing. Shouting is easily heard to be different from the normal voicing even though the intrinsic energies have been equalized.

LARYNGEAL DETERMINANTS OF VOICE

In addition to subglottal pressure, the other major source of voice control is the adjustment of the larynx itself. Changes in the physical dimensions and characteristics of the vocal folds influence the sound that is produced. There are several interrelated properties of the vocal folds that determine the acoustical characteristics of the voice. Here we will focus mainly on how the fundamental frequency of the voice is controlled by changes in the vocal fold length, thickness, mass, and tension. These influences can be summarized by the general rule that the fundamental frequency will rise whenever the vocal folds are changed in some way that will allow them to move faster. That is, whenever the vocal folds can be speeded up, their vibration rate will increase and so, perforce, will the fundamental frequency.

In the aerodynamic-myoelastic theory of voice production the tension of the vocal fold is considered to be one of the important forces for restoring the glottal closure. This force results primarily from stretching the vocal fold between its attachments at the thyroid cartilage in front and the arytenoid cartilage in back. Since the force is directed mainly along the length of the vocal ligament, it is referred to as the *longitudinal tension* of the vocal fold (van den Berg and Tan, 1959). By analogy with springs or rubber bands, it is evident that stretching the vocal ligament will increase its longitudinal tension. In turn, the greater longitudinal tension will accelerate the vocal fold movement more and the rate of vocal fold vibration will increase to raise the fundamental frequency.

Longitudinal tension is increased by stretching the vocal folds. Numerous experimental observations (Sonninen, 1954; Moore, 1937; Arnold, 1961; Fink, 1962; Hollien, 1960; Hollien and Moore, 1960; Luchsinger and Pfister, 1961) confirm that the fundamental frequency of the voice increases as the vocal fold length is increased. There is, in addition to the effect on longitudinal tension, a further significant aspect of vocal fold lengthening. As the folds are lengthened they become thinner. A similar type of thinning can also be observed easily when a rubber band is stretched. The thinning of the vocal fold decreases its effective mass and so the vocal fold becomes easier to move and it is accelerated more rapidly to increase the rate of vibration. Experimental observations (Hollien, 1962) confirm that the rate of vibration is indeed increased as the vocal folds become thinner. Thus theoretically, the lengthening of the vocal folds should be particularly effective in increasing the fundamental frequency because of its double function to increase the longitudinal tension and to decrease the effective vocal fold mass.

Longitudinal tension is a force that acts along the length of the vocal folds. There is another possible force in the larynx that can be applied to the folds. During voicing the arytenoid cartilages are completely adducted to close the glottis. To maintain the adduction the arytenoids are squeezed together. This squeezing force is directed toward the midline and is called

Figure 4-16 The effect of medial compression in shortening the vibrating part of the vocal folds. The structures are seen from above with the front toward the top.

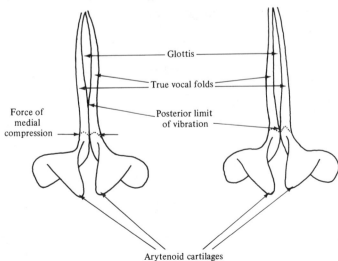

Glottis

True vocal folds

Force of medial compression

Posterior limit of vibration

Arytenoid cartilages

medial compression (van den Berg and Tan, 1959). There is some experimental evidence (van den Berg and Tan, 1959) that increased medial compression can raise the fundamental frequency of the voice. It is thought that this is accomplished indirectly by shortening the portion of the fold that participates in the vibration. This leaves the longitudinal tension mostly unchanged and effectively decreases the mass of the vibrating folds by excluding a part of their total mass from the movement. This is illustrated in Figure 4-16. As the vocal processes of the arytenoid cartilages are pressed together, the contact between the adjacent mucosal surfaces becomes firmer and the effective rear closure of the glottis moves forward. A physical analogy to this phenomenon is the increase in the pitch of a guitar string when it is pushed against a fret: the tension of the string remains essentially the same but the mass is decreased by excluding the part of the string above the fret.

The variables that determine the vocal fold vibration are summarized in Table 4-2 along with their demonstrated or theoretically presumed influence on the fundamental frequency of voicing. From the above discussion it is obvious that not all these variables are independent of one another. In particular, the vocal fold thickness and tension are believed to depend on the vocal fold length. The effective mass of the vibrating part of the folds is thought to depend on both the vocal fold length and the medial compression. The vocalis muscle tension shown in the last line of the table will be discussed below.

It is a matter of common observation that adult males tend to have lower pitched voices than adult females. It is also an anatomical fact that males tend to have longer vocal folds than females. This is due to the more forward projection of the thyroid angle in males: the front attachment of the vocal fold is farther away from the back attachment so that the vocal ligament spans a greater distance. The lower fundamental frequency of vibration in the male larynx can be largely attributed to the greater mass of the vocal folds in the male. Other things equal, the longer, heavier folds will vibrate more slowly than the lighter ones.

Table 4-2   Physiological determinants of the fundamental frequency of voicing.

Variable (*increasing*) *effect on fundamental frequency*	
subglottal pressure	increases
vocal fold length	increases
longitudinal tension	increases
vocal fold thickness	decreases
medial compression	increases
mass of vibrating folds	decreases
vocalis muscle tension	(not conclusively known)

Earlier, we noted that lengthening the vocal folds increases their frequency of vibration. But, paradoxically, we have also just noted that persons with longer vocal folds have lower voices than those with shorter folds. How is it that in one instance we associate longer folds with higher frequency and in another instance we apparently associate them with lower frequency? Actually, this is not paradoxical because the two instances really concern two different aspects of vocal fold length. In the case of vocal fold lengthening or stretching we implicitly refer to the *increase* in vocal fold length from the resting length within a given individual. In the case of individual or sex differences, we are concerned with the resting length itself.

We have just seen some ways that changes in the vocal fold dimensions can affect the sound produced in the larynx. Our next step is to see how these changes are effected by the laryngeal mechanism. The vocal fold dimensions are determined largely through the motions in the cricoarytenoid and crico-thyroid joints. The width of the glottis is determined mostly by the adductory and abductory movements of the arytenoid cartilages. The medial compression of the vocal folds is determined by the adductory squeeze of the arytenoids. These actions of the arytenoid arise from the rocking and gliding motions allowed by the cricoarytenoid joints. The vocal fold length, on the other hand, is determined primarily by the rotation in the cricothyroid joint. As illustrated in Figure 4-7, this rotation carries the arytenoid cartilages backward, away from the thyroid angle stretching the vocal ligament. Since they depend on the vocal fold length, the vocal fold tension and thickness are also determined largely by the relative rotation between the cricoid and thyroid cartilages. Of course, the laryngeal cartilages do not move by themselves. The motions are actively controlled by the laryngeal muscles which we will consider later.

VOICE REGISTERS

If you start singing as low a pitch as you can and gradually ascend to the highest possible pitch, there will typically be two points within the range at which the transition to the next higher pitch cannot be made easily and smoothly. These are the transitions between the different voice *registers*. From lowest to highest, the registers are usually denoted as chest voice, head voice, and falsetto voice. The notable transitions between the registers is perhaps the main reason that we need the concept of voice register; the changes are so obvious that it seems apparent that more than an ordinary pitch change is taking place.

There is some overlap between the registers, e. g., a person's lowest falsetto pitch may be somewhat lower than his highest pitch in head voice.

One of the goals of voice training for singing is to minimize the effects of the abrupt register changes so that the singer can effectively use the full pitch range of the voice. In view of the massive practical knowledge of voice registers that we have from voice training, it is perhaps surprising that we really know relatively little about the physiological and acoustic mechanisms that are involved. In fact, there is not even general agreement about how many registers there are, or about how one register can be reliably distinguished from another. Even though we are using a three-register system in this discussion for the sake of concreteness, this does not mean that more registers do not exist, or that there may not be other legitimate ways of classifying registers. Indeed, several other ways of looking at registers are actually in use and appear to have some merit. One of the difficulties here is that at present we have no good way of relating what we know about the physical mechanisms of phonation to the extensive subjective experience we have about registers. For example, singers may report that chest voice "resonates in the chest" and that head voice "resonates in the head." This appears to be a rather definite report on the singer's experience. At the same time, however, we have virtually no physical evidence to explain this experience. This is perhaps the greatest point of divergence between the views of voice production held by present day voice scientists and voice performers, and the need for a more unified and complete understanding of phonation becomes especially evident here.

At least two different types of physical explanations for the voice registers are conceivable. The first might be called a laryngeal *control* type of explanation and the second a laryngeal *response* type of explanation. A control theory would be based on the observation that there are several different mechanisms for changing the pitch of the voice, as discussed above. Different combinations of mechanisms would be expected to be effective over certain ranges; to go beyond this range would require a different selection of the available mechanisms. Thus the selection of a register would amount to the selection of a certain set of mechanisms for changing pitch, much in the same way that moving an automobile at a certain speed requires the selection of a certain gear. In this sense transitions between registers would amount to "shifting gears" in the larynx; to raise the pitch beyond a certain point would require "shifting" the control of the larynx.

A response theory, on the other hand, might postulate that there exist certain critical values of the laryngeal variables, such as vocal fold length, that determine different basic *modes* or *states* of vocal fold vibration. Below the critical value one mode would prevail, and above it another would. This is analogous to the response of water to continuous temperature changes— above the freezing point it is liquid until the boiling point is reached, beyond which it is steam. One response theory formulated by van den Berg (1960) uses the nonlinear elastic properties of the vocal ligament to explain registers.

This theory treats head voice as a mixed combination of the more extreme modes of chest voice and falsetto voice. Some dramatic support for this theory is that the abrupt register change between head voice and falsetto voice can be produced artificially in a cadaver larynx by gradually increasing the longitudinal tension of the vocal folds while the other variables are held constant (van den Berg et al., 1960).

INTRINSIC LARYNGEAL MUSCLES

The arrangements of the laryngeal cartilages permitted by the cricothyroid and cricoarytenoid joints are effected by muscles that connect between the cartilages. Muscles that have both their origins and insertions on the laryngeal cartilages are called *intrinsic* laryngeal muscles to distinguish them from the

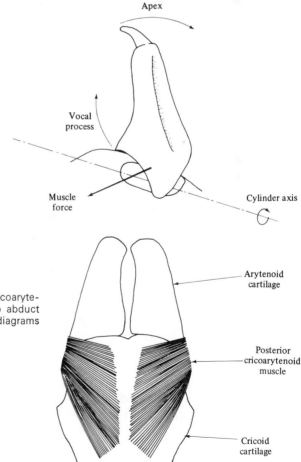

Figure 4-17 The posterior cricoarytenoid muscle and its action to abduct the arytenoid cartilage. Both diagrams are posterior views.

extrinsic laryngeal muscles which have one attachment within the larynx and the other attachment to some nonlaryngeal structure. There are four pairs of major intrinsic laryngeal muscles arranged symmetrically on the left and right sides of the larynx. Each half of the larynx has a posterior and a lateral cricoarytenoid muscle, a cricothyroid muscle, and a thyroarytenoid muscle. There is also an unpaired intrinsic laryngeal muscle, the interarytenoid muscle (transverse and oblique), which courses between the two arytenoid cartilages.

Figure 4-17 shows the posterior cricoarytenoid muscle, a fairly massive muscle that arises from a broad surface on the back of the cricoid lamina and which converges upward and laterally to insert onto the muscular process of the arytenoid cartilage. The posterior cricoarytenoid muscle pulls the muscular process diagonally downward and toward the midline. This direction is very nearly perpendicular to the axis of the cricoarytenoid joint. As a consequence, the posterior cricoarytenoid muscle has good leverage on the muscular process to abduct the arytenoid cartilage by pulling it back through its rocking motion. This is shown schematically in Figure 4-17. As the muscular process is pulled down and medially, the vocal process is rotated outward and upward. The posterior cricoarytenoid is the primary abductory muscle of the arytenoids. It is typically active during the inspiratory phase of the respiratory cycle when the abduction of the arytenoids opens the glottis quite widely.

Figure 4-18 shows the lateral cricoarytenoid muscle. This muscle arises from the upper rim of the side of the cricoid cartilage and courses upward and backward along the rim to insert onto the muscular process of the arytenoid cartilage. The lateral cricoarytenoid pulls downward and forward on the muscular process to rotate the arytenoid forward in an adductory rocking motion as is shown in Figure 4-18. The lateral cricoarytenoid muscle is thus mainly an adductory muscle of the arytenoid. In rocking the arytenoid in an adductory motion, the forward and downward pull of the lateral cricoarytenoid may also move the arytenoid a small distance in its gliding motion. The direction of this gliding motion would be abductory, but the gliding motion is so limited in its range that the dominant effect of the lateral cricoarytenoid muscle is the adductory rocking movement of the arytenoid. When the arytenoids are adducted for phonation, the lateral cricoarytenoids may have the additional function of increasing the medial compression of the vocal folds.

Figure 4-19 is a posterior view of the larynx showing the transverse arytenoid muscle. This is a horizontally directed mass of fibers that arises from the concave posterior surface of one arytenoid cartilage and inserts on the corresponding surface of the other arytenoid. As with the lateral cricoarytenoid, the transverse arytenoid muscle effects an adductory rocking

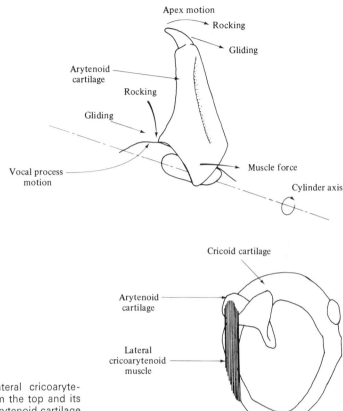

Figure 4-18 The lateral cricoarytenoid muscle seen from the top and its action to adduct the arytenoid cartilage seen from the right side.

motion of the arytenoids. This action is illustrated schematically in Figure 4-19. It may also effect a slight adductory gliding motion by drawing the arytenoids together along the axes of their joints. In addition, the transverse arytenoid may even bend the arytenoids somewhat in a relatively powerful adductory squeeze. This action would increase the medial compression of the vocal folds.

There also exists a pair of oblique arytenoid muscles. These muscles are fairly thin and narrow fibers that course over the surface of the transverse arytenoid from their origins on the muscular processes to their insertions at the apices of the opposite cartilages. The two oblique arytenoid muscles cross each other at the midline and form an X-shaped pattern on the posterior surface of the transverse arytenoid muscle. Since they are rather weak in relation to the other muscles that attach to the arytenoid cartilages, it appears doubtful that the oblique arytenoids have any remarkable function in the

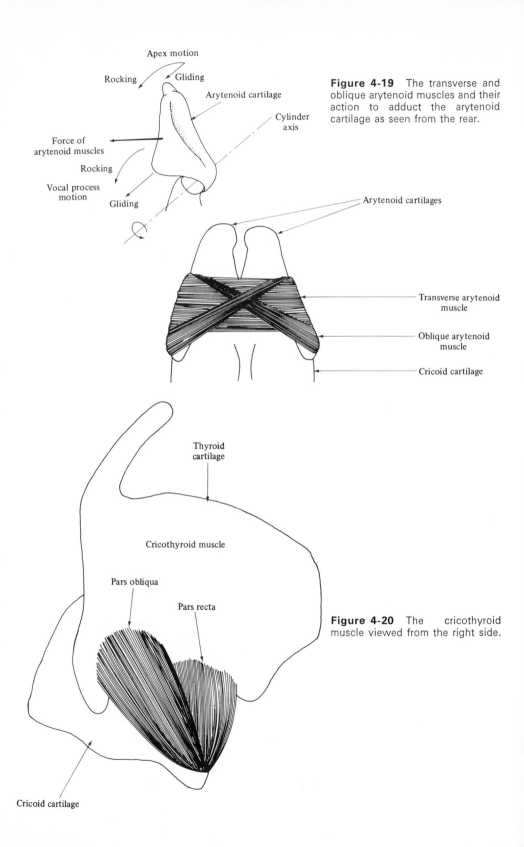

Figure 4-19 The transverse and oblique arytenoid muscles and their action to adduct the arytenoid cartilage as seen from the rear.

Apex motion

Rocking

Gliding

Arytenoid cartilage

Cylinder axis

Force of arytenoid muscles

Rocking

Vocal process motion

Gliding

Arytenoid cartilages

Transverse arytenoid muscle

Oblique arytenoid muscle

Cricoid cartilage

Thyroid cartilage

Cricothyroid muscle

Pars obliqua

Pars recta

Figure 4-20 The cricothyroid muscle viewed from the right side.

Cricoid cartilage

larynx. The net effect of the two oblique arytenoid muscles acting together would be to supplement the effect of the transverse arytenoid muscle.

There appears to be some degree of reciprocal innervation between the posterior cricoarytenoid muscle and the adductory muscles of the larynx in the sense that when the arytenoids are actively abducted the adductors are inhibited and vice versa.

Figure 4-20 shows the cricothyroid muscle. It arises from the lower rim of the thyroid lamina and thyroid angle and inserts onto the upper rim of the cricoid arch. Arnold (1961) has investigated this muscle extensively. The cricothyroid consists of two fairly distinct groups of fibers: the *pars recta* is the more forward group that courses straight down from the thyroid angle; the *pars obliqua* is the more posterior group that courses forward and downward from the thyroid angle. The inferior thyroid tubercle lies between the two parts of the muscle. The cricothyroid muscle draws the cricoid arch closer to the thyroid angle. In this action it rotates the cricothyroid joint, as shown in Figure 4-7. The cricoid arch is drawn upward toward the thyroid angle while the superior rim of the cricoid lamina is rotated backward. Since this carries the arytenoid cartilages posteriorly as well, the effect of cricothyroid contraction is to stretch the vocal folds. For this reason the cricothyroid is sometimes called the *tensor* of the larynx. The cricothyroid muscle is the primary muscular element for adjusting the cricothyroid joint and through this action it is also the main muscle for lengthening the vocal folds.

As shown in Figure 4-21, the thyroarytenoid muscle arises from the inner surface of the thyroid angle just lateral to the vocal ligament. It courses backward, generally parallel to the ligament, to insert broadly over the lower part of the anterolateral surface of the arytenoid cartilage. Two separate parts of this muscle are distinguished functionally, though anatomically the

Figure 4-21   The external thyroarytenoid muscle viewed from above with the front toward the top.

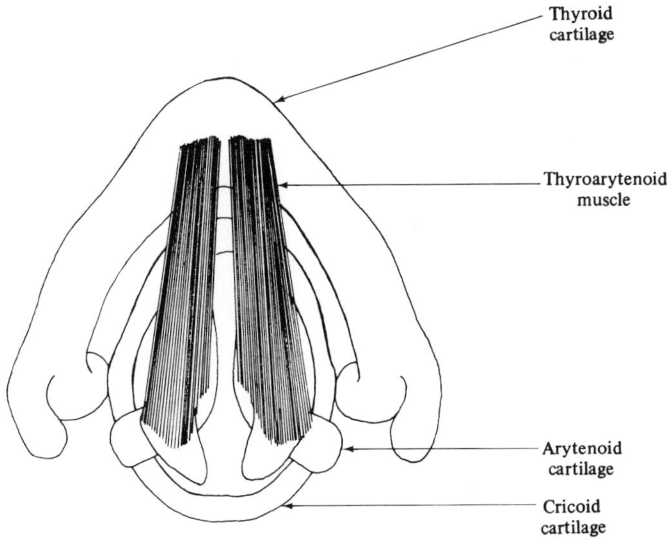

Thyroid
cartilage

Thyroarytenoid
muscle

Arytenoid
cartilage

Cricoid
cartilage

muscle appears to be a single muscle mass. The external part of the thyroarytenoid muscle has its broad insertion on the arytenoid above the vocal
process. This part of the thyroarytenoid is roughly parallel to the lateral
cricoarytenoid muscle and is often anatomically continuous with it. Like the
lateral cricoarytenoid, the external thyroarytenoid muscle can pull forward
on the arytenoid cartilage and move it in an adductory rocking motion.
There may also be some slight abductory gliding component in the muscle's
action. The external thyroarytenoid muscle may also be an antagonist to the
cricothyroid muscle. It would oppose the action of the cricothyroid muscle
by pulling forward on the arytenoid cartilages. This would have the equivalent effect of pulling forward on the cricoid lamina to rotate the cricoid
arch downward away from the thyroid angle. This action would shorten the
vocal fold and lengthen the cricothyroid muscle.

In Figure 4-22 the external thyroarytenoid muscle has been dissected
away to reveal the less massive internal thyroarytenoid or *vocalis* muscle.
(This drawing is based on Sonneson's (1960) study of the vocalis muscle.)
The vocalis arises from a thin vertical region on the thyroid angle just lateral
to the vocal ligament. It courses back to insert along the lateral margin of
the vocal process, just inferior to the broad insertion of the external thyroarytenoid muscle. Thus the vocalis runs parallel to the rest of the thyroarytenoid muscle and may be considered to be the lower medial layer of that
muscle. From its vertical origin on the thyroid angle to its more or less
horizontal insertion on the vocal process, the vocalis muscle twists somewhat
in its backward course. The uppermost fibers from the thyroid angle are
directed almost straight back to insert near the vocal ligament on the vocal

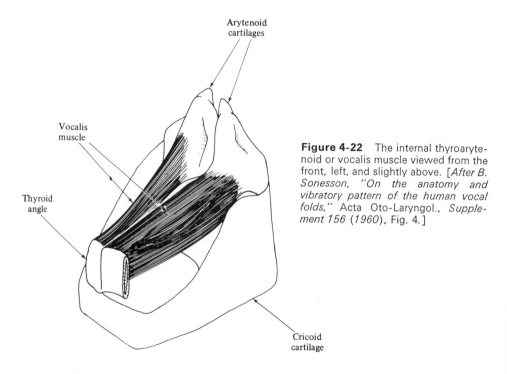

Arytenoid
cartilages

Vocalis
muscle

Thyroid
angle

Figure 4-22 The internal thyroarytenoid or vocalis muscle viewed from the
front, left, and slightly above. [*After B.
Sonesson, "On the anatomy and
vibratory pattern of the human vocal
folds,"* Acta Oto-Laryngol., *Supplement 156 (1960),* Fig. 4.]

Cricoid
cartilage

process. These fibers run adjacent to the vocal ligament along its entire length. The lowermost fibers from the thyroid angle are the ones that insert farthest back on the lateral curve of the vocal process.

The vocalis muscle courses alongside the vocal ligament and, like the vocal ligament, it is also enclosed by the mucosa of the true vocal fold. In this sense the true vocal fold may be considered to consist of the mucosa, the vocal ligament, and the vocalis muscle. As a component of the vocal fold itself, the vocalis muscle is thought to have some special function in voice production and at the very least it must vibrate along with the rest of the vocal fold during voicing.

Theoretically, there are at least two distinct functions that the vocalis might have in phonation. As a part of the thyroarytenoid muscle, the vocalis could act as an antagonist to the cricothyroid. By contracting and shortening the vocal fold it could contribute to a decrease in the fundamental frequency of phonation. On the other hand, since the vocalis is a physical component of the vocal fold itself, its tension is a part of the total vocal fold tension so that increased vocalis activity could act to raise the pitch of the voice. Hence, as an antagonist to the cricothyroid, the vocalis could lower the voice pitch, while as a mechanical part of the vocal fold it could act to raise it. The question of which of these two possible functions is the dominant one has not been clearly answered experimentally. There is actually some limited observational evidence to support either point of view. It is also possible that the vocalis can regulate voice quality and it may even have a function in determining voice register.

There are good reasons to believe that the vocalis muscle does serve some important function in voice production. Fink (1962) has discussed some of them. First, the vocalis tends to be more fully developed in the human larynx than in most other mammals. This coincides with the special function of the larynx in humans for speech production. Conversely, it is difficult to imagine how a finely-developed vocalis muscle would significantly assist the primary biological function of the larynx in protecting the lower respiratory tract. Beyond its actual muscular development, the vocalis muscle is controlled by a relatively abundant set of motor nerves. Rich innervation is usually associated with muscles that are under very rapid and very fine control as, for example, the muscles of the eye. This leads to a second reason for believing that the vocalis muscle, along with the other intrinsic laryngeal muscles, has a significant part in voice production: the behavioral complexity of the voice source would appear to require some highly accurate and rapidly adjustable form of muscular control and the muscular and neural structures that would be required for this exist in the vocalis muscle. Arnold (1961) has suggested that the vocalis muscle is important for the very fine control of the voice. The precise elucidation of the nature of this function is a significant problem for research.

ANCILLARY LARYNGEAL STRUCTURES

The parts of the larynx that we have described so far are the ones that are most essential to an understanding of the primary mechanisms of phonation. Above the true vocal folds the larynx continues as a tube that projects into, and terminates in, the pharyngeal cavity. The supraglottal parts of the larynx probably participate in significant, albeit secondary, ways that are not at present clearly understood. For example, the upper laryngeal passageway can often be observed to constrict during an [ɦ] sound, but the functional significance of this is not clear. Most plausibly, it may be that the constriction results in some way from the intrinsic [h] gesture and is not essential *per se* to the production of a turbulent glottal efflux. For an understanding of the total structure of speech production, nevertheless, we should be acquainted with at least the main features of the supraglottal part of the larynx. It is important to realize that the primary structures for phonation are not isolated anatomically, and that their function may be modified by the forces exerted by neighboring structures, particularly the other parts of the larynx.

Figure 4-23 shows a posterior view of the larynx in two different levels of dissection. The *epiglottis* is a thin, flexible cartilage, shaped approximately like a leaf. From its broad, concave-posteriorward *leaf* the epiglottis tapers to a thin stalk, the *petiole*, that attaches to the inner surface of the thyroid

Figure 4-23   Posterior view of the larynx in two levels of dissection.

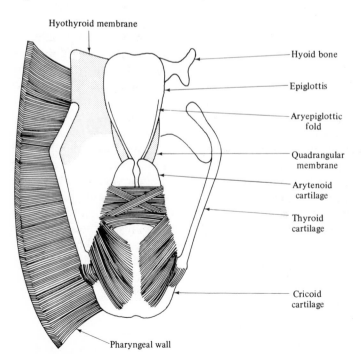

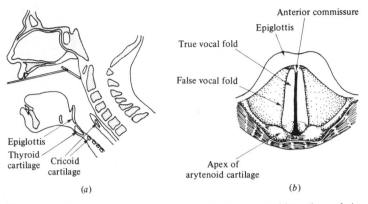

Figure 4-24 Placement of the mirror (left) and resulting view of the larynx (right) in indirect laryngoscopy.

angle just above the true vocal folds. The *vestibular* or *quadrangular membrane* on each side spans the space between the epiglottis and the arytenoid cartilages. Mucosa covers both sides of the quadrangular membrane. The mucosa folds around the upper free border of the membrane to form the *aryepiglottic fold*. Usually each aryepiglottic fold contains a small, elongated *cuneiform* cartilage. Also, it usually contains a few fibers of an *aryepiglotticus* muscle which is actually a continuation of the oblique arytenoid muscle into the aryepiglottic fold. Also enclosed in the fold are the two small *corniculate* cartilages that are fixed on the apices of the arytenoid cartilages. Inferiorly the quadrangular membrane funnels medially to form the *false vocal fold*. The false vocal fold is just above the true vocal fold. The space between the two pairs of folds is the *laryngeal ventricle* (ventricle of Morgagni).

As shown in Figure 4-23, the larynx juts into the pharyngeal cavity and its superior free surface is formed by the aryepiglottic fold, the superior border of the epiglottis, and the superior border of the mucosa covering the interarytenoid muscle. Since the larynx projects into the pharynx, there is some space on either side of the pharynx. These lateral spaces are the *piroform sinuses*.

The superior cornua of the thyroid cartilage are coupled with the greater cornua of the *hyoid bone* through the *posterior thyrohyoid ligaments*. The horseshoe-shaped hyoid bone is unique in that it has no direct connection to any other bone but is suspended under the tongue by muscles and ligaments. The *hyothyroid membrane* spans the space between the hyoid bone and the superior edge of the thyroid cartilage.

The larynx can be observed visually from above by means of indirect laryngoscopy in which a small mirror is placed in the oropharynx as shown in Figure 4-24(*a*). When light beamed into the mouth is reflected down the throat an image of the larynx can be seen, such as is shown in Figure 4-24(*b*). This method is used for examining the larynx and for taking motion pictures of laryngeal motions, especially the vibrations of the true vocal folds. Special care or training is required to inhibit the gag reflex and, in order to get a good view, it is also necessary to produce an [e]-like vowel that leaves both the mouth and throat passages fairly open. Under ideal conditions one can see an image like the one in Figure 4-24, though usually the more anterior parts of the true vocal folds are hidden from view by the epiglottis.

EXTRINSIC CONTROL OF PHONATION

The intrinsic laryngeal muscles exert the primary active forces that control the vocal folds during phonation. There are, in addition, forces exerted on the larynx by other structures. These forces can influence the adjustments of the vocal folds and hence can influence the sound produced in the larynx. Zenker and Zenker (1960) have discussed the extrinsic mechanisms of voice control in some detail. The extrinsic laryngeal muscles actively regulate the position of the larynx within the neck. The larynx can be moved vertically by the so-called *strap* muscles. These muscles, shown in Figure 4-25, include the *sternothyroid*, *thyrohyoid*, and *sternohyoid* muscles. The first two muscles, in particular, are believed to help stabilize the position of the thyroid cartilage. It is also possible that the strap muscles may directly cause some rotation in the cricothyroid joint.

A passive extrinsic force on the larynx is the elasticity of the trachea, and, through its mechanical connections, the elasticity of the entire subglottal system of which it is a part. When the cricothyroid muscle pulls the cricoid arch up and stretches the vocal folds, the force of the muscle is exactly balanced by the passive elastic forces of the cricothyroid joint, the vocal folds, and the trachea. The trachea would be bent backward in this action. The

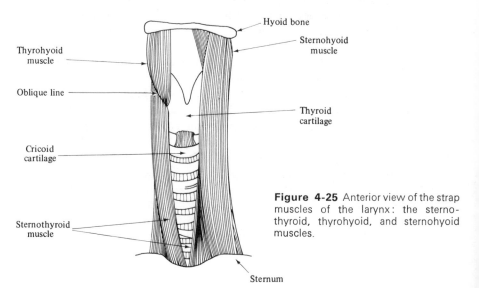

Figure 4-25 Anterior view of the strap muscles of the larynx: the sternothyroid, thyrohyoid, and sternohyoid muscles.

passive tracheal force also opposes the raising of the larynx by the thyrohyoid muscle. As the larynx is raised, the tracheal force should increase and further limit the range of motion in the cricothyroid muscle, i. e., as the cricothyroid's force is exerted more against bending the trachea it has less available force for stretching the vocal folds. It is tempting to speculate that the reduction of tracheal pull is the physical reason that voice students are taught to maintain a relatively low position of the larynx in the neck.

There are, of course, a number of other extrinsic mechanisms that could be important. These include the forces exerted by the pharyngeal muscles, particularly the *cricopharyngeus* and *thyropharyngeus*, the changing forces resulting from tongue movements and the forces resulting from different postures of the head and neck. An additional type of extrinsic influence on phonation is the acoustic loading on the voice source that changes with the movements of the supraglottal articulators. It is believed that the resonances of the vocal tract have some measurable influence on the sound produced at the glottis (Flanagan, 1968).

SOME UNSOLVED PROBLEMS

One has only to listen attentively to the human voice in all its variety of expression to realize that the physical mechanisms of phonation must be complex and under exceedingly delicate control. We know the main mechanisms that determine the fundamental frequency and intensity of the voice, but we do not know very much about the interplay among these mechanisms during speech. What mechanisms, for example, does a speaker employ to stress a syllable, to ask a question, or to express a certain attitude? For that matter, what resultant pitch and intensity patterns correspond to these concepts? These are important and difficult problems for research.

The physical mechanisms for the voice registers of chest voice, head voice, and falsetto need to be elucidated. We can hear the differences between these registers and we can tell when we are producing them, but we still do not have an adequate understanding of how they are actually produced in the larynx.

At the physical level, we need to know more about how the vocal folds vibrate and how the airflow through the glottis generates different types of sound. We know the general mechanisms, but the exact details are still not clear. For example, the mucosa of the vocal folds obviously must vibrate in a different way from the vocal ligament. The mucosa can move like a jelly in relation to the ligament and it would be interesting to know how the interaction between the ligament and mucosa determines the beautiful and complex vibrations of the vocal folds. It would also be interesting to know more about the generation of turbulent airflow in the larynx. We are all familiar with the fact that there are many ways to whisper. How do different laryngeal adjustments lead to different patterns of turbulent flow and how do these different flow patterns result in different types of quasi-random noise? These are some challenges for research.

REFERENCES

ARNOLD, G. E. 1961. Physiology and pathology of the cricothyroid muscle. *Laryngoscope* 71: 687–753.

BERG, J. VAN DEN 1956. Direct and indirect determination of the mean subglottic pressure. *Folia Phoniatrica* 8: 1–24.

BERG, J. VAN DEN 1958. Myoelastic-aerodynamic theory of voice production. *J. Speech Hearing Research* 1: 227–44.

BERG, J. VAN DEN 1960. Vocal ligaments versus registers. *Current Problems in Phoniatrics and Logopedics* 1: 19–34.

BERG, J. VAN DEN and TAN, T. S. 1959. Results of experiments with human larynxes. *Practica Oto-Rhino-Laryngologica* 21: 425–50.

BERG, J. VAN DEN, VENNARD, W., BERGER, D. and SHERVANIAN, C. C. 1960. *Voice Production.* (Black and white, sound, 16 mm). Utrecht, The Netherlands: SFW-UNFI.

CAVAGNA, G. A. and MARGARIA, R. 1965. An analysis of the mechanics of phonation. *J. Appl. Physiol.* 20: 301–7.

FINK, B. R. 1962. Tensor mechanism of the vocal folds. *Annals Oto. Rhinol. Laryngol.* 71: 591–99.

FLANAGAN, J. L. 1968. Source-system interaction in the vocal tract. *Annals N.Y. Acad. Sci.* 155: 9–17.

HIROTO, I. 1966. Patho-physiology of the larynx from the standpoint of vocal mechanism [in Japanese]. *Practica Otologica Kyoto* 59: 229–92.

HOLLIEN, H. 1960. Vocal pitch variation related to changes in vocal fold length. *J. Speech and Hearing Research* 3: 150–56.

HOLLIEN, H. 1962. Vocal fold thickness and fundamental frequency of phonation. *J. Speech and Hearing Research* 5: 237–43.

HOLLIEN, H., COLEMAN, R. and MOORE, P. 1968. Stroboscopic laminagraphy of the larynx. *Acta Oto-Laryngol.* 65: 209–15.

HOLLIEN, H. and MOORE, G. P. 1960. Measurement of the vocal folds during changes in pitch. *J. Speech Hearing Research* 3: 157–65.

ISHIZAKA, K. and MATSUDAIRA, M. 1968. What makes the vocal cords vibrate? *In* Y. Kohasi (ed.) *The 6th International Congress on Acoustics*, Vol. II. New York: Elsevier. B-9–B-12.

ISHIZAKA, K. and MATSUDAIRA, M. 1972. Fluid mechanical considerations of vocal cord vibration. *SCRL Monograph No. 8*. Santa Barbara: Speech Communications Research Laboratory.

ISSHIKI, N. 1964. Regulatory mechanism of voice intensity variation. *J. Speech Hearing Research* 7: 17–29.

LADEFOGED, P. and MCKINNEY, N. P. 1963. Loudness, sound pressure, and subglottal pressure in speech. *J. Acoust. Soc. Amer.* 35: 454–60.

LUCHSINGER, R. and PFISTER, K. 1961. Die Messung der Stimmlippenverlängerung beim Steigern der Tonhöhe. *Folia Phoniatrica* 13: 1–12.

MAYET, A. and MÜNDNICH, K. 1958. Beitrag zur Anatomie und zur Funktion des M. Cricothyreoideus und der Cricothyreoidgelenke. *Acta Anatomica* 33: 273–88.

MOORE, P. 1937. Vocal fold movement during vocalization. *Speech Monographs* 4: 44–55.

PETERSON, G. E. and SHOUP, J. E. 1966. A physiological theory of phonetics. *J. Speech Hearing Research* 9: 5–67.

PRESSMAN, J. J. and KELEMEN, G. 1970. *Physiology of the Larynx*, rev. by J. A. Kirchner. Rochester, Minnesota: Amer. Acad. Ophthamol. Otolaryngol. 1970.

SONESSON, B. 1959. Die funktionelle Anatomie des Cricoarytenoidgelenkes. *Zeitschrift für Anatomie und Entwicklungsgeschichte* 121: 292–303.

SONESSON, B. 1960. On the anatomy and vibratory pattern of the human vocal folds. *Acta Oto-Laryngol.* Suppl. 156.

SONNINEN, A. A. 1954. Is the length of the vocal cords the same at all different levels of singing? *Acta Oto-Laryngol.* Suppl. 118.

VON LEDEN, H. and MOORE, P. 1961. The mechanics of the cricoarytenoid joint. *Arch. Otolaryngol.* 73: 541–50.

WENDAHL, R. W., MOORE, G. P. and HOLLIEN, H. 1963. Comments on vocal fry. *Folia Phoniatrica* 15: 251–55.

ZENKER, W. and ZENKER, A. 1960. Über die Regelung der Stimmlippenspannung durch von aussen eingreifende Mechanismen. *Folia Phoniatrica* 12: 1–36.

5

NORMAL ARTICULATION PROCESSES

Raymond G. Daniloff

INTRODUCTION

The production of speech sounds involves the active movement of various structures within the vocal tract. In conjunction with the flow of air at varying pressures through the vocal tract, movements of the articulators give rise to those acoustic vibrations called speech sounds. The structure of the vocal tract and the structure of the language being spoken determine in large degree the nature of speech articulation. The following is a short description of the structure and functioning of the vocal tract during speech production.

VOCAL TRACT

The *vocal tract* is that tube-like series of cavities which begins at the vocal folds and ends at the opening of the lips. The nasal cavities provide an alternate outlet to the vocal tract. Figure 5-1 is a schematic view of the vocal tract cavities and certain of the structures which form its walls. The vocal tract is a complex system that is involved in a variety of functions. Among these are the processes of speech production, respiration, olfaction, mastication, etc. It is possible that the human vocal tract was selected for and thus evolved into a system uniquely adapted for speech (Lieberman et al., 1969), as well as for nonspeech functions.

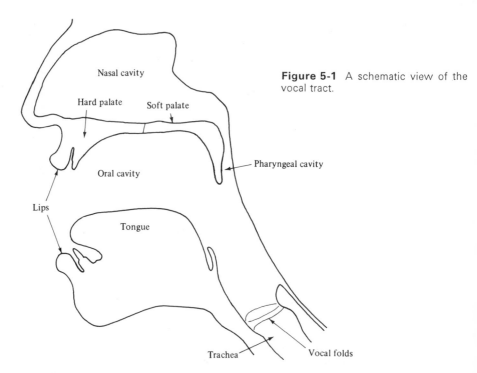

Figure 5-1 A schematic view of the vocal tract.

Speech sounds are those mixtures of acoustic vibration and/or silences which result when a vibrating source of energy sets the air inside the vocal tract into vibration. The major source of energy for speech sound production is usually provided by the egressive (outward) flow of air from the lungs. The potential energy present in the form of flowing air is converted into vibrational or kinetic energy at the vocal folds, or at any point along the vocal tract which is tightly or completely constricted by the articulators.

The *articulators* are those movable structures (such as the tongue and the lips) which directly form a portion of the walls of the vocal tract, or are directly attached to the walls of the tract. Articulator movements serve a dual function; they alter the shape (and to a lesser degree, the length) of the vocal tract, and they create sources of vibrational energy at locations within the vocal tract above the vocal folds. For example, by partially constricting the vocal tract, the air stream flowing through the constriction may become turbulent and serve as a source of noise. If the vocal tract is completely blocked, air pressure may build up behind the blockage; sudden release of the blockage results in a burst of air, a plosive noise. Differing speech sounds are associated with differing vocal tract shapes and/or differing sources of vibrational energy.

Respiratory System

The respiratory or pulmonic system provides the body with a supply of oxygen, carries away carbon dioxide, and functions as the major source of energy which is used to set the air within the vocal tract into vibration. In simplistic terms, this system can be viewed as an air pump, sucking air into or blowing air out of an air pipe (vocal tract). The flow of air in the pipe can be valved, stopped, or allowed to escape through such partial obstructions as are created within the vocal tract by the articulators. The vocal folds, which are an essential part of the larynx or phonatory mechanism, form the poster-ior-inferior boundary of the vocal tract. Complete vocal fold closure stops airflow. Opened vocal folds allow either inward or outward airflow. During voicing, or phonation as it is called, the respiratory muscles and mechanical forces of the pulmonary system create a subglottal air pressure (below the vocal folds) which exceeds the supraglottal air pressure (above the folds). This difference in air pressure above and below the folds, under appropriate conditions, sets the folds into a periodic, vibratory pattern of opening and closing such that puffs of air escape through the glottal (interfold) opening and give rise to acoustic vibrations. There, vibrations (laryngeal tone) set the air column within the vocal tract into sympathetic vibration as discussed in Chapter 4.

Vocal Tract Cavities

Oral cavity

Figures 5-2(*a*) and 5-2(*b*) are frontal views of the oral cavity. The hard palate and a portion of the soft palate form the roof; the tongue dorsum forms the floor of the oral cavity. The maxillary and mandibular teeth and alveolar ridges form the lateral walls of the oral cavity in conjunction with the walls of the cheeks. The lips and the central incisors form the anterior wall of the cavity, while posteriorly, the anterior faucial pillar (*palatoglossus* muscle) marks the posterior limit of the oral cavity. The small pockets between the cheeks, gingiva (gums) and teeth are called the buccal (cheek) cavities.

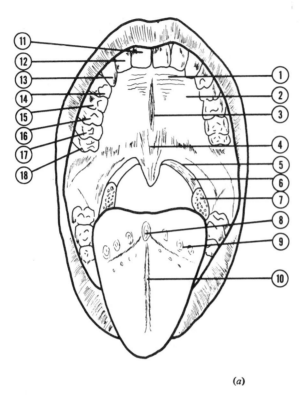

1. Rugae
2. Hard palate
3. Median raphe
4. Soft palate
5. Anterior faucial pillar
6. Posterior faucial pillar
7. Palatine tonsil
8. Sulcus terminalis
9. Papillae vallatae
10. Median sulcus
11. Central incisor
12. Lateral incisor
13. Cuspid
14. 1st bicuspid
15. 2nd bicuspid
16. 1st molar
17. 2nd molar
18. 3rd molar

(a)

Figure 5-2   (a) and (b). Schematic and photographic frontal views of the oral cavity. [*Willard R. Zemlin*, Speech and Hearing Science: Anatomy and Physiology, © *1968* (*Englewood Cliffs, N.J.: Prentice-Hall, Inc.*). *Reprinted by permission.*]

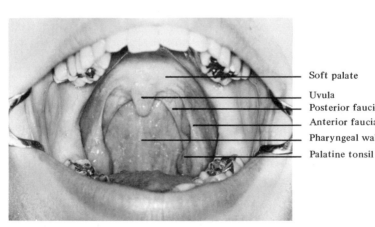

Soft palate

Uvula
Posterior faucial pillar
Anterior faucial pillar

Pharyngeal wall

Palatine tonsil

(b)

Pharyngeal cavity

The pharyngeal cavity is a muscular, horn-shaped tube which arises inferiorly at the level of the glottal opening. It extends superiorly to the base of the skull, and opens into the oral and nasal cavities. It is divided into three divisions (see Figure 5-3).

The nasopharynx. The soft palate forms the floor of the nasopharynx, while the rostrum of the sphenoid bone and pharyngeal protuberance of the occipital bone form the roof of the nasopharynx. The nasopharynx shares an anterior boundary with the posterior nares (*choanae*) of the nasal cavity.

The oropharynx. The soft palate forms the superior border of the oropharynx, the posterior faucial pillar (*palatopharyngeus* muscle) marks the anterior boundary, while the rear of the tongue dorsum marks the inferior border. The oropharynx is considered to terminate inferiorly at the level of the hyoid bone.

The laryngopharynx. The laryngopharynx is bounded by the laryngeal and esophageal openings inferiorly, and is considered to terminate superiorly with the oropharynx at the level of the hyoid bone.

Figure 5-3   A schematic view of the articulators, vocal tract cavities, and places of articulation.

Some places of articulation

1. Labial
2. Dental
3. Alveolar
4. Pre-palatal
5. Palatal
6. Medio-palatal
7. Velar
8. Uvular
9. Pharyngeal
10. Retroflex (curled tongue tip)

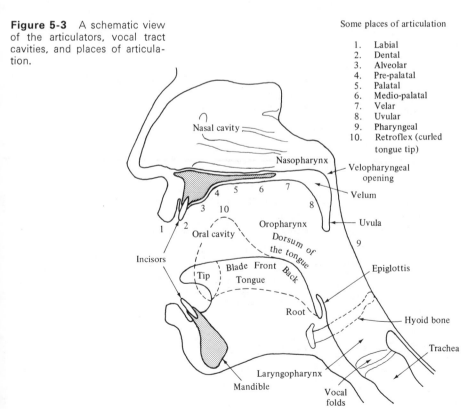

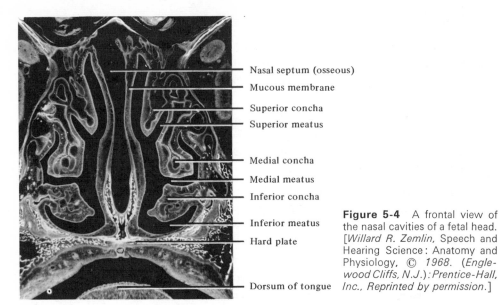

Nasal septum (osseous)

Mucous membrane

Superior concha

Superior meatus

Medial concha

Medial meatus

Inferior concha

Inferior meatus

Hard plate

Dorsum of tongue

Figure 5-4   A frontal view of the nasal cavities of a fetal head. [*Willard R. Zemlin*, Speech and Hearing Science: Anatomy and Physiology, © *1968. (Englewood Cliffs, N.J.):Prentice-Hall, Inc., Reprinted by permission.*]

Nasal cavity

The nasal cavities are comprised of two narrow, rather tortuous channels separated by a nasal septum (see Figure 5-4). These two channels run from the nostrils to the nasopharynx in an anterior-posterior direction. The lateral walls of the nasal channels are invaginated by three sets of openings (*meatuses*) which ramify into a labyrinthine maze. The large surface area of the nasal passages and associated conchae allows for the warming and humidifying of air breathed into the nasal cavity.

Articulators and Associated Structures

The size and shape of the vocal tract cavities may be systematically altered by articulator movements. The size and shape of the vocal tract and the column of air within dictate at which frequencies energy from the sound source(s) will be transmitted to the lip opening. Each different vocal tract shape alters, in a unique manner, the vibratory pattern of the air column. These differing vocal tract shapes or "postures" are used to create distinctively different speech sounds.

The lips

The lips form the anterior boundary of the vocal tract. They are two fleshy, muscular folds which are continuous with the cheeks. If closed they shut the vocal tract. If opened, the size of the opening is greatest when the mandible is low and the lips are spread, the corners of the mouth pulled back against the teeth. The lip opening is smallest when the lips are protruded, that is, thrust outward and bunched or puckered. The lower lip has considerable freedom of movement and easily effects contact with the upper incisors or upper lip.

Mandible

The lower lip, lower teeth, tongue, and a host of muscles attach to the mandible. The complex structure of the *temporomandibular joint* allows elevation-depression, side to side, and protruding-retracting movements of the mandible. Mandibular movements can alter lip opening, tongue position, laryngeal position, and the size and shape of the vocal tract.

Teeth and hard palate

The domed surface of the hard palate is fringed on three sides by the alveolar processes or ridges into which are set the upper teeth. The above structures form the roof and side walls of the oral cavity. Against these fixed structures, lips and tongue may make contacts or partial constrictions for the production of many consonant sounds.

The lower lip and the tongue can be pressed against the upper incisors to form obstructions to air flow useful for the production of certain consonants. Tongue contacts or airway constrictions between the tongue and the inferior surface of the hard palate, on or near the alveolar ridge, occur for a large number of consonants.

The tongue

The highly mobile tongue is a singularly important articulator because it participates in the production of many different speech sounds. The tongue forms the floor of the oral cavity and the anterior wall of the pharyngeal cavity. Tongue movement may simultaneously alter the shape of both oral and pharyngeal cavities, thus changing the resonance properties of the vocal tract. Because of its great complexity of muscle structure, the tongue can adopt a wide variety of shapes, move quickly, and can make contacts and constrictions along the greater part of the vocal tract.

Figures 5-5(a), (b) and 5-6 are views of the tongue and its associated musculature. Descriptively, the tongue can be divided into four parts. These include the tip, blade, dorsum, and root. The tip or frontmost edge is usually nearest to the upper incisors; the blade or front part of the tongue (including the tip) is that portion below the alveolar ridge; the dorsum or upper surface can be separated into a front portion beneath the hard palate and back portion beneath the soft palate; the root is that most posterior portion of the tongue mass which is most directly attached to surrounding structures (see Figure 5-3).

Tongue muscles are attached to such surrounding structures as the epiglottis, soft palate, hyoid bone, styloid process, mandible, etc. Thus, tongue movements affect the position of the soft palate, hyoid bone, mandible, pharynx, etc. (and vice versa).

Intrinsic tongue muscles. Intrinsic muscles have both points of attachment (origin and insertion) within a structure, in contrast to *extrinsic* muscles which have one attachment to a structure, and another attachment outside it. The intrinsic muscles are shown in Figures 5-5(*a*),(*b*) and 5-6. The *vertical* muscle fibers arise from the mucosal lining of the tongue dorsum and run vertically downward to insert into the inferior surface of the tongue. Contraction of this muscle flattens the tongue. The *transverse* muscle fibers

Figure 5-5 (*a*) Frontal sections through the tongue of a fetus. [*From Willard R. Zemlin, Speech and Hearing Science: Anatomy and Physiology, © 1968 (Englewood Cliffs, N.J.: Prentice-Hall, Inc.). Reprinted by permission.*]

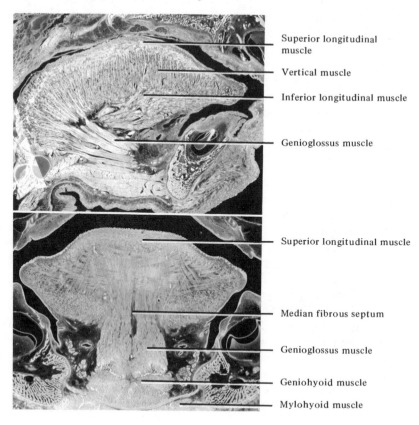

Superior longitudinal muscle

Vertical muscle

Inferior longitudinal muscle

Genioglossus muscle

Superior longitudinal muscle

Median fibrous septum

Genioglossus muscle

Geniohyoid muscle

Mylohyoid muscle

originate on the medial (middle) fibrous septum of the tongue and run laterally to insert into the lateral edges of the tongue. Contraction of this muscle narrows and elongates the tongue mass. The *superior longitudinal* muscle fibers, which form a layer near the surface of the tongue dorsum, originate near the root of the tongue, coursing anteriorly along the length of the dorsum whereupon they insert into the edges of the tongue. Contraction of this muscle can curl the tip and edges of the tongue upward in a bowed fashion, and may also shorten the tongue. The *inferior longitudinal* muscle fibers are deep in the tongue, near the inferior surface. The fibers originate with the muscle mass of the root of the tongue and course forward toward the tongue tip. Contraction of this muscle may pull the tongue tip down or shorten the tongue. In general, the intrinsic muscles are potent in affecting tongue shape as well as effecting tongue movement.

Figure 5-5 (*b*) Parasaggital (above) and frontal (below) sections through a fetal tongue. [*From Willard R. Zemlin*, Speech and Hearing Science: Anatomy and Physiology, © *1968* (*Englewood Cliffs, N.J.: Prentice-Hall, Inc.*). *Reprinted by permission.*]

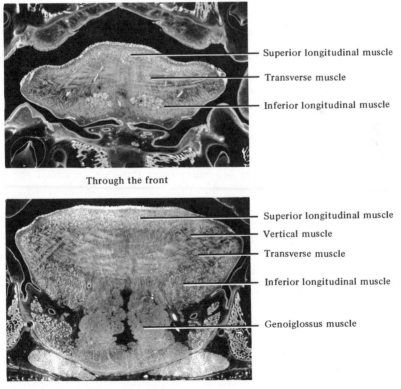

Superior longitudinal muscle

Transverse muscle

Inferior longitudinal muscle

Through the front

Superior longitudinal muscle

Vertical muscle

Transverse muscle

Inferior longitudinal muscle

Genioglossus muscle

Through the blade

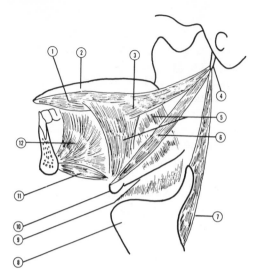

1.	Inferior longitudinal
2.	Dorsum of tongue
3.	Styloglossus
4.	Styloid process
5.	Hyoglossus
6.	Stylohyoid
7.	Stylopharyngeus
8.	Thyroid cartilage
9.	Greater cornu
10.	Hyoid bone
11.	Geniohyoid
12.	Genioglossus

Figure 5-6 A schematic view of the extrinsic tongue muscles.
[*From Willard R. Zemlin*, Speech and Hearing Science : Anatomy
and Physiology, © 1968. (*Englewood Cliffs, N.J.: Prentice-Hall,
Inc.*). *Reprinted by permission.*]

Extrinsic tongue muscles. The extrinsic muscles, shown in Figure 5-6, move the tongue mass to and fro, and to a lesser extent, affect tongue shape.

The *genioglossus* muscle is the largest muscle of the tongue, and it contributes most to the bulk of the tongue. This fanshaped muscle originates from the posterior surface of the inferior edge of the mandible and its fibers extend upward into the tongue from root to tip. The lowermost fibers course to the hyoid bone. When the genioglossus muscle fibers are contracted in various ways, they protrude the tongue tip or pull the tongue down into the trough of the mandible, imparting a concave shape to the tongue profile.

The *styloglossus* muscle originates from the anterior tip of the styloid process of the temporal bone and runs downward and anteriorly, fanning out into a flat sheet of muscle which intermingles with the main mass of superior longitudinalis and hyoglossus muscles. When contracted, this muscle lifts the tongue upward and backward, as well as lifting the tongue edges.

The *hyoglossus* muscle originates from the upper edge of the greater cornu of the hyoid bone as well as from the main body of the hyoid. It runs in a thin, flat, rectangular sheet upwards to insert in the submucosal tissue of the back half of the tongue, mixing with the fibers of the palatoglossus. The hyoglossus serves to lower and retract the tongue body.

Finally, the *palatoglossus* muscle originates in the anterior surface of the soft palate running laterally downward where it inserts into the sides of the tongue, blending with fibers of the styloglossus, hyoglossus, and transverse muscles (Figure 5-7). Contraction of the palatoglossus may raise the tongue or lower the palate, depending on the relative fixation of the two ends of the muscle.

Tongue movement

During speech production, all or part of the tongue can move up or down (high-low) or front-to-back simultaneously. It is not unusual to observe the tongue tip curling upward even while the rear of the tongue dorsum moves down and back. The body of the tongue can be shaped in various ways—concave, convex, flat, curled, etc.

For consonant productions, rapid tongue movements in many directions and swift changes of tongue shape occur as partial or complete occlusions of the vocal tract are created. Figure 5-3 shows points of contact for the tongue at the lips, upper incisors, alveolar ridge, hard palate, soft palate, and even the posterior pharyngeal wall, and at many spots between these points. The constrictions are very open for vowels, moderately open for sounds like [r], [l], [w], relatively tightly constricted for [s] or [f], and closed off for [p] or [g].

Although the tongue may adopt relatively fixed (quasi-static) positions during vowel production, it is in almost constant motion during the production of certain consonants. For example, during the production of the [r] sound as in the word "right," the tongue moves continuously. The tongue dorsum rises to a broad hump in the rear even as the tongue tip curls upward (retroflexes) toward the alveolar ridge, and then moves downward smoothly.

The velum

The *velum* or soft palate is a muscular flap of tissue which, when relaxed, hangs downward into the oropharynx, almost touching the tongue dorsum. When the velum is relaxed, the *velopharyngeal port* is open, allowing the passage of air and acoustic vibrations into the nasal cavities. The velum is typically open during quiet breathing, and closed for the production of oral speech sounds. The velum is open and the oral cavity closed off for the production of nasal sounds. Normally, oral sounds can be "nasalized" if the velum is partially opened so that air passes out both nasal and oral cavities. Recent research (Willis and Stutz, 1969) indicates that patterns of velopharyngeal closure vary among speakers. In some, the velum alone rises to close the velopharyngeal port. In others, the lateral and posterior pharyngeal walls may move medially toward the sides of the rising velum to assist in closure.

The *palatal levator* muscle, shown schematically in Figure 5-7, can contract and raise the velum in a superior, posterior direction. This paired muscle, arising from the petrous portion of the temporal bone, courses downward and medially to insert into the palatal aponeurosis at the midline of the velum. It is the primary muscle for velopharyngeal closure.

The *palatoglossus* muscle, when contracted, may depress the velum if the tongue is fixed, or raise the tongue if the palate is fixed in position.

The *palatopharyngeus* muscle arises from the sides of the velum and courses downward and laterally, blending into the stylopharyngeus muscle,

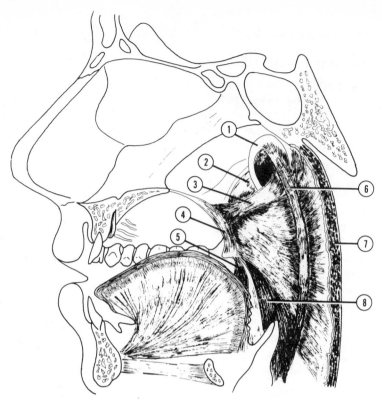

1.	Orifice of Eustachian tube	5.	Glossopalatine muscle
2.	Tensor palatine muscle	6.	Salpingopharyngeus muscle
3.	Levator palatine muscle	7.	Superior constrictor muscle
4.	Uvular muscle	8.	Palatoglossal muscle

Figure 5-7 A schematic view of palatal musculature and adjacent structures. [*Willard R. Zemlin*, Speech and Hearing Science: Anatomy and Physiology, © *1968* (*Englewood Cliffs, N.J.; Prentice-Hall, Inc.*). *Reprinted by permission.*]

and thence into the side walls of the pharynx (see Figure 5-8(*b*)). When contracted, this muscle, like the palatoglossus may serve to lower the pelum, or may act in a sphincter-like fashion, pulling the posterior faucial yillars toward each other.

The *palatal tensor* muscle originates on the base of the medial ptervgoid plate of the sphenoid and lateral wall of the *eustachian tube*. The muscle fibers course downward, ending in a tendon which winds around the *hamulus* of the medial pterygoid plate and passes medially to insert along the palatal aponeurosis of the velum. Contraction of this muscle flattens and tenses the velum.

Velar elevation is accompanied by simultaneous activity in the palatal levator and palatal tensor muscles (Fritzell, 1969), while rapid opening movements of the velum during speech production involve palatoglossus activity.

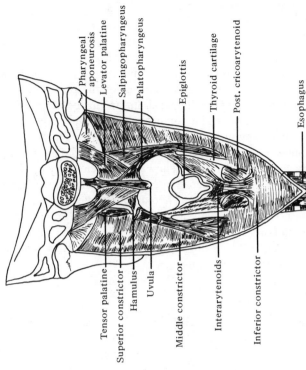

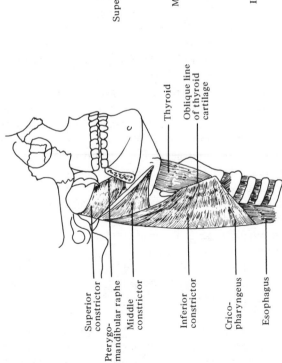

Figure 5-8 (a) A view of the pharyngeal constrictor muscles. (b) A posterior view of the pharynx and palate. [Willard R. Zemlin, Speech and Hearing Science: Anatomy and Physiology. © 1968 (Englewood Cliffs, N.J.: Prentice-Hall, Inc.). Reprinted by permission.]

Pharynx

The pharyngeal cavity, although not previously considered to be an active articulator, has been shown to engage in active movement (Kelsey et al., 1969). These movements alter the diameter of the pharyngeal airway. The pharyngeal muscles shown in Figures 5-8(*a*),(*b*) include the superior, middle and inferior constrictors. The topmost muscle, the *superior constrictor*, consists of a small ring of muscle fibers enclosing the superior portion of the pharynx. It may be the contractions of this muscle which move the pharyngeal walls inward at the level of the velum during velopharyngeal closure. The *middle constrictor* is a large, fan-shaped muscle which encloses the pharynx, originating from the cornua of the hyoid bone and encircling the pharyngeal airway to insert into the pharyngeal aponeurosis. The *inferior constrictor* arises from both the cricoid cartilage and the oblique line of the thyroid cartilage. The muscle fibers fan out posteriorly and meet each other at the midline raphe of the pharynx.

Articulation as Motor Behavior

Motor behavior (movement patterns of the body) can be characterized by the intensity, rate, and time patterns of such movements. Movements of the articulators can be recorded directly. One can make inferences about articulator movements by examining the muscles involved, their size, their neural innervation, and the tasks which they perform. Articulator movements associated with speech production are governed, in part, by the structure of the language, and also by the structure of the vocal tract.

Speech articulation demands the coordinated, simultaneous contraction of many muscle groups. Consider the swing of a golfer as an analogy to the complex movements needed to articulate a speech sound. Swinging a golf club involves simultaneous movements of calves, knees, thighs, hips, shoulders, arms, wrists, fingers, and neck. For a good swing, these movements must be coordinated both in time and intensity. Timing of muscle contraction is important; too much or too little movement too early or too late and the intended shot is not well accomplished. The beginner slowly learns to produce this complex set of movements automatically, or almost unconsciously, as his swing becomes truly precise. If, by some chance, one component gesture of the swing becomes deviant or disordered (e. g., excessive bending of the wrists) it takes much practice to alter the single gesture because it is embedded in a complex of gestures, and to change one is to change all in a subtle way.

The development of the complex, language-directed articulator movement arises during infancy when children initially move their articulators in an exploratory non-language way, during crying, babbling, feeding, or breathing. At birth, the respiratory system and much of the vocal tract are coordinated at a reflex level, to produce distress and pleasure cries. This coordination includes the diaphragm, intercostal muscles, larynx, tongue, jaw, lips, etc. The latter structures produce the open vocal tract for vowel-like cries, and the rapid lip and tongue movements which create consonant-like noises. Conscious language-directed articulation develops from this initial repertoire or substratum of early vocal tract behaviors.

Importance of the ear to articulation

Speech is difficult to acquire naturally and to maintain if the speaker suffers severe hearing loss. Speech quality and intelligibility are usually abnormal when such hearing anomalies exist. During language learning, the child models his utterance upon what he hears others speak. The speaker listens to himself as he talks. If he misarticulates a sound, he hears it and proceeds to correct his ongoing articulation, or, he can correct his articulation the next time that the particular sound occurs. The total time elapsed from the moment a speaker's articulators move, to when he hears the sound and can move his articulators to correct it, is from about $\frac{1}{6}$ to $\frac{1}{4}$ of a second (Kozhevnikov and Chistovich, 1966).

Speakers may be able to correct some of the longer speech sounds, vowels and some fricative consonants, as they are articulating them. Other sounds of short duration like the stop consonants are completed before speakers perceive them and can alter their articulation. Because utterances are usually as long as several words in length, speakers can monitor the loudness, pitch, stress, and rate of articulation and can alter them as well as the overall precision of articulation.

Tactile and proprioceptive feedback

The vocal tract is lined with receptors sensitive to pain, touch, temperature, muscle stretch, etc. The tactile receptors are responsible for the senses of light touch, surface pressure, and deep pressures. The kinesthetic and proprioceptive receptors within muscle bodies, tendons, and joints provide feedback indicating the positions in space which the various structures have achieved. Thus, information is provided to the speaker about articulator movements, positions, contacts, and pressures throughout the vocal tract. Each articulator and the surfaces which it touches have differing kinds and numbers of feedback receptors. For example, the tongue is liberally endowed with tactile and kinesthetic receptors and hence is very sensitive to changes of position, movement, or pressure. On the other hand, the inferior surface of the soft palate is relatively insensitive because of the lack of such receptors. Articulators whose movements are precise and well controlled are rather well endowed with tactile-kinesthetic receptors.

These sources of feedback information on articulation are used in conjunction with auditory feedback to control articulation. Malfunctioning in these feedback systems may trigger severe impairment of articulation. There is some evidence (Shriner et al., 1969) to suggest that speakers who suffer disorders of their feedback systems display more articulation errors, and a reduced level of articulation development (Weiner, 1967). MacNeilage et al. (1967) examined a girl who had suffered severe congenital loss of tactile-proprioceptive feedback of the oropharynx. They observed severe misarticulation of speech indicating that her loss had interfered with normal articulation development.

Articulator movements

When muscle fibers are activated, they shorten in length. If not allowed to shorten (contract) because the points of muscle attachment are fixed, the muscle remains at its original length, exerting a strong, steady bracing pull on both points of attachment. The former manner of contraction is referred to as *miometric*, while the latter is called an *isometric* contraction. Fine and precise articulation movements result from a few, well-timed muscle contractions (a few motor units firing) while strong, fast, and less well-controlled movements result from the rapid sustained contraction of many muscle fibers (many motor units firing). The faster the rate of neural discharges and the more motor units involved, the greater is the force of muscle contraction.

Each movable speech articulator contains one or more muscle bodies, each with a particular innervation ratio. The innervation ratio is defined as the number of muscle fibers attached to a single motor neuron. Muscles with a high innervation ratio (many muscle fibers per motor neuron) respond rather wholistically, producing large, abrupt movements as a result of a few stimulating neural impulses. Such rapid, abrupt articulator movements are produced by intense, unchecked muscle contractions. Once set into motion, an articulator can be stopped or controlled by the force of gravity, by contact with other structures, by reaching the elastic limits of the articulator's attachments, or by the antagonistic (opposing) contractions of muscles which oppose the ongoing movement. It is the usual case that the rather well-controlled articulator movements result from the simultaneous controlling muscle contractions of antagonistic muscles which regulate the movement of articulators produced by the agonistic muscles of propulsion.

The size and nature of the nerve which innervates a given muscle influences muscle contraction speed and other operating characteristics. Kaiser (1934) observed a relationship between speed of movement and the neural innervation for different muscles. Lip and facial structures whose muscles are innervated by the facial nerve move at a maximum rate of 2.5–3 syllables per second; the tongue, supplied by the hypoglossal nerve, moves at a maximum rate of 8.2 syllables per second (during the production of the syllable "tat") at the tip, and 7.1 with the back of the tongue (Hudgins and Stetson, 1937). The mandible can move at 7.2 syllables per second, faster than the lips, more slowly than the tongue. For fast lip closures, the lower lip is carried upward by the mandible. Miller (1951) estimates the average rate of syllable production for conversational speech to be about five syllables per second which is roughly 12½ speech sounds per second.

Articulator speed is largely a function of neural innervation, articulator mass, and articulator structure. For example, the tongue tip probably moves a little faster than the back of the tongue because of the tip's smaller mass; the velum rises faster than it falls because the muscles which close it are more powerful and faster acting than those which act to open it.

During speech, six of the twelve cranial nerves and many of the spinal nerves are simultaneously active, producing and coordinating activity in muscles ranging from the abdominals to the orbicularis oris of the lips. Shankweiler and Harris (1966) and Huntington et al., (1968) have shown that one of the characteristics of the speech of aphasic and hearing impaired speakers is a muscular discoordination with respect to timing and amount of muscle activity. This is not surprising in view of the complex requirements for normal articulation.

THE SOUNDS OF SPEECH

Speech production involves the creation of a stream of speech sounds or *phones*. Individual speech sounds are indicated in brackets, such as the sound [s], as in the word "sit." Speech sounds which involve vocal fold vibration are voiced (sonorant). Those not involving vocal fold vibrations are voiceless (surd). If air and vibration during sound production escape only from the oral cavity, the sound is called "oral," in contrast to "nasal" sound where all air escapes through the nose.

Speech sounds may be classified according to the articulatory movements/ vocal tract shapes used to generate them. They may also be classified according to the nature of the acoustic vibrations associated with each speech sound, or according to the way(s) in which listeners perceive them. The physiological-articulatory classification will be emphasized herein. In the descriptions which follow, speech sounds will be classified according to the *place* along the vocal tract where the articulator(s) involved perform their movements. It should also be noted that not every movement of the articulators results in a distinct sound or change in a speech sound.

Vowel Sounds

Vowel sounds, in almost all languages, are produced with a relatively open vocal tract. They are voiced, and acoustically, they are rather longer in duration and more intense than consonants. The quality of vowel sounds depends on the shape/size of the vocal tract above the vocal folds. The two articulators which most effectively change the shape of the vocal tract are the tongue and lips, hence it is the shape and position of tongue and lips which are used to classify the vowels. Before proceeding to the description of the vowels, a note of caution. The shape of the vocal tract varies continuously along its entire length, from vocal folds to lips. Vowel quality depends very largely upon the total pattern of vocal tract shape. To simplify the description of vocal tract shape, phoneticians have claimed that tongue-lip positions are the major determinants of vocal tract shape. The location of the high point of the tongue dorsum is taken to be the major descriptor of vocal tract shape. This is akin to saying that the high point of a hill, irrespective of the irregularities of the shape of the hill, is the most important aspect of the hill.

The first of the major parameters describing vowel production is the height of the high point of the tongue dorsum. Figures 5-9(a), (b) show that the vowels [u] as in "new" and [i] as in "he" are high vowels, [ɛ] as in "get" and [ʌ] as in "hut" are mid vowels, and [æ] as in "had" and [a] as in "Tom" are low vowels.

The second major parameter of vowel description is the front-to-back position of the high point of the tongue. For example, [o] as in "toe" is a mid-back vowel, [ʊ] a high back vowel, and [i] a high front vowel, etc. It should be noted that the point of maximum vocal tract constriction may be a more relevant descriptor of tongue position for vowels. This is especially true for back vowels such as [o] where it can be seen (Figure 5-9(a)) that the high point of the dorsum and the point of greatest constriction are widely separated. For the vowel [ɝ] as in "heard," the tongue tip curls upward toward the hard palate, which results in a vowel which shows two points of maximum vocal tract constriction (see Figure 5-10(a)).

The third articulatory parameter of import is the degree of lip opening. Notice in Figure 5-9(a) that the lip opening is smallest and protruded outwards most for the vowel [u], whereas for [æ] the lip opening is largest and the lips are retracted maximally toward the teeth. The size of the lip opening and the length of the lip channel, from the teeth to the outer edge of the lip, are important determinants of how a vowel will sound. In certain languages, such as Swedish, lip opening is a very crucial variable of vowel production.

There are a number of secondary articulatory dimensions or parameters which affect the production of certain vowels. The position of the velum is critical in this respect. If the velum shuts off the velopharyngeal port, then a normal, orally produced vowel results. If the velopharyngeal port is deliberately or accidentally opened, air passes through both oral and nasal cavities, and the resultant vowel is physically "nasalized." Listeners can sometimes detect a nasal quality in such nasalized vowels. The height of the larynx may affect vowel quality by altering the length of the vocal tract, and the movements of the pharyngeal walls, sometimes inward and outward, can alter the diameter of the vocal tract along its length.

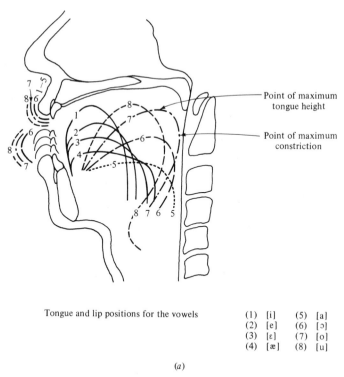

Tongue and lip positions for the vowels

(1)	[i]	(5)	[a]
(2)	[e]	(6)	[ɔ]
(3)	[ɛ]	(7)	[o]
(4)	[æ]	(8)	[u]

(a)

Figure 5-9 (a) A schematic drawing of tongue and lip positions for certain vowels. (b) Location of the high point of the tongue for various vowels.

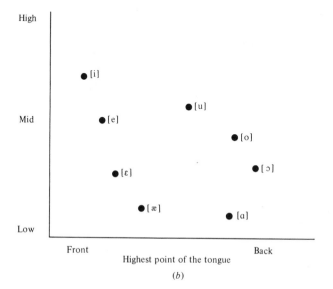

(b)

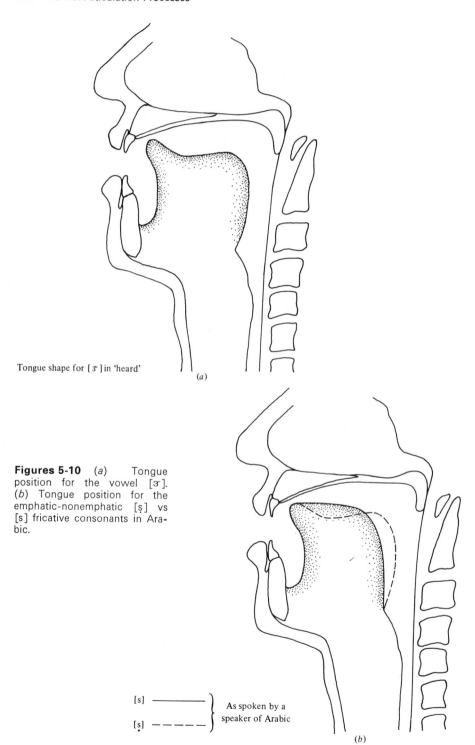

Tongue shape for [ɝ] in 'heard'

(a)

Figures 5-10 (a) Tongue position for the vowel [ɝ]. (b) Tongue position for the emphatic-nonemphatic [ṣ] vs [s] fricative consonants in Arabic.

[s] ———
[ṣ] – – – – –
} As spoken by a speaker of Arabic

(b)

Consonant Sounds

The distinction between vowel and consonant sounds is a major one. During consonant production, the vocal tract is completely or quite closely constricted or obstructed, whereas vowels are made with a much more open vocal tract. Vowels are usually made without noise occurring at the point of greatest constriction whereas noise usually occurs at the tight or complete consonant constrictions. Consonant sounds are usually classified along the dimensions of *place* of articulation: labial, dental, alveolar, palatal, velar, uvular, etc., and *manner* of articulation: voiced vs voiceless, nasal vs non-nasal, stop vs continuant, etc. Figure 5-3 illustrates some of the various places of consonant production.

Consonants differ rather markedly from vowels in that many consonants involve rather rapid movements of one or more articulators such that the acoustic vibrations change rapidly during the consonant. For example, the stop consonant [t] in "pretty" involves a rapid movement toward a closure of the vocal tract during which the vibrations emitted from the mouth rapidly change in quality and then disappear. Subsequently there is a noise burst after which voicing reappears and rapidly grows in intensity. This pattern of acoustic change accompanies the rapid closing-opening movements of the tongue tip for [t], which is a "stop" consonant. For the sound [s], the tongue tip forms a tight slit at the alveolar ridge through which air is forced in a swift stream which creates noise as the air stream escapes from the slit and strikes the upper incisors. The production of [s] can be maintained rather steadily, thus the manner classification of [s] is a fricative-continuant.

Both vowel and consonant productions may involve the simultaneous activity of many articulators. For vowels, the tongue, velum, lips, and larynx are all in operation simultaneously and it is difficult to say that one articulator's movements are more important than another's. Certain speech sounds seem to be "multiply" articulated. For example, for the consonants [p] and [t], there can be simultaneous oral and glottal stoppages. In languages other than English the lips and tongue may form such simultaneous vocal tract stoppages. Multiple articulation is important in Arabic, for example, in contrasts such as [s] and [ṣ]. In the second, or emphaticized sound, in addition to a slit formed by the tongue tip at the alveolar ridge, the tongue dorsum moves toward the posterior pharyngeal wall, creating a narrow airway which contributes to the distinctive character of the [s] sound (see Figure 5-10(*b*)).

A Listing of Speech Sounds

A variety of symbols based on the Latin alphabet have been used to signify various speech sounds. The most commonly used system is that of the

International Phonetic Alphabet (IPA). In Table 5-1 is found a list of some commonly occurring consonant sounds. The places of articulation (see Figure 5-3) are listed across the top, and manners of articulation at the side. This list does not include all the consonants used in other languages or by speakers of English. In fact even the place and manner divisions might be better differentiated. For example, the French alveolar (apical) consonants [t], [d], and [n] are made with a more forward tongue position than their English counterparts.

Table 5-1   A table of consonants.

	Bilabial	Labio dental	Lingua- dental	Alveolar	Palatal	Velar	Glottal
Stop	p,b			t,d		k,g	
Fricative		f,v	θ, ð	s,z	∫(s), Z(z)		h
Affricate					t (c)		
Nasal	m			n		ŋ	
Liquid (lateral)				l		ɫ	
(retroflex)				r			
Semi-vowel (glide)	w				j (y)	w	

Place of Production is listed across the top columns; *Manner of Production* is listed down the rows.

The "stop" consonants, or stop-plosives as they are called, are given in the first row in Table 5-1. The voiceless stops [p, t, k] are considered to be "aspirated," and are written [pʰ], [tʰ], [kʰ] if there is a time delay between the release (opening) of the stop-closure and the onset of voicing. Often during the aspiration, there is release of a slight puff of air at the moment of release. Stop consonants are of relatively short duration, acoustically of low intensity, and involve dynamic articulator movements toward and/or away from closures. They demand relatively high intraoral air pressure and hence a tight velopharyngeal closure for successful production. Acoustically, they are characterized by swiftly changing resonance patterns as the vocal tract is rapidly opened and closed. There has been some suggestion that the changing acoustic patterns or transitions which occur during the opening or closing phases of stop consonants are the chief cue to their perception.

The fricative consonants listed in row two of Table 5-1 are created by having an articulator move to form a slit or constriction of precise dimensions. When air is forced through the slits, it picks up speed and, as it emerges, undergoes turbulent flow which causes the "hissy" noise associated with fricatives. Fricatives, or sonorant-continuants as they have been called, are quasi-static articulations which are made by having the articulators maintain the slit precisely. Certain of the fricatives are of high intensity, and all fricatives involve high intraoral breath pressure for proper production. In certain sounds not ordinarily classified as fricatives, such as the semivowel [j], or a very high vowel, fricative-like noises may be made.

The affricate class of consonants listed in row 3 can be characterized either as a combination of stop and fricative consonants, or, as a single multiply-articulated sound in which a stop-phase is gradually and smoothly opened into a gradually increasing slit from which an air stream emerges to create a fricative-like noise.

The nasal consonants are characterized by a closed oral cavity and an open velopharyngeal port through which the air and vibrations make their exit. The closed-off oral cavity acts as a side branch resonator. Nasals are characterized by a strong, well-defined, relatively intense acoustic pattern which is rather vowel-like in nature. However, in contextural speech, the rapid opening and closing of the oral cavity for the nasals leads to their being characterized in part by stop-like acoustic transitions.

The lateral consonant [l] as in "lip" is characterized by a tongue tip contact on the alveolar ridge, with openings over the sides of the tongue through which air and vibration escape to the lips. Thus the vocal tract passage through the lips is quite complex for [l], as is the tongue shape necessary for this sound. Acoustically, the [l] is rather vowel-like in character, intense, and of relatively long duration. The "dark" [l] as in "fool" vs the clear [l] in "lip," is articulated in such a way that the tongue dorsum is raised toward the velum, in addition to there being tip contact.

It is difficult to assign a manner of production to the [r] sound. There are many sounds which partake of the [r] quality although they are made differently. In the production of the [r] consonant the tongue dorsum and the tongue tip are usually elevated so that there are two points of constriction, one between tongue dorsum and soft palate, another between the retroflexed, upward curled tip and the alveolar ridge (see Figure 5-10(a)). The constrictions are not tight enough to cause friction-type noise. Some [r] type sounds demand brief or repeated (trilled) contacts between the tongue tip and hard palate.

Finally, the semivowels can be considered as high vowels which become consonantal because of additional constriction. For example [j] is in "yet" is even higher than the vowel [i], while [w] as in "witch" shows tight constriction at the lips and between tongue dorsum and soft palate.

The table of consonant sounds omits many descriptive features of sound production. When great care is taken to listen to speech sounds and record them in all of their nuances, diacritical markings are added to the symbols to indicate certain fine aspects of how the sounds are articulated. For example, if a sound such as the [l] is produced voicelessly, it is written as [l̥]. If [s] is produced with lip protrusion, it is recorded as [sʷ]. Such articulatory features as aspiration, devoicing, shortening, lengthening, nasalization, palatalization pharyngealization, etc., may be indicated by adding the appropriate diacritical marking to the phonetic symbols.

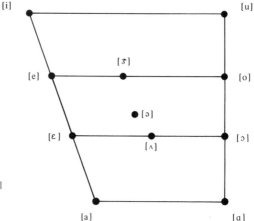

Figure 5-11 The Cardinal vowel diagram.

As stated previously, vowel sounds can be classified on tongue height, front-to-back tongue position, and lip rounding dimensions. In most languages, front unrounded and back rounded vowels are most common. In general, vowels can be described as points on a continuum, in the sense that the tongue and lips can move continuously along the three dimensions and produce a vowel sound at each point. The Cardinal Vowel System was established as a convenient way to classify vowel sounds. Figure 5-11 is a diagram of the eight Cardinal vowels. The vowel are [i] is the highest and farthest forward vowel which is made with spread lips. The cardinal vowel [a] is made with the tongue as low and to the rear as possible with spread lips. The Cardinal vowels [e], [ɛ], and [a] were chosen to be "perceptually equidistant" in such a way that the distance between any two adjacent cardinal vowels is as great as the distance between any other adjacent pair. Similarly, [ɔ, o, u] are back vowels which continue the vowel series up to the highest, most lip-protruded back vowel, [u], possible. X-ray pictures and acoustic recordings of these vowels were made. Thus, students the world over can use these standardized vowels as points of convenient reference when they analyze the vowel sounds of particular speakers. To complete the list of IPA vowel symbols, there is an [I] vowel between [i] and [e] and [æ] between [ɛ] and [a], an [ʊ] between [o] and [u]. The central vowels are [ə], [ʌ], and [ɝ].

One factor useful in classifying consonant and vowel sounds is the concept of *fortes* (tense) and *lenis* (lax). The term tense has been associated at times with the term long, and lax with short. Speaking of consonant sounds, the voiceless stops [p, t, k] have been called tense, and the voiced sounds [b, d, g] lax. A similar dichotomy holds between most other voiced/voiceless cognate sounds. In English, certain vowel pairs have been differentiated on a tense-lax basis; [i] is tense and [ɪ] lax, [u] tense and [ʊ] lax. It has been argued that when tense sounds are spoken, more energy is used in the articulatory musculature for a longer period of time so that tense productions tend to be longer in duration, involve greater air pressures, greater forces of articulator contact, and even greater precision of articulation.

Diphthongs are vowel-type sounds which have traditionally been considered to be a combination of two vowels forming one syllable. Acoustic and cineradiographic observations reveal that diphthongs can be characterized by an initial steady-state portion, a smooth transition, and a final, somewhat shorter steady-state portion (Gay, 1968). As a speaker talks more rapidly, the steady-state portions shrink, and the entire duration of the diphthong is occupied by the transitional movement of the tongue. Although diphthongs can be written as if they were combinations of two vowels, such as [aʊ] in "how," it is known that the tongue positions generally achieved during the initial and final portions of the diphthong are not exactly the tongue positions for [a] and [ʊ] taken separately. There is some evidence to support the claim that diphthongs deserve recognition as single, dynamically articulated vowel-type sounds. The following diphthongs are among those observed in English: [aʊ] as in "how," [aɪ] as in "high," [ɔɪ] as in "ahoy," [eɪ] as in "pail."

The Relationship of Phonetics to Phonemics

Phonetics involves the description and classification of speech sounds relative to a set of standardized sounds such as the Cardinal vowels, or the place/manner schemes of the IPA descriptions of consonants. *Phonology*, on the other hand, involves the study of phonemes and rules for the distribution of phonemes. *Phonemes* can be defined as abstract sound units which convey semantic differences. For example, the words "Bill, kill, sill, till, shill, fill, mill, hill, etc.," all have different meanings. Upon examination, it can be observed that the initial sounds [b, k, s, t, ʃ, f, m, h, etc.] are perceptually distinctive, that is, the speech sounds contrast with each other in such a way that the meaning of the word "ill" changes as the initial sounds change. Speech sounds which contrast with each other are placed in phonemic classes, and are called members of that phonemic class. Phoneme(s) are written in slash marks. For example, the sounds [æ], [æ̥], [æ̃], [æ:] are all speech sounds belonging to the phoneme class /æ/. The first /æ/ differs from the second which is voiceless, the third which is nasalized, and the fourth which is lengthened. Despite these real, physical-acoustic-articulatory differences, all belong to the same phonemic class because they do not change the identity of the word "sam' → /sæm/ even if articulated in these four different ways. Not all differences in sounds contribute to changes in a word's meaning. Which sound differences make a phonemic difference varies with languages. English speakers do not hear the [p] vs [pʰ] (non-aspirated vs aspirated stop) sounds as different phonemes although speakers of other languages *do!* It is a subtle and exacting task to ferret out those differences between sounds which regularly occur, and in some cases do and in other cases do not contribute to differences in word meaning.

When all speech sounds made in approximately the same way (and which do not contrast with each other in signifying the meaning of a word) are grouped together under a single phonemic classification, they are called *allophones* of a phoneme.

The process of discovering phonemes in a language demands that one determine which speech sounds contrast. In doing this linguists make use of two rules of allophonic variation: complementary distribution and free variation. To illustrate complementary distribution, suppose that the sound [k] is always produced by a palatal contact when following a high front vowel, e.g., "leak, ' and by a velar contact when following a back vowel, e.g., "Luke" (see Figure 5-12). Thus the difference in the two [k] sounds or /k/ allophones is dictated or constrained by the phonetic environment, that is by the position of the sounds or by the identity of the surrounding sounds. Thus the fronted [k̪] is an allophone of the phoneme /k/ which is in complementary distribution with the back variant of [k̪]. Speech sounds which are

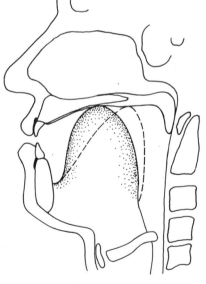

Figure 5-12 Schematic drawing of tongue position for [k] as spoken in the words "leak" and "Luke."

Different tongue positions for [k] as spoken in different words

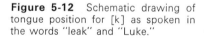

——————— [k] as spoken in "leak"

– – – – – – – [k] as spoken in "Luke"

not in complementary distribution are mutually substitutable for one another. For example, one can say the word "stop" in two ways: [stap] vs [stap^h]. That is, [p] may be nonaspirated [p] or aspirated [p^h]. Thus the [p] and [p^h] are said to be in free variation. The phonetician who seeks to establish phonemic classifications uses the above two principles. Sounds which are in free variation, which are made in dissimilar ways, and which convey a difference in meaning very often are members of differing phonemic classes.

It is theorized that when a speaker is producing speech sounds, he translates his knowledge of phonemic classes on the psychological level of competence into actual articulatory movements and acoustic vibrations which result in speech sounds or phones. The listener's task may very well be the process of reextracting the encoded phonemes from the perceived string of speech sounds.

THE ORGANIZATION OF ARTICULATION

Frequency of Occurrence of Speech Sounds

Speech sounds do not occur equally often, either in the speech of children or adults. Nor are speech sounds misarticulated equally often or learned equally soon. French et al. (1936) have shown that consonants occur nearly twice as often as vowels and diphthongs. Sounds like [n, t, r] occur very often, [a, ɔɪ, θ, dʒ] very infrequently. Miller (1951) speculated that the more frequently occurring sounds might be easier to produce and/or easier to discriminate. In defense of this, he notes that the first eight most frequently occurring written consonants of Dewey (1923) are lingua-alveolar, sounds made with the agile, easily used tongue tip.

The least frequently used consonants involve, ". . . the cooperation of the less agile articulatory muscles." The preference for lingua-alveolar consonants, says Miller is, ". . . convenient for both the listener as well as for the talker . . ." since intelligibility tests show that the principal confusions occur among sounds formed in the same manner. Consonants produced in the same place but in a different manner are seldom confused. For example, [p] is often confused with other voiceless plosives [t] and [k] (made in different places). The [p] is not often confused with the voiced plosive [b], the nasal continuant [m], or the continuant [f], all formed in the same position (but with different manners of articulation).

It has been observed that children misarticulate consonant sounds disproportionately often compared to vowels (Templin, 1957). Among the most commonly misarticulated sounds for primary school children are [s, t, l, d, θ, tʃ, dʒ, w, etc]. It may be that consonants involve more difficult articulatory maneuvers than do vowels. Since consonants are presumed to demand greater use of auditory-tactile-kinesthetic feedback for successful production, it may well be that young children have insufficiently matured feedback systems, and hence misarticulate consonants more often than vowels because the necessary feedback is deficient or inefficiently used.

The Role of Vowels and Consonants

It has been observed that consonants and vowels tend to alternate in the stream of speech sounds. Vowels involve a relatively open vocal tract excited into vibration by the larynx, while consonants involve a relatively closed vocal tract produced by certain articulator movements. Miller (1951) says, "This tendency is so marked that one is tempted to think of laryngeal and articulatory muscles (supralaryngeal) as antagonistic muscle groups."

Dudley (1940) and Öhman (1966) speculated that speech production consists fundamentally of one long vowel-like utterance. Vowels function as a relatively powerful acoustic carrier signal; they are the basic material of utterance. Take for example, the sentence, "He saw Tom," [hi sɔ tam]. The vowels involved are [i-ɔ-a]. The speaker moves his tongue and lips smoothly between one vowel position and another in diphthong-like gliding movements. The consonants in the sentence [h-s-t-m] function as sudden modulations or interruptions of the steady vowel movements. These modulations involve sudden complete or partial closures of the tract. The consonant articulations break the steady lip and tongue movements for the vowels into syllabic units which have specific rhythmic, timing, and junctural patterns. When two, three, or even four consonant sounds are mutually adjacent they are called clusters. Such clusters, from an articulatory point of view, form a single, multiply-articulated, complex consonant. The term cluster is useful insofar as the consonants do seem to merge together—that is, the articulator movements (gestures) for each consonant are subtly and smoothly integrated with those of the other consonants. Certain clusters occur in only certain word or syllable positions. For example, [ts] as in "pots" occurs only in final positions, whereas [sp] can occur initially or finally as in "speak" or "lisp."

Although tongue movements for vowels can be rapid, they are not the fast, "ballistic" movements typical of many consonantal closures such as that for /t/. MacNeilage and Scholes (1964) observed electrical activity of tongue muscle contractions during articulation and noted that, "The impression (of tongue activity) is not one of ballistic movements. . . . It is rather a complex pattern of finely graded changes in activity as a function of time, in which one or two of the muscles produce most of the movement, and others cooperate in movement, stabilize adjacent structures, or actively oppose the movement."

Articulation Targets

The stream of articulatory movements and of speech sounds during speech production is very nearly continuous and constantly changing. How to describe the steady flow of gestures is a difficult task. Certainly, listeners have little trouble in listening to the speech stream, and segmenting or cutting the stream into "phonemes," psychological-abstract sound segments. Viewed in this way, then, articulation may be considered as "a collection of articulator movements" for each speech sound. Consider an isolated [t] sound. Articulation of [t] involves a movement of the tongue tip toward the alveolar ridge, a closure, and an opening with a noise burst. Production of [t] involves open lips, a partially lowered jaw, and no voicing. Aside from the tongue tip, the remainder of the tongue is free to vary during production of [t] insofar as it does not obstruct the vocal tract. The situation can be summarized by listing the functionally "important" articulators in Table 5-2 with the articulations they perform. However, as MacNeilage (1970) says, it is difficult at times to tell which articulators are important to the production of a typical sound.

Table 5-2   Some articulators involved in /t/ articulation and the articulations performed.

	Possible articulations	*Targets*
Articulator 1	Articulation A Articulation B Articulation C	"ideal" position, contact shape, airflow, etc. Target B
Articulator 2	Articulation D Articulation E Articulation F	Target E
Articulator 3	Articulation G Articulation H	Target H
etc.	Articulations –, –, –	
	Choose one articulation per articulator, or more, if multiple articulations are not contradictory	All three or more targets are achieved simultaneously or in some defined pattern

The list of important articulators in Table 5-2 is a static one; to make a satisfactory [t], the tongue tip must make a gesture, i.e., move in, make contact, and release contact.

The only fixed position or "target" which can be talked about is that closure must be made and held for a short period of time. A more complete description of [t] articulation might include the dynamic movement of the tip toward and away from closure including speed and force of contact. When the tongue tip makes contact for [t], all other tip gestures such as making a slit, depressing or rolling upwards are contradictory, impermissible. The vocal folds must not vibrate during approach to [t] closure, or during and slightly after closure. The lips must be open, but how far open is not crucial. That is, the lips are given a "neutral," unassigned value or position for [t] production. The mandible may be a "secondary" articulator for [t] in that it can assume any number of positions (neutral specification); only full closure is prohibited. The dorsum of the tongue is more interesting to consider. A satisfactory [t] can be articulated with the tongue dorsum high or low, and forward or in the middle of the oral cavity, but not when very far back in the mouth, nor must there be a closure other than at the tip. The tongue is relatively free to vary its position, as is the mandible and to some degree the lips, hence the label secondary articulator-articulations. The vocal folds and tongue tip have very precise tasks and, unless executed properly, the [t] production is unsatisfactory. Also a part of the articulation is the necessity for the closure to be made with a particular speed, for the air pressure to build up at a particular rate so that a noise burst is produced when the closure opens, and for the force of tip contact to be sufficient. From this discussion, the reader should deduce that some articulations are relatively fixed in nature, while other articulations have more freedom to vary. Equally necessary is the need to view all articulations as dynamic. Even if the tongue tip ceases movement after contacting the alveolar ridge, the muscles of the tip continue to contract, holding it there while necessary air pressure is built up for the stop explosion.

Speech articulations seem to have targets, ideal places of contact, forces of contact, particular shapes, particular airflows, and particular patterns of movement necessary for a given speech sound. Targets can be defined as those final, ideal values of position, shape, etc., achieved when the speech sound is spoken in isolation, slowly, and in a prolonged fashion. Alternatively, the speech sound could be spoken carefully in a "neutral" environment. The above definitions of target are artificial because speakers do not usually produce isolated, sustained sounds. Perhaps targets should be redefined as those positions and shapes, etc., achieved during conversational speech.

The danger in this is that although "targets" may be convenient for describing an articulation, they may not be the way articulation is controlled or organized. At any rate, suppose that the view of articulation as a succession of targets to be achieved is valid. Then, the vocal tract contains a collection of movable articulators, such as vocal folds, larynx, mandible, lips, tongue root, tongue blade, tongue tip, velum, upper pharynx, lower pharynx, etc. Each articulator can perform a number of articulations, e.g., the tongue root and blade together can move up and down, forward and backward, and the lips may protrude, retract, or rest in a neutral position, and open or close. The tongue tip can retroflex (curl upward) to make contact in a number of places, form a slit, or be depressed downward. Some articulators can perform only one articulation at a time; the tongue tip cannot make a contact and slit simultaneously. Some articulators can perform more than one gesture at a time—the tongue body can move forward and upward simultaneously, and the lips can retract and open simultaneously. Some targets may be "stronger" or more necessary than others. An [u] sound can be made with immobile lips, and with an immovable jaw but it cannot be made without moving the tongue high and backwards in the oral cavity.

A description of articulation would demand specification of:

(1) Every structure which can perform articulations.
(2) Every articulation which an articulator can perform.
(3) Which articulations cannot be performed simultaneously, that is, which "contradict" each other.

If articulatory targets can be called articulatory features, then speech sounds are collections of features, e. g.:

Speech sound, [t]

	Articulatory features	Voiceless
		Open lips
		Velopharyngeal port
		    closed
		High intraoral
		    pressure
		Tongue tip elevation, etc.

Targets		

Allophonic Variation

It is a truism to say that individual productions of a given speech sound vary both randomly and systematically. Speech articulation is motor behavior involving coordinated, rhythmical sets of muscular movements produced at a variable rate and rhythm. The way any two speakers produce a sound is different because of differences in articulator structures and motor coordination. Successive articulations of a sound by the same speaker result in variations in the speech sounds because conditions are never the same twice. Another factor influencing variations is that speech sounds occur and are articulated in different linguistic, phonetic, social, psychological, and emotional environments. Variations in these environments and of the physiological status of the speaker are responsible for those changes in articulation which produce allophonic "variants" of a given phoneme. Listeners and phoneticians seem capable of chopping the speech stream into separate, independent, nonvarying phonemes. However, it is very difficult to observe anything like an invariant phonemic pattern in either the muscle contractions, discharges, the articulatory movements, or in the speech acoustic wave (Liberman et al., 1967). Consider, for example, the two allophones of /1/, the clear [l] in "light" and dark [ł] in "pull." The two allophones which are in complementary distribution sound very different, but both are classified as an /1/ phoneme. There is some controversy as to whether or not listeners store a mental image of the phoneme as an idealized perception, or whether they store the major allophones of the phoneme and try to match their perceptions to them (Wickelgren, 1969). The same holds for the articulation process. Do speakers store rules for producing the major allophones and deliberately articulate them? Or, do speakers have rules only for an idealized phoneme, the production of allophones occurring because of contextual differences?

Phonetic Context as
a Source of Allophonic Variation

There are numerous phonetic contexts (or environments) which cause speech sounds to vary allophonically in a known way. For example, vowels are longer or shorter, and have greater or lesser intensity depending on whether the consonants around them are stops or fricatives, voiced or voiceless. In English sentence or phrase-final positions, stops like [p] in "Hit the top" are rarely aspirated; the closure is formed, but is not released with a noise burst. Aspirated stops are expected medially and initially, and when followed by a vowel.

A classic example of allophonic variation occurs when a voiceless stop like [t, p, k] occurs in the [s-V] (V = vowel) context. When it does, the [p] in "spit" [spɪt] sounds like a [b]. If the [s] is spliced or cut away from tape recordings of "spit," the remaining [pɪt] segment sounds like [bɪt]. The intended [p] is heard as [b] because the voiceless fricative-vowel environment alters the closure duration and voicing onset time for the vowel. Different sounds occurring before or after a given sound will often cause predictable variations in that sound. These variations often occur because articulators have past "histories." In the sequence *ABC* or *CBA*, articulators must move from target positions at *A* to those of *B* and then *C*. In the other case, they move from *C* to *B* to *A*. The two paths are different, little wonder that *B* in these two environments exists as two allophones, when the movements toward *B* closure and away from it are so very different. An example of this occurs when [it] and [ɔt] are spoken. Tongue tip movement from the low back position of [ɔ] vs the high front position of [i] involves a different path, a

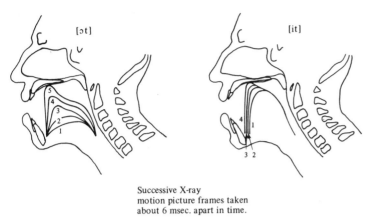

Successive X-ray
motion picture frames taken
about 6 msec. apart in time.

Figure 5-13 Tongue movement toward [t] contact in two phonetic environments.

different distance, a different amount of time. The tongue tip travels only a small distance from [i] to [t] closure. Notice also that the shape of the tongue during [t] contact is different in both cases (Figure 5-13). To reemphasize, articulation processes consist of more than movements and vocal tract shapes. Articulation involves articulator speeds, forces of contact, air flows and pressures, and timing and rhythm of movements. Such factors vary widely when a speech sound is placed into different environments.

*Coarticulation as
a Source of Allophonic Variation*

Coarticulation (or assimilation as it is sometimes called) is a major source of allophonic variation. It is that process which occurs when two or more speech sounds overlap in such a way that their articulatory gestures intermingle, i.e., occur simultaneously. Take for example the nonsense words [tiku] and [tuki]. In one case the vowel sequence is [i-u] front to back, and in the other [u-i], back to front. If speech production consists of one long vowel utterance which is slurred from vowel to vowel, then tongue positions will shift from front to back and vice versa as the two words are spoken. This means that even as the [k] is being articulated via tongue dorsum contact with the palate, the tongue root will be moving toward the following vowel position. The simultaneous presence of the moving tongue root (a vowel gesture) and the consonantal contact gesture is coarticulation. The new result of this coarticulation is an allophonically varied [k] production.

X-ray films of a speaker producing the two words are schematized in Figure 5-14. For [tuki] the tongue starts in the [u] position, and all the while

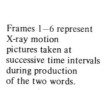

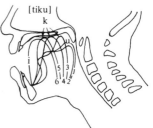

Figure 5-14   Tracing of successive tongue shapes during the production of [tuki] and [tiku].

Frames 1–6 represent X-ray motion pictures taken at successive time intervals during production of the two words.

it moves upward toward [k] contact, it also moves forward in anticipation of [i]. While [k] contact is made, the tongue root moves, sliding the [k] contact forward toward [i] position. For [tiku], the opposite occurs; the tongue moves backward toward [u] even while [k] is being articulated. This overlap of articulatory gestures occurs because the backward tongue root movement does not conflict with (contradict) the upward tongue dorsum movement toward [k] closure. Data like these led Öhman (1966) to suggest that the tongue consists of three articulators which, though physically connected, can act semi-independently of one another.

The above results demonstrate that the target for [k] contact does not specify a very strict tongue placement. Rather, tongue contact at any of a number of points along the hard palate produces a satisfactory [k]. Because tongue contact position for [k] varies widely, the tongue root may coarticulate by moving in the direction demanded by the surrounding phonemes. To illustrate the extent to which phonemic context affects a phoneme production, observe the position of [k] contact in the symmetrical [i-i] and [u-u] environments of Figure 5-15. The two points of tongue contact on the palate are separated by as much as $1\frac{1}{2}$ cm. Obviously, the two [k]'s are different allophones. They are articulated in different places, and on careful listening, sound different.

The study of coarticulation phenomena has led some observers to speculate that the basic unit of speech production is larger than the phoneme. If an articulatory gesture appropriate to one sound segment is spread over several adjacent sounds, perhaps the production unit is a group of sounds, syllabic in size.

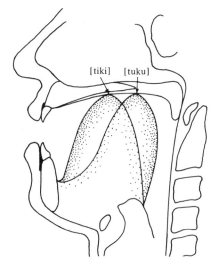

[tiki]   [tuku]

Figure 5-15 Differences in position of [k] contact in an [i-i] and an [u-u] environment.

Mechano-Inertial Timing
Sources of Coarticulation

Each of the articulators is of different size and mass, from the relatively small tongue tip to the more massive tongue body and mandible. The tongue and mandible are required to move quickly during speech, therefore large muscular forces must act upon them. Each articulator contains a particular amount of mass, and therefore shows inertial properties. Articulators resist attempts to start moving when muscle force is suddenly applied, and they resist slowing down or stopping when the accelerating force is removed. This means that there is a time delay between arrival of motor commands at the muscles and the time when the articulators begin to move. The more massive the articulator the longer the delay. The inertial properties account for time delays (in starting or stopping movement) built into articulation. Stevens and House (1963) have discussed the effects which various mechano-inertial factors have upon articulator movements. They point out that rate of articulation is an important factor in determining the extent of coarticulation.

If motor commands for the sounds in a word occur very rapidly, the commands may overlap, or the commands for one sound may reach an articulator while the articulator is still attempting to achieve target values for a previous articulation. Because of the articulator inertia and possible overlapping of neural commands to an articulator at fast rates of production, an articulator cannot move instantly from one position to another. As a result, the articulator movements and positions and vocal tract shapes at any one time may reflect the influence of instructions from two or more sounds. Note in Figure 5-16 that the commands for sound two arrive at a time when the articulators are still approaching target for sound one. Shortly after commands for sound two arrive, the vocal tract shape and articulator positions reflect the presence of commands for both sounds; thus, the vocal tract shape is co-articulated. This means that when any two speech sounds are immediate neighbors when spoken, there will usually be simple structural, inertial, and rate induced coarticulatory overlap between them and resulting allophonic variation of both. Another example occurs in the word "runs" [rʌnz]. When spoken quickly, the velum opens for [n], and is still open and attempting to close when the tongue is already in position for [z], thus coarticulation of "nasality" occurs within the [z̃].

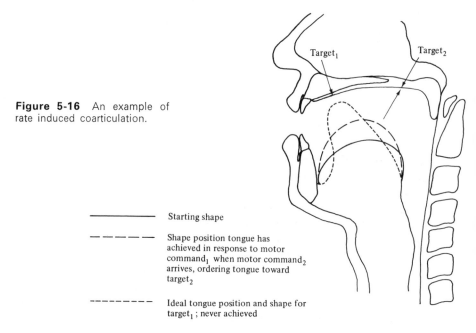

Figure 5-16   An example of rate induced coarticulation.

—————— Starting shape

— — — — Shape position tongue has achieved in response to motor command$_1$ when motor command$_2$ arrives, ordering tongue toward target$_2$

– – – – – – Ideal tongue position and shape for target$_1$; never achieved

Neurally-Programmed Coarticulation

Notice, in Figure 5-13, the shape of the tongue during [t] contact for the VC syllables [ɔt] and [it]. The tongue shape, except for the tip, looks like that for the preceding vowel. Therefore, what has already been articulated and is past (the vowel) affects the later production of [t]. This is so-called left to right coarticulation. It commonly results from structural, rate, and inertial effects. There are, however, right to left coarticulation effects which seem to be caused by the structure of the articulatory code in the brain.

As an example of right to left coarticulation, Fujimura (1961) observed that during the articulation of /CV/ type words, the tongue was moving into position for /V/ even when the jaw prepared to elevate for /C/. Amerman et al. (1969) observed that when speaking sequences such as $[C_1 C_2$ æ], the jaw began lowering for the low vowel [æ] during the movements of lips and tongue toward the closure for Consonant$_1$. In these two cases and in countless others, what is observed is that when given the chance, articulator movements are often initiated far in advance of the sound in which they are crucial (anticipatory positioning). This is the so-called right-to-left coarticulation.

Kozhevnikov and Chistovich (1965) noted that a speech articulator gesture will coarticulate as long as it is not contradictory in $[C_1 C_2 V]$ type syllables. For example, let us examine the syllable [nsu] from the word, "monsoon.' During the production of [n] and [s], the lips are not especially involved; thus they can be protruded without preventing satisfactory [n] and [s] production. Hence there is a neutral (0) articulatory value for these two sounds.

Speech Gesture: Lip Protrusion

n	s	u
0	0	+

0 = Neutral, unspecified with respect to lip protrusion
+ = Lip protruded
− = Lip retracted

But the lips are generally protruded for [u], hence the specified or (+) value. What seems to occur during production of the [nsu] or [CCV] syllable, is that the lips are being protruded as far in advance of [u] as is physically practical. As long as the protrusion gesture is neutral or noncontradictory, lip protrusion for [u] can be initiated. If, however, one of the consonants had lip retraction as an articulatory feature or gesture, then the lip protrusion and retraction would be contradictory because lips could not do both simultaneously. In this case lip protrusion coarticulation would be inhibited; lip protrusion could not start until the contradictory gesture was finished.

At this point, it is useful to ask why "anticipatory" right-to-left coarticulation occurs. Cooper (1966) noted that speakers can easily produce 12–18 sounds/second during conversation, a fast rate indeed. If each sound were produced separately, speakers would have to turn the speech musculature on/off once for each sound—twelve to eighteen times per second. This is an impossibly high rate—a finger can't be tapped that fast. Listening to speech produced in such an on/off manner would be difficult; instead of a smooth flow of sounds, listeners would hear interrupted, abrupt, buzz-like sequences of sounds. The fastest moving controllable articulator, the tongue tip, will, at maximum, perform only eight or more closures per second. The essence of speech production is that it is easy, smooth, flowing, and unforced. The articulators are relatively independent of each other i. e., the velum can rise independently of the jaw, and the lips can open without influencing the tongue. Thus, Cooper proposed that the speech articulators can be controlled semi-independently of each other i. e., they can operate in "parallel."

As a useful analogy, imagine each articulator as a light bulb on a Christmas tree. When lights are in parallel, some lights can be on, some off, at the same time. The lights can function together or separately. In the same way, the speech articulators probably function in a parallel fashion. Articulators are free to move at their preferred rates of movement from target to target.

Consider the succession of targets which the tongue tip achieves during production of the word "[strɪp]" illustrated in Figure 5-17. The tip moves first to a slit for [s], a contact for [t], then an apical position for [r], a neutral position for [ɪ], and to a neutral position for [p]. The articulating tip moves smoothly, rhythmically, and at its own rate between each of these targets. Examination of the movement pattern shows that it consists of a series of glides toward and away from each target to the next.

Figure 5-17 A schematic diagram showing articulator movement between successive target positions for the sequences [strɪp] and [stu].

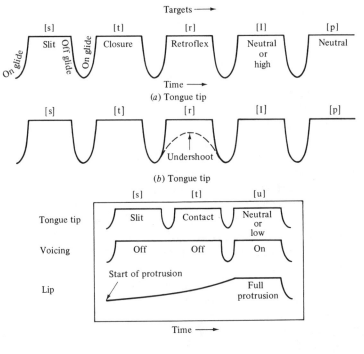

If rate of articulation is particularly fast, the articulator may never reach target (it undershoots it) because the articulatory gesture is interrupted by a neural command ordering it to smoothly progress toward the next target position. Therefore before the tongue tip can reach the [r] apical target, it is ordered on to [ɪ] target position. The early, anticipatory start of an articulatory gesture may occur because it is easier to take a longer time, moving more slowly, to reach target than to move quickly and abruptly. The result is that lip protrusion gesture occurs over two phonemes in advance of [u] in "[stu]." Such coarticulation eases the work load of the articulatory system. Lower speeds of movement mean less strain.

Another example of right-left anticipatory coarticulation was observed by Moll and Daniloff (1971). They hypothesized that the velum performs a single articulation—velar closure/opening. What they observed seemed to be three degrees of closure:

(1) Open (−) for nasal consonants [n, m, ŋ].
(2) Neutral (just barely closed) (0) for vowels.
(3) Closed tightly (+) for stops, fricative consonants, etc.

Take, for example, the words "free Ontario" in which the sequence [fri + an] occurs, [CCVVN], where N = nasal. The velum articulations are:

			a	n
(+)	(+)	(0)	(0)	(−)

As soon as the velum moves toward target for the vowel [i], which has a neutral velar position, it is free to begin lowering in anticipation of the open (−), non-neutral position for the nasal consonant. This happened for every sequence examined. With sequences like [sn], the velum could not begin to lower for [n], or coarticulate, until the [s] was complete. This is apparent because [s] production demands tight velopharyngeal closure.

AFTERTHOUGHTS

Speakers and writers of a language implicitly recognize the continuous nature of language production despite the segmentations into letters or phonemes which are forced upon it. In its written form, periods, commas, semicolons, colons, exclamation marks, question marks, quotes, etc., are placed within and around sentences to indicate the prosodic and flowing nature of speech along with its natural pauses. Phonemes as abstract or psychological "elements" of the language code are useful because they represent the minimum units of sound differences. But speech may be perceived and encoded in larger units. Perhaps when a child hears "ba" and "pa" he distinguishes the entire syllable to be different in the two. Language units of different sizes may be used during speaking (encoding) and listening (decoding). Articulation processes run together and overlap the phoneme-sized units so that the phonemes are allophonically varied and changeable. From this shifting, continuous stream, listeners can decode speech and extract the phoneme units, even though it is difficult to observe independent, nonoverlapping sounds in the speech acoustic wave (Liberman et al., 1967). It is this seeming divergence between production and perception (Kozhevnikov and Chistovich, 1965) and between larger, perhaps syllable-sized, production units and smaller perceptual ones, which puzzles students of articulation.

Thus, much future work in phonetics and articulation will be aimed at solving the problem of how allophonic variations occur, how they are perceived, and how they are neurally programmed. It is, at this time, difficult to explain how speech sounds, which by their nature are separate and independent events, are serially ordered into a continuous, overlapped stream of movements and sounds.

REFERENCES

AMERMAN, J. D., DANILOFF, R. G. and MOLL, K. L. 1970. Lip and jaw coarticulation for the phoneme /æ/. *J. Speech Hear. Research* 13 : 147–61.

COOPER, F. S. 1966. Describing the speech process in motor command terms. Status Report on Speech Research SR-516. Haskins Laboratories.

DEWEY, G. 1923. *Relative Frequency of English Speech Sounds.* Cambridge, Mass: Harvard Univ. Press.

DUDLEY, H. 1940. The carrier nature of speech. *Bell Syst. Tech. J.* 19: 495–515.

FRENCH, N. R., CARTER, C. W. and KOENIG, W. 1930. The words and sounds of telephone conversations. *Bell Syst. Tech. J.* 9: 290–324.

FRITZELL, B. 1969. The velopharyngeal muscles in speech: An electromyographic and cineradiographic study. *Acta Oto.* Suppl. 250.

FUJIMURA, O. 1961. Effects of vowel context on the articulation of stop consonants. Paper read at the program of the 61st meeting of the Acous. Soc. Amer.

GAY, T. 1968. Effect of speaking rate on diphthong formant movements. *J. Acoust. Soc. Amer.* 44: 1570–73.

HUDGINS, C. V. and STETSON, R. H. 1937. Relative speed of articulatory movements. *Arch. Neerl. Phon. Exper.* 13: 85–94.

HUNTINGTON, D. A., HARRIS, K. and SCHOLES, G. 1968. An electromyographic study of consonant articulation in hearing impaired and normal speakers. *J. Speech Hear. Research* 11: 147–58.

KAISER, L. 1934. Some properties of the speech muscles and the influence thereof on language. *Arch. Neerl. Phon. Exper.* 10: 121–33.

KELSEY, C. A., MINIFIE, F. D. and HIXON., T. J. 1969. Applications of Ultrasound in Speech Research. *J. Speech Hear. Research* 12: 564–75.

KOZHEVNIKOV, V. A. and CHISTOVICH, L. 1965. *Rech: Artikulyatsia i Vospriyatiye.* [transl. *Speech: Articulation and Perception.*] Moscow-Leningrad: Nauka. [Transl. by U.S. Dept. of Commerce, Joint Publications Research Service (JPRS)] Washington, D.C. No. 30, p. 543.

LIBERMAN, A. M., COOPER, F. S., SHANKWEILER, D. P. and STUDDERT-KENNEDY, M. G. 1967. Perception of the Speech Code. *Psychol. Rev.* 74: 431–61.

LIEBERMAN, P. C., KLATT, D., and WILSON, W. A. 1969. Vocal tract limitations on the vowel repertoires of Rhesus monkey and other non-human primates. *Science* 164: 1185–88.

MACNEILAGE, P. F. 1970. The motor control of serial ordering of speech. *Psychol. Rev.* 77: 182–96.

MACNEILAGE, P. F., ROOTES, T. P. and CHASE, R. A. 1967. Speech production and perception in a patient with severe impairment of somesthetic perception and motor control. *J. Speech Hear. Research* 10: 449–67.

MACNEILAGE, P. F. and SCHOLES, G. N. 1964. An electromyographic study of the tongue during vowel production. *J. Speech Hear. Research* 7: 209–32.

MILLER, G. A 1951. Speech and Language. *In* S. S. Stevens (ed.) *Handbook of Experimental Psychology.* New York: John Wiley & Sons, Inc.

MOLL, K. L. and DANILOFF, R. G. 1971. An investigation of the timing of velar movements during speech. *J. Acoust. Soc. Amer.* 50: 678–84.

ÖHMAN, S. E. G. 1966. Coarticulation in VCV utterances: Spectrographic measurements. *J. Acoust. Soc. Amer.* 39: 151–68.

SHANKWEILER, D. P. and HARRIS. K. 1966. An experimental approach to the problem of articulation in aphasia. *Cortex* (II): 277–92.

SHRINER. T. H., HOLLOWAY, M. S. and DANILOFF, R. G. 1969. The relationship between phonological errors and syntax in speech defective children. *J. Speech Hear. Research* 12: 319–25.

STEVENS, K. N. and HOUSE, A. S. 1963. Perturbation of vowel articulation by consonantal context: An acoustical study. *J. Speech Hear. Research* 6: 111–28.

TEMPLIN, M. E. 1957. Certain Language Skills in Children. Institute of Child Welfare Monograph Series. Minneapolis: Univ. Minnesota Press. No 5.

WEINER, P. S. 1967. Auditory discrimination and articulation. *J. Speech Hear. Dis.* 32: 19–28.

WICKELGREN, W. A. 1969. Auditory or articulatory coding in verbal short-term memory. *Psychol. Rev.* 76: 232–35.

WILLIS, C. R. and STUTZ, M. L. 1969. Patterns of velopharyngeal closure in normal subjects. Paper read at Amer. Speech Hear. Assoc. Convention, Chicago, Ill.

ZEMLIN, W. R. 1968. *Speech and Hearing Science: Anatomy and Physiology.* New Jersey: Englewood Cliffs, Prentice-Hall Inc.

6

SPEECH PHYSIOLOGY

Ronald Netsell

INTRODUCTION

The preceding three chapters have described the functioning of three subdivisions of the speech producing apparatus: the respiratory pump, the
laryngeal valve, and the upper airway system. Although conceptual partitioning of the apparatus is helpful in appreciating some of the intricacies of these
respective subdivisions, it is misleading to view any one of them as functioning independently of any other. Indeed, it is the concerted activity
of many body parts distributed throughout the torso, neck, and head that is
responsible for the movement patterns which produce the acoustic events of
speech. This chapter has two goals with respect to understanding the physiology of speech: to provide (1) a conceptual framework from which to
appreciate various physiological events, and (2) descriptions of the major
physiological mechanisms underlying the production of speech.

A CONCEPTUAL FRAMEWORK

In developing a framework from which to appreciate speech production, it will be helpful to delineate: (1) conceptual levels of the production process, (2) functional components of the production apparatus, and (3) muscular and nonmuscular forces that operate on the various components of the apparatus.

Levels of the Speech Production Process

The speech production process can be thought of as a chain of events originating in the brain and ending in the formation of an acoustic signal. It is possible to divide this process into the five conceptual levels represented by the large blocks in Figure 6-1. Arrows that connect the blocks from the top of the figure downward indicate the sequencing of this production process. Level (*a*) represents the central nervous system (CNS) organization that is necessary to produce speech; that is, the neural result of linguistic processes. Moving downward, Level (*b*) depicts the nerve impulses that travel the various pathways to the muscles. The combination of muscular events and resultant structural movements are reflected in the block at Level (*c*). While muscular events and structural movements might be thought of as separate levels, they are lumped here, since they are inseparable in cases where the structure being moved is mainly muscle (e. g., the tongue, velum, or lips). In terms of

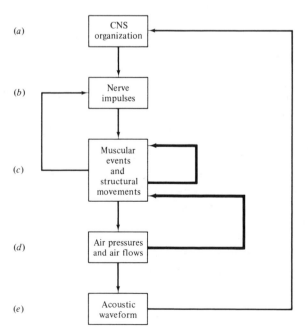

(*a*)

(*b*)

(*c*)

(*d*)

(*e*)

Figure 6-1 A block diagram of five conceptual levels of the speech production process. (See text for explanation.)

muscular forces, the innervation of as many as 100 muscles results in the movements of the speech structures (viz., muscle, bone, and cartilage). Level (d) emphasizes the fact that the air pressure and air flow events associated with speech are the direct result of the structural movements. Finally, the *acoustic waveform* level represents the acoustic result of the interactions between the (1) air pressure-air flow events, and (2) size and shape of the vocal tract.

Several lines are shown to connect various blocks of the diagram. In deference to the probable differences between the maturing and fully developed neuromuscular systems (Hardy, 1970), the following speculations about these connecting lines apply to the fully developed production apparatus of the normal speaker. The thick solid lines refer to clearly established influences, and the thin solid lines to probable influences. It should be stressed that all of these lines do not represent *feedback* (i.e., the return of information in neural form to some higher level of the process). And even in the feedback cases, it is not implied that the motor activity is necessarily modified by the returning information.

The thin solid line moving from the acoustic waveform level to the CNS organization level suggests that the disruption of speech output by electronically delaying the return of the acoustic signal to the speaker's ears (*delayed auditory feedback*) is probably initiated by disturbing the CNS organization of the time program for speech production. The line of influence moving from the air pressure-air flow block back to the muscular events and structural movements block is shown as a thick solid line. This boldness is to indicate that the interaction is definitely established, as evidenced most obviously by the Bernoulli effect (sucking force) in the vocal fold region. Recall that once the lateral edges of the vocal folds are sufficiently approximated, they are quickly sucked together by the air rushing past them. It is not known if air pressures commonly recorded in the vocal tract during speech are large enough to passively move such large structures as the tongue. The line of influence within the muscular events and structural movements block simply represents the passive influence that the movement of one speech structure may have on another. An obvious example is the influence that jaw position in speech has on the degree of lip opening simply due to the attachment of the lower lip musculature to the jaw. The final interconnecting line suggests that the muscular events and structural movements might influence the nature of nerve impulses along the peripheral nerves. The question as to whether or not these returning impulses effect major influences on the motor control for speech remains largely unanswered. However, recent data implicate the muscle spindle system as a necessary feedback mechanism for normal sensorimotor control of the speech movements (Abbs, 1971). More will be said about this system in a following section.

Functional Components of the Speech Apparatus

We stated earlier that the speech producing apparatus is often divided into respiratory, laryngeal, and upper airway parts. Unfortunately, this division does not emphasize the working of these parts as a whole. In order to view the numerous parts of the speech apparatus as constituting a single mechanism, consider Figure 6-2. Figure 6-2 is a mid-sagittal line drawing of the chest, head, and neck with numbers referring to the approximate location of nine functional components. A component in this context is defined as a structure or combination of structures working to generate or value the speech air stream. Component 1 includes the abdomen and diaphragm. Component 2 is made up of the rib cage and its muscles. Component 3 consists of all the structures involved in the speech operations of the larynx while Component 4 is defined as the muscles of the mid-lower pharynx and posterior aspect of the tongue that shape and valve the pharyngeal cavity. Component 5 consists of the muscles of the velopharyngeal valve. Components 6 and 7 involve the muscles that regulate the movements of the middle and anterior aspects of the tongue, respectively. Component 8 is defined by the jaw and the muscles that move it during speech. Finally, component 9 contains all the facial muscles that are responsible for lip rounding, spreading, opening, and closing. In a sense, all we have done to this point is to divide the apparatus into nine components as opposed to three. To illustrate the value of the nine part segmentation, we'll briefly outline the role of these components in developing the air pressure-air flow patterns of speech. As we will see in a subsequent section of this chapter, these pressure-flow patterns reflect a great deal about the various structural movements used in speech.

The speech apparatus can be thought of as a large air container that is always closed on the bottom end (by the lungs). The only two openings to the atmosphere on the container are the nostrils and mouth. However, within the container there are several valves that can be opened or closed to various degrees, thus changing the shape of the container. These valving actions are performed by components 3 through 9 as represented in Figure 6-2. As we saw in Chapter 3, the basic role of components 1 and 2 is to actively regulate pressure inside the lungs. Through the actions of components 1 and 2, the air pressure build-up in the lungs effectively pushes an air column up and out of the container. The rate at which, and openings through which, the air escapes from the pressurized container is regulated to a great extent by the coordination of movement in components 3–9. The respiratory system is very much responsible for the rather constant driving pressure (subglottal air pressure, P_s) recorded in the lungs.[1] The effect of the coordinated move-

---

[1] As pointed out in Chapter 3, certain respiratory muscles also execute brief contractions to add pulse-like increases to P_s for stressed or emphasized sound segments. More will be said about this later in this chapter.

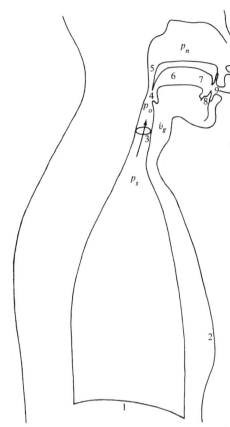

Components
1. Abdomen-diaphragm
2. Rib cage
3. Larynx
4. Tongue-pharynx
5. Velopharynx
6. Tongue (middle)
7. Tongue (anterior)
8. Jaw
9. Lips

Figure 6-2 A mid-sagittal line drawing of the vocal tract showing the location of nine functional components (see text) and points where air pressures and air flows are typically recorded. The pressures include those recorded in the nasal tract (P_n), oral tract (P_o), subglottal region (P_s), and atmosphere (P_{atm}). The volume velocities of air flow that are of interest include those crossing the glottis ($\dot{V}_g$) and those leaving the nasal and oral tracts ($\dot{V}_n$ and $\dot{V}_o$, respectively).

ments of these nine functional components is to create a series of rapidly changing air pressures and air flows at various points along the vocal tract. In addition to the subglottal air pressure (P_s), the values of air pressure in the nasal cavity (P_n) and behind the smallest opening in the oral cavity (P_o) are requisite to understanding the aerodynamics of speech. P_{atm} refers to atmospheric pressure. The rate at which air flows ($\dot{V}$) through any of these valves is determined by the resistance to flow offered by the valve and the magnitude of the pressure drop (ΔP) across the valve. Thus, the rate of air flow through the glottis ($\dot{V}_g$) is determined by the resistance of the glottal chink and the pressure drop across the glottis (P_s–P_o). Air flow through the nasal channel ($\dot{V}_n$), in turn, is regulated by the combined series resistance of the (1) velopharynx, nasal cavities, and nares, and (2) associated pressure drop (P_o–P_{atm}). Finally, air flow through the oral channel ($\dot{V}_o$) is a function of the resistance (as formed by the channel which is bounded by the tongue, teeth, and lips) and pressure drop across these structures (P_o–P_{atm}).

In summary, the speech apparatus can be viewed as a series of component parts that generate and valve the speech air stream. The position of the components at any point in time determines the size and shape of the vocal tract and, thereby, influences the magnitudes of air pressures and flows in the tract. The acoustic consequences of the physiological pressure-flow interactions with the size and shape of the vocal tract are the subject of Chapter 7.

Muscular and Nonmuscular Forces

The third part of this conceptual framework involves the consideration of muscular and nonmuscular forces in speech production. Both muscular and nonmuscular forces are responsible for the movement of any one of the nine functional components depicted in Figure 6-2. Recently there has been a host of studies attempting to establish the nature of central nervous system (CNS) events from the analysis of peripheral activity. This strategy is represented schematically in Figure 6-3. Moving from left to right, we see the input of neural signals to our machine (the speech apparatus) with the output being the movements of the various structures. There are at least two basic reasons why such CNS interpretations of peripheral events are confounded: (1) the presence of the speech apparatus with its inherent response characteristics, and (2) the probable influences of output feedback on the nature of the controlling neural inputs. In other words, the movements themselves are not direct reflections of the neural events because of the contributions of both muscular and nonmuscular forces to the movements.

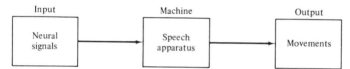

Figure 6-3 A block diagram depicting the sequence of events from neural signals to movements of the speech structures. The middle block represents the various muscle, bone, and cartilage parts that make up the speech apparatus.

Muscular forces

The term *muscular force* is used here in reference to the strength of contraction developed within the muscle. The strength of contraction, or muscular force, developed within a muscle is influenced basically by two factors: (1) the magnitude of the applied neural signal, and (2) the length of the muscle at the moment the neural signal is applied. For a given neural input, muscles develop a maximum force when at resting length or somewhat shorter (Wilke, 1956). That is, a muscle stretched beyond its resting length will not

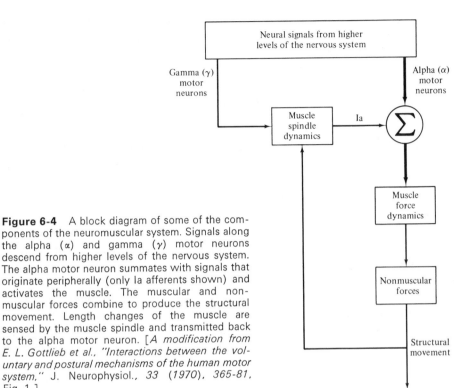

Figure 6-4 A block diagram of some of the components of the neuromuscular system. Signals along the alpha (α) and gamma (γ) motor neurons descend from higher levels of the nervous system. The alpha motor neuron summates with signals that originate peripherally (only Ia afferents shown) and activates the muscle. The muscular and nonmuscular forces combine to produce the structural movement. Length changes of the muscle are sensed by the muscle spindle and transmitted back to the alpha motor neuron. [*A modification from E. L. Gottlieb et al., "Interactions between the voluntary and postural mechanisms of the human motor system,"* J. Neurophysiol., *33* (1970), 365-81, Fig. 1.]

develop as much force when excited by the same neural signal as will a muscle at resting length. The movements of many speech structures are realized by varying the strength of contraction in antagonistic muscles.[2] Examples of this are seen in the *palatolevator* muscle versus *palatoglossus* muscle actions that determine velar movements, and *orbicularis oris* muscle versus *quadratus labii inferior* muscle actions in closing and opening the lips for bilabial consonants. In these cases, the muscular force, or strength of contraction, of the prime mover(s) is only minimally opposed by its antagonist counterpart(s).

Even though some very fundamental operations of nerve and muscle in simple motor acts are not fully understood, it is possible to speculate about some neuromuscular events that may underly speech production. Figure 6-4 shows a representation of the nervous system signals, viz., alpha (α) and gamma (γ) motor neuron impulses that originate in the higher nervous centers

[2] The muscle that contracts to move the structure along a given path is called the prime mover, or *agonist*, while those in opposition to that movement are called *antagonists*. Muscles working with the prime mover are called *synergists*. To reverse the direction of the movement, the muscles involved simply reverse roles with the former becoming the antagonist and the latter becoming the prime mover.

and impinge on the muscles. Cortical representations of both the alpha and gamma system do exist (Mortimer and Akert, 1961). Therefore, it may be that as the child learns to produce speech the alpha-gamma central control system generates a set of neural events that cannot be functionally ascribed to either the alpha or gamma motor neurons. Neural signals that arise in response to structural movements are represented by the gamma signal (Ia) leaving the muscle spindle and returning to impinge on the alpha motor neuron.[3] This arrangement suggests that gamma motor neurons can modify the alpha signals at the periphery due to movement-induced impulses coming from the muscle spindles. Thus, it is conceivable that the gamma system has a dual role in speech production: (1) as part of the alpha-gamma central control signals, and (2) as part of a peripheral feedback mechanism.

Nonmuscular forces

The nonmuscular forces that contribute to the movement of the various speech structures can be grouped into four categories: (1) physical properties, (2) mechanical restraints, (3) aerodynamic influences, and (4) gravity.

Each of the speech structures has its own inherent physical properties. Mass and elasticity are probably the most obvious. Their contribution as a nonmuscular force is acutely evident in vocal fold vibration. The elasticity of the folds contributes to their restorative closing forces that are necessary to maintain the oscillations. Their effective vibrating mass determines, in part, the fundamental frequency of fold vibration (Hollien and Curtis, 1960).

An example of mechanical restraint occurs when the position of one structure presents a restraining force to the movement of another structure because of their anatomical connections. Due to the numerous attachments (muscle to muscle, muscle to bone, muscle to cartilage, etc.) the various structures simply are not free to move to the position that the muscular forces might specify. Consider the obvious example that the lower lip and tongue assume positions during speech that are, in part, related to the position of the jaw.

The third category of nonmuscular forces is labelled aerodynamic influences. The extent to which structures are passively moved by air pressures and flows during speech is largely undetermined. However, such influences are undoubtedly present as is clearly illustrated by movements of the vocal folds during phonation. The only laryngeal muscular forces necessary to initiate phonation are those which serve to adduct the medial edges of the folds. From

---

[3] It is appreciated that tendon and joint receptors may provide similar peripheral feedback. The gamma feedback is exemplary here, since this is the only such system to be empirically implicated in speech production to date (Abbs, 1971).

this muscular adduction, the individual vocal fold vibrations are generated by the air pressure-air flow events. For example, the folds are sucked together due to the air rushing past them; and they are effectively blown open by the increase in air pressure.

A fourth category of nonmuscular force that must be considered is that of gravity. An example of a major gravity effect is seen in the differential influence of the abdominal contents on diaphragm action that occurs as a function of posture (see Chapter 3). In particular, the gravitational force acting on the abdomen in the upright posture opposes the abdominal expiratory muscle forces used in speech, while it aids the speech expiration by the abdominal system in the supine posture. Thus, adjustments in the forces applied by specific respiratory muscles must be made according to the speaker's posture. The effects of gravity on such things as the tongue-jaw mass can only be guessed at in the absence of good estimates of the mass.

Summing Up

In reviewing what has been said to this point in this chapter, it must now strike the reader that the production of speech may well be the most intricate and complex behavior that man performs. Conceptually speaking, the chemical and neural events that generate our thoughts and spoken language are almost inconceivable. Even at the peripheral levels of nerve and muscle the picture is far from clear. However, once the speech process has reached the muscular level, we are able to make physical measurements of it. In so doing it is helpful to view the peripheral machinery that produces the acoustic events of speech as a number of components that coordinate to generate and valve the speech air stream. Moreover, it is important to realize that the movements of the various parts of these components are the result of muscular and nonmuscular forces.

SOME PHYSIOLOGICAL MECHANISMS

Considering the foregoing remarks about a conceptual framework from which to view speech production, we now turn to a consideration of some of the actual physiological mechanisms. It should be emphasized that the research referred to here represents descriptive studies in the main, and the explanations of the underlying physiological events are really no more than hypotheses about how speech is produced. To this point we have not mentioned such words as *consonant, vowel,* or *syllable.* Instead we have referred only to speech sounds, or segments. In order to describe the physiological and acoustic events of speech, it is convenient to make some rather arbitrary segmentations of larger speech parts (e. g., sentences, phrases) into smaller divisions (e.g., consonants, vowels, syllables). For example, rather than describe the entirety of the sentences "That's fine" and "That's mine" in physiological-acoustic terms, we might say the sentences are perceptually different according to the differences between the two smaller segments /f/ and /m/. It should be underscored that the use of these smaller segments is simply a descriptive convenience.[4] With these words of caution, we'll now review and interpret some research findings under the headings of: (1) phonetic aspects, (2) prosodic aspects, and (3) physiological aspects of speaking effort.

Phonetic Aspects

The sound segments that have been mentioned to this point (viz., consonants, vowels, and syllables) are usually referred to as *phonetic*, or *segmental* features. As was pointed out in Chapter 5, consonant productions can be distinguished from vowels according to the degree of openness of the upper airway. Moreover, the laryngeal muscles always bring the vocal folds together for vowels, and various states of vocal fold approximation are hypothesized for certain consonant types (Chapters 4 and 5). The objective of this section is to point out the temporal-spatial coordination of the entire speech apparatus that is used to generate the various phonetic segments. This coordination will be illustrated via changes in air pressure and air flow which reflect net forces and movements of the speech apparatus. These pressure-flow events are also relatively easy to record and, thus, are widely used in the evaluation of speech functions. Locations where these pressures and flows are typically recorded are shown in the mid-sagittal line drawing of Figure 6-2. The air pressures and air flows for a speaker saying, "Phonetic aspects," are shown in Figure 6-5. Intraoral air pressure (P_o) is shown as a solid line and the hypothetical subglottal air pressure (P_s) has been drawn as the dotted line. It should also be pointed out that the oral and nasal air flows are on different scales, with a 100 cc/sec flow rate from the nose appearing much larger on the figure than a similar flow from the oral channel. Finally, the vertical lines drawn on the figure delineate boundaries of the various phonetic segments as defined by changes in the air pressure and air flow magnitudes.

---

[4] The size of the segments used in assembling the speech output has been the subject of much research and speculation. The issue has focused around the question, "Is *it* of syllable size, or smaller?" No compelling answer has evolved from any data or argument presented to date. Indeed, it is conceivable that the question is unanswerable. In any event, further discussion of this point is outside the purposes of this chapter.

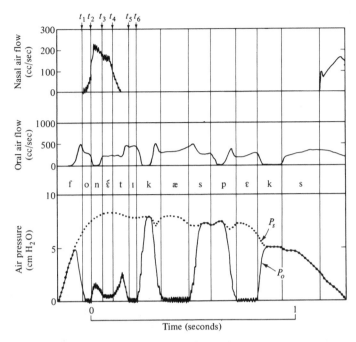

Figure 6-5   Oral and nasal air flow ($\dot{V}_o$ and $\dot{V}_n$, respectively), and intraoral and subglottal air pressure (P_o and P_s, respectively) for a speaker saying "Phonetic aspects." Time markers (t_1–t_6) are shown as boundaries for the various phonetic segments. (See text for explanation.)

The respiratory system

The respiratory system does not appear to develop different magnitudes of subglottal air pressure (P_s) for specific phonetic segments of the English language. Accordingly, the bumps and dips recorded on the P_s trace of Figure 6.5 are believed to be reflections of structural movements in the glottal and upper airway regions.[5] The rapid decrease in P_s during the [k] and [s] segments at the end of the sentence is typically seen when such sentences are spoken in a conversational, declarative manner.

Recent studies (Netsell, 1969 a, b; McGlone and Shipp, 1971) have shown that voiced and voiceless consonants are produced with essentially identical magnitudes of P_s. Moreover, the peak P_s and P_o levels used in production of voiceless consonants (viz., [p], [t], and [s]) are identical. This is shown in the [f], [k], [s], and [p] segments of Figure 6-5. Therefore, results of earlier studies

---

[5] An exception to this is the P_s level achieved during the [ɛ] segment in [fonɛtɪk]. More will be said about P_s increases that accompany stressed or emphasized segments in a following section.

(Arkebauer et al., 1967; Malecot, 1968) that found no statistically significant difference between the peak P_o magnitudes of the various voiceless consonants support the hypothesis that the respiratory system develops an essentially constant P_s level with respect to the phonetics of the sentence. However, the reader should recall (from Chapter 3) that maintenance of this essentially constant P_s level throughout the sentence requires rather precise adjustments in the balance of muscular forces against non-muscular forces.

The larynx

There are several indications of glottal activity in Figure 6-5. The very small and rapid fluctuations on the P_o trace reflect the vocal fold vibrations associated with phonation. Notice also that toward the end of the [æ] segment the oral air flow is beginning to increase. In the absence of a P_o increase, this oral flow increase probably reflects the increase in glottal aperture that is requisite for the forthcoming [s] segment. The glottis apparently does not reach a maximum opening until approximately 30 msecs into the [s] segment as evidenced by the continuing (1) small, rapid vibrations on the P_o trace and (2) increase in oral air flow. The events described above illustrate the speed and precision with which the laryngeal muscles must adduct and abduct the vocal folds during speech. Indeed, these major adjustments of the glottal area are effected within one-tenth of a second (100 msecs). Thus, the larynx must be viewed as an articulator (i. e., a valve of the air stream) in the same sense as are the velopharynx, tongue, front teeth, and lips.

The upper airway

Many of the valvular actions of the upper airway structures are reflected in the $\dot{V}_n$, $\dot{V}_o$, and P_o variations of Figure 6-5. Although a segment by segment analysis of the entire figure demonstrates the descriptive power of speech aerodynamics, we will focus here on just a few events that illustrate the coordination of some of the upper airway parts. It is expected that a slow careful reading of this section is required. However, in the end it should provide a considerable appreciation of the coordinated act of speaking. In particular, we'll examine the $\dot{V}_n$, $\dot{V}_o$, and P_o traces that resulted from the speaker saying "Phonetic," [fonɛ́tɪk]. The [f] segment is defined by the build-up of P_o to 5 cm H_2O pressure, followed by a burst of $\dot{V}_o$ that peaks at about 500 cc/sec. The rapid fluctuations on the $\dot{V}_n$ and P_o traces that occur at the first vertical time marker (t_1) reflect the onset of vocal fold vibrations for the vowel [o]. The presence of $\dot{V}_n$ during the [o] segment indicates that the velopharynx has already opened for the oncoming [n]. At time marker two

(t_2), both P_o and $\dot{V}_n$ make an abrupt increase and $\dot{V}_o$ quickly falls to zero. This represents the movement of the tongue tip to the alveolar ridge and the complete closure of the oral channel (zero $\dot{V}_o$) for the [n] segment. Time markers three and four (t_3 and t_4) bound the vowel [ɛ] and the continuing $\dot{V}_n$ reveals that the velopharynx is still open. It is apparent that the velopharynx does not close until half way through the [t] segment as evidenced by the fall of $\dot{V}_n$ to zero in the presence of the increasing P_o. At this point (viz., half way between t_4 and t_5) the $\dot{V}_o$ shows a rapid increase as P_o falls to zero. This reflects the fast shift (30–40 milliseconds) of the tongue tip from the alveolar ridge to a lower position for the vowel [ɪ]. It is particularly interesting to note that $\dot{V}_o$ does not go to zero, nor do the rapid pressure fluctuations disappear from the P_o trace during the [t] segment. This suggests that the oral channel was not completely sealed and that the vocal folds continued to vibrate. In all probability, then, the acoustics actually produced sounded more like a [d]. The open velopharynx during the first half of the [t] segment may have been partially responsible for the continuing transglottal air flow and vocal fold vibrations.

The aerodynamic events that occurred within and around the [n] segment boundaries clearly illustrate the multiple movements of the upper airway parts. It is also clear that these movements must be precise and adhere to a very close time schedule in order for the various phonetic segments to be accurately produced. Moreover, in order to produce speech sounds at a conversational rate, a particular structure must often simultaneously execute movements for at least two phonetic segments. For example, even as the tongue tip was moving for the [t] in "phonetic" (Figure 6-5), the body of the tongue was undoubtedly forming a shape for the production of [ɪ]. This is an example of the activity termed "coarticulation" in the preceding chapter.

Summing up

In brief, then, we can suggest that the respiratory system provides an essentially constant air pressure and the laryngeal and upper airway structures move to modulate the escaping air stream so as to form the several phonetic segments of the English language. The transitions from segment to segment are so rapid (e.g., often within 50 milliseconds) that the structures must often participate in movements for more than one segment at a time.

The foregoing has only touched upon the surface of the events that lead to a particular sequence of speech sounds. Even so, however, a particular phonetic sequence would remain linguistically meaningless without the addition of the so-called prosodic aspects of the language. We'll see in the following section that these prosodic characteristics require neuromuscular activity that is, in part, independent from the physiology of phonetics.

Prosodic Aspects

Now that we have some understanding of the physiological activity that is associated with consonant and vowel production, we are in a better position to appreciate some of the physiological events that produce the acoustic correlates of the *prosodies*. A host of terms has been applied to the *prosodic* (or *suprasegmental*) features; including pitch, intonation, loudness, intensity, stress, duration, rhythm, juncture, tempo, and voice quality. In addition to disagreeing about what to label these suprasegments, we often wrongly interchange perceptual and acoustic levels of description (e. g.; people often talk about the "pitch and intensity" of the voice). Regardless of the labels used, it seems that the designation of particular speech events as prosodic has been helpful in various linguistic descriptions. It might be inferred that these suprasegmental events are independent of, and of longer duration than, the segmental events. The independence of the suprasegment is exemplified by our ability to stress, or add emphasis to, any syllable of speech. The extension of suprasegmental features over many segments is evidenced by the intonation contour of a sentence; i. e., the perceptual correlate of the time course of the fundamental frequency of vocal fold vibrations. However, evidence that a prosodic feature can be restricted to a very small phonetic segment (viz., a vowel) is revealed in the many meanings that can be given to "oh" (e. g., "oh?," "oh!," etc.).

To facilitate the following discussion of physiological mechanisms, it will be helpful to operationally define three prosodic features: intonation, stress, and rhythm. *Intonation* is the perception of changes in the fundamental frequency of vocal fold vibration (fo) during speech production. Thus defined, intonation can apply to fo shifts within a given vowel. When these fo shifts are viewed over several consecutive segments, we have a visual display of the acoustic determinant of the *intonation contour*. *Stress* is the perception of syllable emphasis, relative to the emphasis perceived on other syllables in the same sentence, or phrase. Therefore, the degree of stress for a given syllable is relative to the stress perceived on the other syllables. For example, in saying "That's a boy," "That's" is more strongly stressed than "boy," and, "boy" is more strongly stressed than "a." Various combinations of (1) fo and sound intensity shifts, and (2) time components of pause and syllable duration give rise to the perception of stress. *Rhythm* can be defined as the perception of the time program applied to the phonetic events. This definition allows the rhythm of the English language to be "stressed-timed" (Allen, 1969) in that the relative degrees of stress in a sentence, or phrase, establish the variations in time (pauses, syllable duration) of the remaining segments.

Intonation

Intonation was just defined as the perception of changes in the fundamental frequency (fo) of vocal fold vibration. These variations in fo occur around some average level fo used by the particular speaker. Many factors enter into what this average level might be. For example, the higher overall pitch used by females appears to be related, in part, to their smaller anatomy. Also, the average pitch can vary considerably within the speaker according to his emotions of the moment. Thus, the laryngeal muscles must set a given level of overall tension for this average fo level. While this basic background tension is being maintained, selected laryngeal muscles undergo rather rapid contractions to effect the variations of fo that are perceived as intonation.

There is not a great deal of research available from which to speculate about the physiological specifics used to generate these fundamental frequency variations. Moreover, it should be pointed out that not all variations in the fo contour are the result of laryngeal muscle adjustments. For example, with laryngeal muscle tension held constant, pulsatile increases in subglottal air pressure will result in an upward shift in fo of less than 5 Hz/cmH_2O (Hixon et al., 1970). It is also apparent that a complete closure of the upper airway by the lips, tongue, and velopharynx will eventually stop the transglottal flow; and, hence, the vocal fold vibrations.

Although systematic study of the laryngeal muscle adjustments used to effect these fo shifts is in an infant stage, the preliminary findings implicate more than a single muscle pair. Hirano, Ohala, and Vennard (1969) concluded from their electromyographic (EMG) study of the cricothyroid, vocalis, and lateral cricoarytenoid muscles that all three of these muscle

Figure 6-6 Integrated electromyographic signals (*cricothyroid, lateral cricoarytenoid,* and *thyrovocalis* muscles) fundamental frequency changes (dashed lines), and associated microphone signals (audio) that were recorded as the speaker said the declarative and interrogative forms (parts *A* and *B* of the figure, respectively) of the sentence "Bev bombed Bob". [*From M. Hirano et al., "The function of laryngeal muscles in regulating fundamental frequency and intensity of phonation,"* J. Speech Hearing Research, *12 (1969), 616-28, Fig. 7.*]

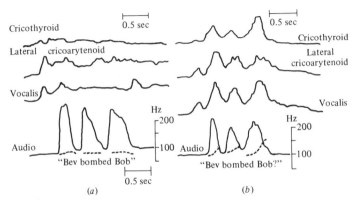

pairs were active in regulating the vocal fold tension changes which vary the *fo*. In particular, these three muscle pairs displayed discrete increases in EMG activity immediately preceding the increases in *fo*. It was assumed that these EMG increases signaled a rise in length and tension of the vocal folds that, in turn, resulted in the *fo* increases. Examples of these electromyographic patterns, *fo* changes, and associated microphone (audio) signals are shown in Figure 6-6. Parts (*a*) and (*b*) of the figure contrast the declarative and interrogative forms, respectively, of the sentence "Bev bombed Bob." The EMG patterns and associated *fo* contour for the declarative sentence are essentially unchanging throughout when compared to the three discrete EMG increases in each muscle that correspond to the three *fo* increases in the interrogative sentence.

While the EMG and *fo* variations shown in Figure 6-6 were critical to forming the perception of intonation and, hence, the distinction in this case of the sentence as a question as opposed to a statement, the meaning of the sentence remains ambiguous; i. e., several meanings are possible depending upon the stress, or emphasis, given to the various words. For example, stressing of the first word would lead to the meaning, "You mean *Bev* bombed Bob?"

Stress

As will be apparent in the following discussion, stress has been more extensively studied from a physiological viewpoint, and an hypothesis concerning its neural basis seems more straightforward than is presently the case with intonation and rhythm. Recall that stress was defined as the perception of a syllable, or word, as emphasized over surrounding speech segments. Acoustically, this emphasis can be manifested by an increase in fundamental frequency, intensity, and/or duration of the particular sound segment.[6]

As will be seen in the following paragraphs, the participation of the various parts of the speech machinery appears to vary as a function of the degree of stress. Moreover, the available data are consistent with the hypothesis that the acoustic correlates of stress result from the application of a transient increase in neural signal strength to the entire speech musculature (Öhman, 1967).

In general, slight increases (0.5 to 1.0 cmH$_2$O) in subglottal air pressure are recorded with stressed vowels as compared with unstressed vowels (Ladefoged, 1967; Netsell, 1969b). In view of the high glottal resistance associated with vowel production, the subglottal air pressure increase may be primarily due to pulse-like contractions of certain respiratory muscles.

---

[6] Although a controversy exists as to whether the duration of the sound segment is of vowel length or longer, the opinion offered here is that existing data do not offer a critical test of the question.

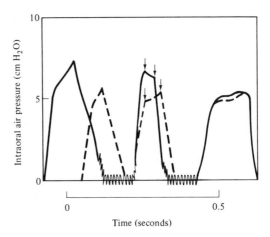

Figure 6-7 Recordings of intraoral air pressure obtained as the speaker said "I proTEST again" (dashed line) and "My PROtest again" (solid line). Arrows on the trace refer to points of assumed oral tract closure during the [t] segments. (See text for explanation.)

A secondary contribution to this air pressure increase may be a narrowing of the glottal aperture during stress. Although the subglottal air pressure recorded during the consonant of stressed speech segments is not always greater than the consonant pressure in an unstressed production, the slope of the pressure curve for a voiceless stop plosive is highly predictive of the vowel that will be perceived as stressed. This is illustrated in Figure 6-7 where intraoral air pressure (P_0) is shown for the contrast of the noun "PROtest" (solid line) with the verb "proTEST" (dashed line). It is important here to recall that during the stop phase of a voiceless stop plosive, the subglottal and intraoral air pressures are equal (Netsell, 1969a; McGlone and Shipp, 1971). Thus, during the [t] stop (as defined by arrows on the (P_0) record in Figure 6-7), a greater (P_0) is recorded in this case when the [t] is associated with the unstressed syllable in "PROtest." However, the air pressure slope during the [t] in "proTEST" points toward the stressed [ɛ], and the slope of [t] in "PROtest" points toward the stressed [o]. The inference here is that the increasing slope of this air pressure during [t] in "proTEST" is a reflection of the rate of change in the net respiratory muscle force applied, and that this force is increasing in preparation for a higher subglottal air pressure on the stressed vowel.

When an increase in fundamental frequency accompanies the stressed vowel (as is usually the case), discrete electromyographic (EMG) bursts are recorded from the cricothyroid, thyrovocalis, and lateral cricoarytenoid muscles (Hirano et al., 1969). This EMG activity presumably reflects an active contraction of these muscles which, in turn, probably results in a slight tensing, lengthening, and thinning of the vocal folds to effect the frequency increase. An additional frequency increase occurs due to the subglottal air pressure increase during the stressed vowel. It was noted earlier that, without a change in muscular forces of the vocal folds, a one cmH_2O pressure increase beneath the folds would increase the fundamental frequency of their vibration by less than 5 Hz. Although it is presently not possible to separate the increase in frequency due to laryngeal muscular adjustments from the increase due to the greater transglottal air pressure drop, there is little doubt that both factors are contributory when the subglottal air pressure increase accompanies the stress, since *fo* increases with stress might be as great as 50 Hz. It has been hypothesized that the perceptions of minimal stress differences are responses to fundamental frequency variations and the primary physiological mechanism is the regulation of these variations by the laryngeal muscles (Netsell, 1969b).

A recent group of studies reveals stress specific modifications in EMG patterns and structural movements of the upper airway (Harris et al., 1969; MacNeilage, 1969; Kent and Netsell, 1972). For example, the muscles regulating bilabial stop consonant movements show electromyographic increases with stress. Also, the opening and closing movements of the jaw are faster for stressed vowels and the tongue moves closer to the so-called idealized position for the particular vowel.

Taken together, these data from these few studies represent the bare beginnings into the understanding of physiological mechanisms involved in generating the acoustic variations perceived as stress. Our best guess at present seems to be no more than a confirmation of Öhman's 1967 hypothesis; viz., the entire speech musculature receives an increment of neural signal strength which is reflected by durational increases as well as increased velocities and displacements of the various structures throughout the vocal tract.

Rhythm[7]

Everyone feels his language to be rhythmic and can give these feelings substance by citing songs or lines of poetry or by simply gesturing "in time" to his speech. Despite this universal intuitive appeal of language rhythm, however, little is known of its exact nature, scientifically speaking. In this section we shall attempt to establish a conceptual framework for language rhythm and to discuss some of the relatively few pertinent experimental results.

We have defined rhythm earlier as the perception of the time program applied to the phonetic events by the speaker. We shall now elaborate on this definition by distinguishing between two kinds of "time," one longer than the other, and between the rhythmic groupings that exist with respect to these two kinds of time.

The longer of these two kinds of time, and the kind we usually think of in talking about language rhythm, is the time extending over phrases. A phrase

---

[7] The author expresses gratitude to George D. Allen, School of Dentistry, University of North Carolina, Chapel Hill, N.C., for contributing this section to the chapter.

is composed of words and syllables, and so the rhythm of a phrase is the manner in which its words and syllables are grouped in time. Such temporal groupings of syllables are closely analogous to the metric feet one encounters in poetry and are the usual structures one thinks of in considering the rhythm of speech.

The shorter kind of time during which important rhythmic groupings exist in speech is the time taken to utter the individual segments that make up each syllable. For example, we articulate the initial consonants of a syllable according to an exact time program that depends upon both the following vowel of that syllable and the final segments of the preceding syllable. It may be confusing at first to think of such segmental time programs, which bear little resemblance to the groupings of syllables into phrases, as "rhythms." We must, therefore, emphasize that we are talking about rhythm and time programs in a very general way; that is, any kind of structure in the time sequence of speech. For, even though we can neither hear nor describe segmental timing as easily as we can the rhythms of phrases, both kinds of temporal structure play an important part in determining the rhythmic character of our language.

Let us put off the treatment of segmental timing for the moment and discuss the phrase rhythm of English. Pike (1945) writes that the rhythm of language can be organized either around all of its syllables or just around the stressed syllables; that is, either (1) every syllable is a "beat" of the rhythm, or (2) just the stressed syllables are beats, and the intervening unstressed syllables are "off beats." Japanese is often cited as an example of the first sort, a so-called "syllable timed" language, and English is felt to be the second kind, a "stress timed" language. Pike notes, however, that English speaking children's taunts often can be syllable timed, as in "Su-zy-is-a-tat-tle-tale." Although there are few, if any, languages in which phonetic units other than the syllables or the stresses are the beats, some languages are hard to classify as either syllable or stress timed. There may, in fact, be a continuum between these two extremes, with all syllables competing for a place in the phrase rhythm, which is eventually determined by sentence structure and, as in English, the existence of strong stresses.

It is hard to know just how phrases come to have the rhythms they do. One reasonable assumption, based on the fact that rhythm conveys very little information in speech, is that speakers impose rhythm on the phrase as they would on any motor behavior. It is well known to psychologists, for example, that people cannot move their muscles in random patterns, but instead organize their movements into rather simple groupings of ones, twos, threes, and fours (Miyake, 1902). There is no reason why the sequence of syllabic gestures that make up a phrase should not become similarly organized.

Additional evidence of this "explanation" of phrase rhythm as deriving from rather general patterns of motor organization is the fact that the resulting rhythm is inexact. That is, we feel when we speak the sentence,

"This is the house that Jack built" (conversationally rather than poetically), that the stressed syllables follow each other at precisely equal intervals. Investigations have shown, however, that this is not true in English and that, in general, the time between two stresses increases as the number of unstressed syllables between the two stressed syllables increases, although not proportionately (c.f., Allen, 1968). The temporal spacing of the stressed syllables is thus irregular and appears to be a combined result of the structure of the sentence and a natural urge to organize the movements associated with stressed syllables into patterns.

Corresponding to this imprecision in temporal spacing of stressed syllables on the part of the speaker is a similar inability on the part of the listener to tell whether or not the rhythm is exact. Again, psychologists tell us that listeners will impose a nonexistent rhythmic structure on a random time pattern of stimuli, and again the patterns are usually ones, twos, threes, and fours (c.f., Woodrow, 1951). Phrase rhythm in English may, therefore, derive primarily from the natural tendencies of speakers to behave in a somewhat organized fashion and of listeners to impose rhythmic structure on any speech they hear.

This hypothesis about the origin of phrase rhythm in English has two major weaknesses. First, there are real differences in phrase rhythm from language to language, differences that are probably not also present in the motor and perceptual systems of the speakers of those languages. Even if these differences turn out not to be very great, they do exist and must be learned along with the rest of the language. Second, the hypothesis ignores the strong feelings which have existed through the ages by students of language and speech that the stressed syllables of English are equally spaced in time. There may, in fact, be substance to these feelings, and some direction has been given toward the discovery of such constraints between stressed syllables in English (Allen, 1968).

Now let us return to the temporal constraints between phonetic segments in English. As an illustration, let us consider the difference between English and French in the way the initial consonants of a syllable are grouped. In English, the two phrases "tense cows" and "ten scows" do not sound the same. If we listen to the [k] sounds in the two phrases, we hear an aspirated [k] in "cows" and an unaspirated [k] in "scows," the difference in aspiration deriving from the time of onset of [au] relative to the release of the [k] closure. The point of this example is not that this difference exists but rather that it exists in English and not in French. That is, the French speaker uttering analogous phrases in French will use an unaspirated [k] in both and the listener will have to derive the difference in meaning from some source other than the temporal relationships between the consonant and vowel articulations.

Another example of segmental timing is the way neighboring consonants and vowels are grouped in a speaker's articulatory time program. In English, vowels are grouped with the following consonant(s) to form higher order time units (Allen, 1970). In Russian, however, vowels form temporal units with preceding consonants (Kozhevnikov and Chistovich, 1965). Such differences in the way segments group themselves into patterns give each language part of its own rhythmic flavor.

We have given only two examples, but the very diversity of possible temporal constraints between segments means that there may be ways to classify the rhythms of language in other than the "stress timed" and "syllable timed" terms discussed above. One has only to listen to the different rhythms of English and German, both of which are definitely stress timed languages, to appreciate the fact that the rhythm and timing of speech are phenomena too complex to be categorized in such broad terms.

In summary, then, we have said that speech rhythm derives from two kinds of temporal structure; namely, the grouping of syllables and stresses into phrases and the grouping of segments into syllables. English phrase rhythm is based on the regular succession of stressed syllables, but much of our intuitive rhythmic "feel" may result simply from the natural tendency of movements to group themselves and of listeners to impose rhythmic structure on what they hear. The organization of segments into syllables can take many forms, and the particular segmental constraints found in English give it further special rhythmic character.

Physiological Aspects of Speaking Effort[8]

The idea that you can use more or less effort when speaking is intuitively meaningful. For example, it seems reasonable to assume that it requires less effort to speak to a person standing next to you than to one across the street. Two things happen quite naturally when we increase our speaking effort: our voice intensity and fundamental frequency increase. The following review of research evidence on this topic points out that, as the speaker is asked to increase the effort with which he is speaking, there is a heightened physiological activity throughout the speech apparatus.

When an increased speaking effort is desired, the respiratory system develops a greater overall subglottal air pressure. This pressure increase is usually achieved through the combination of: (1) a slightly deeper inspiration to begin the speech, and (2) an increased expiratory muscle activity throughout the speech. It will be recalled from Chapter 3 that, by beginning the speech at a higher lung volume level, the static recoil pressure of the system adds a larger component to the subglottal air pressure. It was also

---

[8] Although the term *vocal effort* is most often used in reference to this phenomenon, the word *vocal* implies a restriction to the *vocalic*, or vowel, segments of the speech.

pointed out that as the speech continued into lower and lower lung volumes, the recoil pressure contribution diminished and the expiratory muscles had to contract more forcefully to maintain the desired subglottal air pressure.

It seems that the speaker's internalized perception of the effort he uses in speaking is directly related to the magnitude of subglottal air pressure used in the speech. For example, assume a speaker is using $10\ cmH_2O$ subglottal air pressure in producing his conversational speech, and he is told to assign the number 10 to this effort level. If he is then asked to produce speech with effort levels corresponding to the numbers 20 and 30, his subglottal air pressure will rise to values of 20 and $30\ cmH_2O$, respectively (Prosek and Montgomery, 1969).

Whether or not there are *active* increases in the intrinsic and/or extrinsic laryngeal muscles with increases in speaking effort is very much open to question at this point. There is no doubt that increases in fundamental frequency and intensity of the voice occur with the increased speaking effort. However, the increased subglottal air pressure developed by the respiratory muscles causes an increase in the transglottal pressure drop during vowel productions which could conceivably account for these acoustic changes. The increased electromyographic activity of certain intrinsic laryngeal muscles may represent reflexive tension increases in the presence of the heightened subglottal air pressure as opposed to voluntary muscular contractions. When all the data are in on this point, it may be shown that part of the laryngeal EMG increases reflect the increased neural energizing from higher centers and a lesser part reflects peripheral neuromuscular adjustments in response to the subglottal air pressure increases. We can only conjecture on this point at present.

Several dimensions of the upper airway are seen to change with an increase in the speaker's effort. The effect of these changes is to increase the openness of the oral cavity. When more effortful vowels are contrasted to less effortful ones, the lips are further apart, the jaw and tongue are lowered, and the velum is elevated (Tucker, 1963). The extent to which the greater lip separation and lower tongue position are the result of the lower jaw position has not been quantified. It is also known that the force with which two structures make contact for consonant productions is increased with increases in speaking effort. For example, the contact force between the tongue tip and alveolar ridge in effecting the [t] stop phase becomes greater with increases in speaking effort (Leeper and Noll, 1969). Part of this augmented force may be necessary to oppose increases in subglottal air pressure that result from the effort increases. However, air pressure increases behind the closed valves represent only a small fraction of the contact pressure increases that occur in the valves. Thus, it is probable that the major part of the increase in contact force that accompanies the increase in speaking effort is the result of a greater neural signal strength to the musculature.

Summing Up

We have seen the coordinated way in which the speaker uses all parts of his speech apparatus to form a particular sequence of speech sounds (i. e., the phonetic aspects). We have also described the physiological events that alter the acoustic waveform such that similar sound sequences have different perceptual meanings (i. e., the prosodic aspects). Finally, we have suggested that a person can speak at any one of a number of effort levels without changing the phonetic identity or meaning of the speech. It is as if the physiology associated with phonetic and prosodic segments is super-imposed upon a basic muscular tone, or "energy level," of the speech apparatus.

REFERENCES

ABBS, J. H. 1971. The influence of the gamma motor system on jaw movement during speech. Ph.D. Thesis. Univ. Wisconsin.

ALLEN, G. D. 1968. On testing for certain stress-timing effects. *Working Papers in Phonetics* U.C.L.A. Phonetics Lab. 10: 47–59.

ALLEN, G. D. 1970. Temporal structures in speech production. *J. Acoust. Soc. Amer.* 47.1:(A)58.

ARKEBAUER, H., HIXON, T. J. and HARDY, J. C. 1967. Peak intraoral air pressure during speech. *J. Speech Hear. Research* 10: 196–208.

GOTTLIEB, G. L., AGARWAL, G. C. and STARK, L. 1970. Interactions between the voluntary and postural mechanisms of the human motor system. *J. Neurophysiol.* 33: 365–81.

HARDY, J. C. 1970. Development of neuromuscular systems underlying speech production. *Amer. Speech Hearing Assn.*, Rep. No. 5, 49–68.

HARRIS, K. S., GAY, T., SCHOLES, G. N. and LIEBERMAN, P. 1968. Some stress effects on electromyographic measures of consonant articulations. *Haskins Lab. Report* 1: 137–51.

HIRANO, M., OHALA, J. and VENNARD, W. 1969. The function of laryngeal muscles in regulation of fundamental frequency and intensity of phonation. *J. Speech Hear. Research* 12: 616–28.

HIXON, T. J., KLATT, D. and MEAD, J. 1970. Influence of forced transglottal pressure changes on vocal fundamental frequency. Paper read to the Acous. Soc. Amer., Houston, Texas.

HOLLIEN, H. and CURTIS, J. F. 1960. A laminagraphic study of vocal pitch. *J. Speech Hear. Research* 3: 361–63.

KENT, R. D. and NETSELL R. 1972. Effects of stress contrasts on certain articulatory parameters. *Phonetica* 24: 23–44.

KOZHEVNIKOV, V. A. and CHISTOVICH, L. A. 1965. *Rech: Artikulyatsia i vospri yatiye.* [transl. *Speech: Articulation and Perception.*] Moscow-Leningrad: Manka. [Transl. by U.S. Dept. of Commerce, Joint Publications Research Service (JPRS)] Washington D.C. No. 30, p. 543.

LADEFOGED, P. 1967. *Three Areas of Experimental Phonetics.* London: Oxford University Press.

LEEPER, H. A. and NOLL, J. D. 1969. Pressure measurements of articulatory behavior during alterations of vocal effort. Paper read to the Amer. Speech Hearing Assn., Chicago, Ill.

McGLONE, R. and SHIPP, T. 1971. Comparison of subglottal air pressures associated with /p/ and /b/. Paper read to the Acous. Soc. Amer., Washington D.C.

MacNEILAGE, P. F., HANSON, R. and KRONES, R. 1970. Control of the jaw in relation to stress in English. Paper read to the Acous. Soc. Amer., Atlantic City, N.J.

MALECOT, A. 1968. The force of articulation of American stops and fricatives as a function of position. *Phonetica* 18: 95–102.

MALMBERG, B. 1968. *Manual of Phonetics.* Amsterdam: North-Holland Publishing Co.

MIYAKE, I. 1902. Researches on rhythmic action. *Stud. from the Yale Psychol. Lab.* 10: 1–48.

MORTIMER, E. M. and AKERT, K. 1961. Cortical control and representation of fusimotor neurons. *Amer. J. Phys. Med.* 48: 228–48.

NETSELL, R. 1969a. Subglottal and intraoral air pressures during the intervocalic /t/ and /d/. *Phonetica* 20: 68–73.

NETSELL, R. 1969b. A physiological-acoustic-perceptual study of syllable stress. Ph.D. Thesis. Univ. Iowa.

ÖHMAN, S. E. G. 1967. Word and sentence intonation: a quantitative model. *Quart. Progr. Status Rep.* Speech Transmission Lab, Royal Inst. Techn., Stockholm, 2-3: 20–54.

PIKE, K. L. 1945. *The Intonation of American English.* Ann Arbor: The Univ. of Michigan Press.

PROSEK, R. and MONTGOMERY, A. 1969. Some physical correlates of vocal effort and loudness. Paper read to the Amer. Speech Hearing Assn., Chicago, Ill.

TUCKER, L. 1963. Articulatory variations in normal speakers with changes in vocal pitch and effort. M.A. Thesis. Univ. Iowa.

WILKE, D. R. 1956. The mechanical properties of muscle. *Brit. Med. Bull.* 12: 177–82.

WOODROW, H. 1951. Time Perception, pp. 1224–36. *In* S. S. Stevens (ed.) *Handbook of Experimental Psychology.* New York: John Wiley & Sons Inc.

7

SPEECH ACOUSTICS

Fred D. Minifie

INTRODUCTION

Thus far in this textbook we have concentrated on the physiological aspects
of speech production. It is the dual purpose of this chapter to provide some
descriptive information regarding the acoustical properties of the sounds of
English and to clarify the relationships between speech physiology and
speech acoustics.

Simply stated, speech production involves the generation of more-or-less
noisy sounds somewhere within the vocal tract and the selective modification
of those sounds by the resonance characteristics of the vocal tract (acoustical
filtering). Much of this chapter is devoted to acoustical descriptions of individual speech sounds or sound types. These descriptions are conveniently
partitioned to include discussions of: (1) the physiological mechanisms which
govern temporal variations in air pressure (produce sound); (2) the spectral
properties of the sounds produced (source spectra); and (3) the acoustical
consequences of vocal tract perturbations during speech articulation (i. e.,
the effects on the acoustic spectrum at the mouth opening of alterations in
vocal tract shape).

The latter part of this chapter is devoted to descriptions of the dependency
of acoustical properties of speech sounds upon the phonetic contexts in

which they appear, and the effects of linguistic stress, intonation, etc. An important perspective for the reader embarking on this chapter is to understand that sounds produced in isolation may yield slightly different acoustical patterns than the same sounds produced in dynamic utterance. Chapter 5 provided a comprehensive discussion of the effects of physiological coarticulation during dynamic utterance. In a very real sense, the forces applied to regulate the spatial and temporal patterning of the complex physiological gestures during dynamic speech production also determine the acoustical characteristics of the sounds generated. With this orientation in mind, it is not difficult to appreciate that physiological variations due to coarticulation will produce slight variations in acoustical output.

Further, if we make the assumption that the acoustical signals produced by the talker carry the information-bearing elements of the intended message, we can view speech acoustics as the link between speech production and speech perception. We may conclude, in this restricted sense, that the ease or difficulty with which the acoustical characteristics of speech sounds are perceptually differentiated is lawfully related to the manner in which the sounds are produced. This chapter on speech acoustics provides a description of the "raw materials" for speech perception, and should be understood prior to reading a detailed analysis of how speech is perceived by listeners.

CLASSIFICATION OF SOUNDS

There are many ways in which speech sounds may be classified. Perhaps the most convenient method is through the use of the International Phonetic Alphabet (IPA), described on page 190 in Chapter 5. The IPA provides a single symbol for each distinctively different speech sound. Recall that in Chapter 5 we suggested that there are between forty and forty-five distinctively different speech sounds in English. Phoneticians and linguistics have employed minimal pair comparisons (e. g., *pan* versus *ban*, where only one element in the word differs) to determine the number of distinctively different speech sounds (phonemes) in our language.[1] These observers recognize that some sounds

---

[1] The concept of the phoneme is an abstraction, identifying each distinctively different speech sound with a single symbol. There is a growing concern among many phoneticians as to whether the concept of the phoneme is useful. These phoneticians argue that since the articulatory patterns used to produce speech appear to be regulated by neural instructions that transcend phoneme boundaries and listeners appear to perceive speech sounds in units several phonemes long, the concept of the phoneme may not have either a physiological or perceptual reality. Hence this concept may be misleading; its definition providing a verbal fence within which we compartmentalize our thinking. It is the position of this author that since the arguments for and against the phoneme concept are only now being aired, we will present acoustical descriptions of the various phonemic categories, while recognizing that these descriptions may need modification as our knowledge of the rules which govern the organization of our phonology develops.

are more easily distinguishable than others. For example, it is easier to distinguish the initial /f/ sound in the work "father" from the /ɑ/ sound which follows it, than it is to distinguish the initial sounds in the words "fin" and "thin." From a physiological point of view, the manners of production for /f/ and /θ/ (th sound) are more similar than are the manners of production of /f/ and /ɑ/. Consequently, the acoustical signals at the mouth opening are more similar for /f/ and /θ/ than for /f/ and /ɑ/. As a result /f/ and /θ/ are harder to perceptually differentiate than /f/ and /ɑ/. Although speakers can consistently identify and produce a finite number of distinctively different speech sounds in a language, each attempt at uttering the same phoneme may result in a slightly different acoustical signal. If asked to produce the isolated vowel /æ/ one hundred times in succession, it is questionable that many of the utterances would be *exactly* alike. Also, the same sound in different contexts may be produced with slight variations. For example, the /æ/ sound in the word "pat" /pæt/ is slightly different from the /æ/ sound in the word "pal" /pæl/ and both are different from the /æ/ sound in the word "pan" /pæn/. Yet, all of the vowel sounds produced perceptually fall within the /æ/ "phoneme family." Such nondistinctive variations in speech sounds are called *allophones*.

Speech sounds may be classified under two major categories: *vowels* and *consonants*. Vowels are produced by acoustically energizing the vocal tract at the level of the larynx with a periodic excitation while keeping the vocal tract relatively open or unconstricted. Consonant sounds, on the other hand, are produced with the vocal tract partially or completely occluded. The location of the sound source during consonant production may be laryngeal, supra-laryngeal, or both. A full understanding of the production of vowels and consonants involves the integration of concepts pertaining to various physiological and acoustical events which occur during their production.

VOWELS

The production of vowels may be discussed in terms of the acoustical proper-ties of the sound source and the modification of that source by the acoustical filtering which takes place within the vocal tract. By combining the informa-tion from Chapter 4 on the physiology of phonation, with the information from Chapter 6 on articulatory physiology during speech production, and applying some of the basic principles of acoustics discussed in Chapter 2, we may develop a description of *how* vowel sounds are produced, *what* makes vowels acoustically different from one another, and *why* they are different. Thus, this chapter will proceed along the lines of a source-filter theory of sound production.

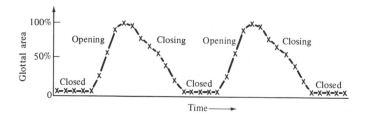

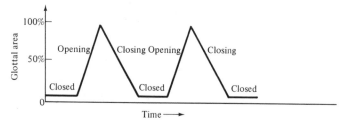

Figure 7-1   Schematic representation of glottal area changes during phonation of vowels produced at medium fundamental frequency and intensity. [*Adapted from R. Timcke et al., "Laryngeal vibrations— Measurements of the glottal wave. Part I: The normal vibratory cycle,"* Arch. Otolaryngol., *68 (1958), 1-19. Copyright 1958, American Medical Association.*]

The Sound Source

All vowel sounds are produced by using a laryngeal sound source. The *glottis* is the aperture or opening between the vocal folds. During normal vowel production, a glottal sound results from the effects of a quasi-periodic vibration of the vocal folds acting upon the air stream escaping from the lungs. All sounds produced with vocal fold vibration are known as voiced sounds. Thus, all normally produced vowels are voiced sounds.[2]

Chapter 4 presents an aerodynamic, myoelastic theory of voice production.[3] This theory attempts to account for the interactions among aerodynamic, muscular and elastic forces which are believed to regulate the opening and closing patterns of the glottis. Recall that during normal phonation the opening and closing patterns of the vocal folds cause the glottal area to vary over time in roughly a triangular manner as is shown in Figure 7-1.

When the vocal folds are closed, a transglottal pressure difference builds up until it overcomes the opposing forces offered by the adducted vocal folds.

---

[2] When vowels are produced in a whisper, the sound source remains at the level of the glottis. During whisper, turbulence is created in the air stream at the glottis but the vocal folds do not undergo periodic vibration. Hence, whispered vowels are aperiodic and voiceless.

[3] For a full discussion, see pages 138–53.

The net driving force of the transglottal air pressure causes the vocal folds to be pushed upward and laterally, thereby increasing the area of the glottal aperture during the "opening phase" of the vibratory cycle. After the vocal folds have been maximally parted and the transglottal pressure difference reduced due to the escape of air through the glottis, a restoration of the adducted state is achieved by the mechanical forces (elasticity) in the intrinsic laryngeal muscles and vocal ligament, aided by the aerodynamic suction force (Bernoulli force) which is associated with the rapid streaming of air particles through the glottis. Complete restoration of the adducted state occurs because the mechanical and aerodynamic restorative forces exceed the transglottal driving forces. Thus, the glottic area is reduced from maximum to zero. The vocal folds remain closed until once again the respiratory mechanism provides sufficient force to overcome the resistance of the vocal folds, and the vibratory cycle repeats itself.

If a somewhat constant driving force is applied, the changing glottal area pattern will regulate the flow of air through the glottis so that small volumes of air will escape during periods of small glottal area, and larger volumes of air will escape during periods of larger glottal area. Indeed, Flanagan (1958) has shown, via electrical analogues of the larynx, that the volume velocity[4] of air escaping through the glottal chink is reasonably proportional to the glottal area.

Figure 7-2 presents an adaptation of Flanagan's graph which shows the relationship between glottal area and the volume velocity passing through the glottis. Note that the volume velocity varies over time and is dependent upon the glottal area.

Since the area of the glottal opening is inversely related to the resistance offered by the vocal folds (opposition to flow), when the vocal folds are closed the resistance is infinitely large and no flow of air occurs. When the

---

[4] *Glottal volume velocity* may be defined as particle velocity integrated over the area of the glottis, which yields the volume flow of air which passes through the glottis per unit time.

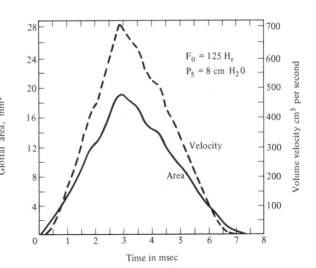

Figure 7-2 Relationship between glottal area and glottal volume velocity during vocal fold vibration of 125 Hz with an assumed transglottal pressure drop of 8 cmH₂O. [*After J. L. Flanagan, "Some properties of the glottal sound source," J. Speech Hearing Research, 1 (1958), 106, Fig. 5.*]

vocal folds are maximally displaced, the resistance is minimal and maximal flow occurs. Thus, the triangular variation in glottal area over time gives rise to a triangular variation in glottal volume velocity. The glottal volume velocity wave (triangular shaped wave) may be analyzed as would any other complex periodic wave.

In Chapter 2 sounds are described as simple or complex. Simple waves are sinusoids with but a single frequency present. Complex waves consist of two or more frequencies. When sound waves are complex and periodic, the frequencies which make up the complex wave are harmonically related (whole number multiples of the fundamental frequency of vibration). One of the properties of triangular shaped waves is that they are rich in harmonic energies, having both odd and even harmonics present in the complex wave. Flanagan (1958) has estimated that the spectral energies in the human glottis during normal vowel production are present in successive harmonics up to about the 40th harmonic.[5] The amplitudes of the energies decrease with an increase in harmonic number, decreasing at a rate of approximately 12 dB/octave above 1,000 Hz (see Figure 7-3). Since there is no way to record and measure the acoustical characteristics of the glottal wave, they must be calculated via computer.

If the vocal folds vibrate at 100 Hz, a Fourier analysis[6] of the resulting triangular shaped volume velocity pattern will show discrete energies present at the harmonics 200, 300, 400, etc. No sound energy is present between the discrete harmonic energies. Thus, if only harmonic energies are present at the sound source, and the vocal tract (resonance system) only serves to alter the

---

[5] It is important at this point to clarify the difference between physiological and acoustic pressure waves. The valving which takes place at the glottis serves to modify the physiological air stream by altering the physiological volume velocity in a triangular manner. However, the glottal wave also serves as an acoustical sound source. It is obvious that the physiological air stream differs from the acoustical stream (radiated acoustical wave). Air particles escape from the lung with a transmission velocity of about 5 cm/sec, while acoustical waves have a transmission velocity of about 34,000 cm/sec.

How then can the complex wave at the glottis be described as an acoustical wave? The answer appears to be that an acoustical wave is set up by the rapid changes in physiological volume velocity in the glottis, so that for an instant the acoustical volume velocity and the physiological volume velocity are proportional. Instantaneously, the two signals separate as the acoustic wave rapidly radiates outward through the vocal tract. It is the acoustical volume velocity changes which energize the acoustical resonance system (the vocal tract).

Consider the analogy of a swimmer diving into a pool. When he enters the water, he disturbs the medium and sets up a wave in the water. His entry into the water also sets up an acoustic wave which will travel either in the water or in the air. If a person is standing at the other end of the pool from the diver, he will hear the acoustical wave (sound) long before the water wave reaches him. In this analogy the same driving force sets up two types of waves within a medium. These waves travel with different velocities, depending upon the nature of the energy in the wave.

[6] A Fourier analysis of a complex periodic wave discloses the frequencies and amplitudes of the constituent simple waves (sine waves) which make up the complex periodic wave.

Figure 7-3 Calculated spectral characteristics of the glottal wave. [*After K. N. Stevens and A. S. House, "An acoustical theory of vowel productions and some of its implications,"* J. Speech Hearing Research, *4 (1961), 302-20.*]

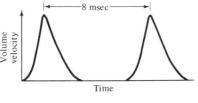

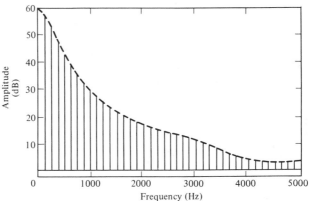

amplitudes of the source energies, then the sound at the mouth opening, although modified in amplitude, must also be made up of energies at the same harmonic frequencies as in the source.

Since it is impossible to record, in man, the unmodified glottal wave, contrasts in glottal spectra can only be appreciated by comparing differences in acoustic spectra at the mouth opening and reasoning back to the glottal contributions to those spectra. The sound energies in vowels produced at conversational levels by male adults will range from roughly 100 Hz to 4,500 Hz. The psychological sensation of *pitch* for a particular vowel will be dependent upon the fundamental frequency of vocal fold vibration. Obviously during high-pitched sounds, the harmonic energies are more widely distributed across the frequency spectrum than during low-pitched sounds. Figure 7-4 shows the sound spectrum at the mouth opening for the same vowel produced with a low pitch and then with a high pitch. For the moment, ignore the changes in the amplitudes of individual components and observe the locations of the components along the frequency continuum. Note that the harmonic energy pattern is dependent upon the fundamental frequency of vibration. When there is a low frequency vibration of the vocal folds (as in 7-4(*a*)), component energies are closer together along the frequency continuum than when there is a high frequency vibration as in 7-4(*b*).

Changes in the intensity of vowel production (perceived as changes in loudness) are achieved by decreasing the duty cycle of the glottal area pattern.

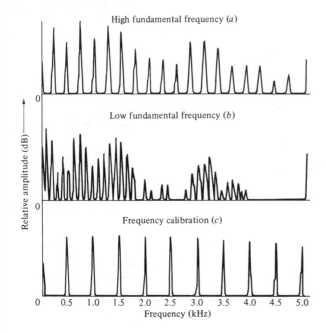

Figure 7-4 Acoustic spectra recorded at the mouth opening of a male speaker during the production of the sustained vowel /æ/. (*a*) Shows the spectrum associated with a high fundamental frequency of vocal fold vibration; (*b*) The spectrum from a low frequency phonation; (*c*), Frequency calibration markers.

The *duty cycle* is the percentage of time the glottis is open during each vibratory cycle. As the duty cycle decreases, the steepness of the slopes on the resulting volume velocity waves increases. The increase in the steepness of the triangular volume velocity waves results in an increase in the amplitudes of all of the harmonic energies in the glottal spectrum as well as a decrease in the dB drop per octave. As a result of increased intensity, there is more energy available at each harmonic and more harmonics are produced (see Figure 7-5).

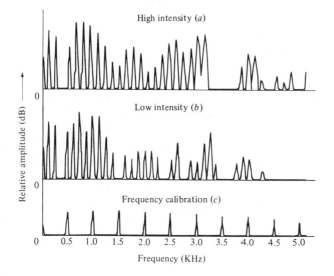

Figure 7-5 Acoustic spectra recorded at the mouth opening of a male speaker during sustained productions of the vowel /ɑ/. (*a*) The spectrum resulting from a high intensity production of /ɑ/. (*b*) The spectrum from a normal production of /ɑ/. Note the larger amplitudes of the harmonic energies in (*a*) as compared to (*b*), particularly at higher frequencies.

The figure shows a marked increase in the number of harmonics present at the mouth opening as a result of increasing the intensity of the glottal tone.

The significant aspects of the discussion to this point are that sound produced at the larynx is a complex sound composed of successive harmonic energies up to about 4,500 Hz in adult males. This broad harmonic spectrum energizes the vocal tract and is modified by the resonant properties of the vocal tube. During vowel production, the nature of the sound at the mouth opening is partially dependent upon the nature of the glottal spectrum. *No other frequencies will appear at the mouth opening than those which are present at the glottis.* The amplitudes of the various harmonic energies from the glottal sound source will be selectively modified by the vocal tract resonators in order to "shape" the distinctive vowel sounds.

The Vocal Tract

During the production of vowels the vocal tract may be viewed as a tortuously shaped tube open at one end (the opening between the lips) and bounded at the other end by a vibrating valve which has the effect of closing off the tube at the larynx. The three-dimensional geometry of this tube may be altered through the contraction of muscles which regulate the movements of the tongue, velum, pharynx, mandible, lips, epiglottis, and larynx. These structures may be moved individually or in various combinations. The combination of structures which move during the production of a particular speech sound will determine the unique vocal tract configuration, and hence, the unique acoustical filter for that sound.

Point of major constriction

At the physiological level vowels may be classified according to whether the major point of vocal tract constriction is in the front, central, or back portion of the oral cavity (see Figure 7-6).

If the major constriction of the airway during vowel production is the result of elevating the tongue tip and blade so that the point of vocal tract constriction occurs near the alveolar ridge, the vowel is called a front vowel. Included in this category are vowels /i, ɪ, e, ɛ, æ, a/. If the major constriction of the airway is between the dorsum of the tongue and velum or between the dorsum of the tongue and the posterior pharyngeal wall, the vowel is called a back vowel. Included in this category are the vowels /u, ʊ, o, ɔ, ɑ/. The remaining vowel sounds are produced with either no obvious points of vocal tract constriction, or with the major point of constriction occurring at the region of the hard palate. These sounds are called central vowels and include /ʌ, ə, ɚ, ɝ/.

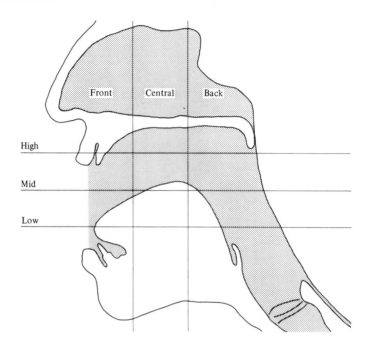

Figure 7-6 Schematic diagram of the vocal tract and the partitioning assumed for classifying the place and degree of constriction of the vocal tract during production of vowel sounds.

Figure 7-7 Tracings of lateral head X-rays showing the vocal tract configurations during the production of /i/ and /æ/.

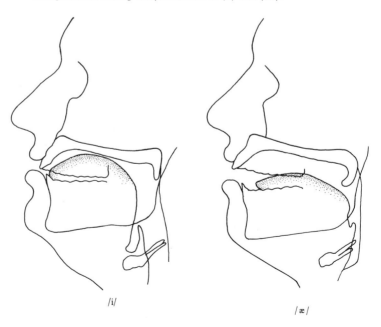

Degree of constriction

A second identifying characteristic of vowels is the degree of constriction within the vocal tract during vowel production. Some vowels are produced with the tongue held high in the vocal tract, thereby increasing the degree of constriction (narrowing the airway), while others are produced with the tongue comparatively low in the mouth which leaves the airway relatively open, even at the point of major constriction. This contrast can be appreciated by comparing the vocal tract configurations for /i/ and /æ/, seen in Figure 7-7.

Vowels produced with relatively constricted vocal tracts are called high vowels (the tongue is held *high* in the oral cavity) or close vowels (the tongue is *close* to the palate). Vowels produced with relatively unconstricted vocal tracts are called low vowels (the tongue is low in the mouth) or open vowels. Intermediate tongue heights are required for the production of mid vowels (see Figure 7-6).

Degree of lip rounding

A third physiological factor which may be used in vowel classification is the degree of lip rounding. A physiological comparison of the high front vowel /i/ with the high back vowel /u/, shows that /i/ is produced with the lips in a spread position, while /u/ is produced with the lips pursed and rounded. The effect of lip rounding is to constrict the airway at the mouth opening. Thus, lip-rounded vowels have two major constrictions within the vocal tract: one between the dorsum of the tongue and the palate (or between the tongue and the posterior pharyngeal wall); and the other at the lips. As a general rule in English only the mid-back and high-back vowels are classified as lip-rounded, with the degree of lip rounding increasing with tongue height. Try saying the following vowels, paying particular attention to the degree of lip rounding: /ɑ, ɔ, o, ʊ, u/.

Degree of muscular tension

The degree of tensity utilized in vowel production is often used as a fourth means of differentiating among vowels which have the same place of constriction, degree of constriction, and degree of lip rounding. For example, the sound /i/ is classified as a high, front, unrounded, tense vowel while the /ɪ/ is classified as a high, front, unrounded, lax vowel. Similar tense-lax distinctions are made between the /e/ and /ɛ/, /ʌ/ and /ə/, /u/ and /ʊ/, and /ɝ/ and /ɚ/. In each case, the tense and lax vowels are similar in regard to the place of vocal tract constriction, degree of constriction, and amount of lip rounding. Tense vowels tend to be longer in duration and carry more sound energy (greater in amplitude) than lax vowels. The physiological mechanisms which contribute to the tenseness or laxness of vowels (independent of those changes which occur during changes in the intensity of sound production such as occur when a sound is stressed) are not well known.

Acoustical Filtering during Vowel Production

The three-dimensional shape of the vocal tract at any instant in time is the primary determinant of the vowel quality being produced. The reason for this is that the vocal tract acts as a mechanical acoustical filter which modifies the sound produced at the larynx. That is, the size and shape of the tube determines what the filtering properties will be.

Perhaps the concept of an acoustical filter may be better understood by drawing upon the well-understood analogy of "sunglasses," an example of an optical filter. Sunglasses allow certain wavelengths in the light spectrum to pass through the glasses to our eyes while other wavelengths are impeded and do not pass through. Just as there are many wavelengths of light energy, the complex periodic sound that is produced at the glottis is rich in harmonic sound energies, covering a broad spectrum of frequencies (wavelengths). The vocal tract acts as an acoustical filter, allowing some of the sound energies from the glottis to pass freely through to the mouth opening. Other sound energies are impeded so that they are reduced in amplitude by the time they reach the mouth opening or are eliminated entirely from the acoustical signal. Thus, the vocal tract serves to selectively modify the acoustical signal from the sound source so that the sound at the mouth opening is dependent upon both the nature of the sound source and the nature of the acoustical filter (see Figure 7-8).

Figure 7-8   Shown is a schematic drawing of the physiological and acoustical characteristics of speech sound production. The triangular volume velocity pulses (*a*) are passed through the vocal tract (*b*) and exit the mouth opening as a complex sound wave (*c*). If this process is viewed from a spectral perspective, we can see that the glottal waveform consists of a harmonic spectrum of the type shown in (*d*). The vocal tract resonating characteristics (*e*) modify the glottal spectrum so that the radiated acoustic wave is dependent upon both the glottal spectrum and the vocal tract transfer function (*f*). [*After G. Fant,* Acoustic Theory of Speech Production (*The Hague: Mouton & Co., Publishers, 1970), p. 19. Reprinted by permission of the author and the publisher.*]

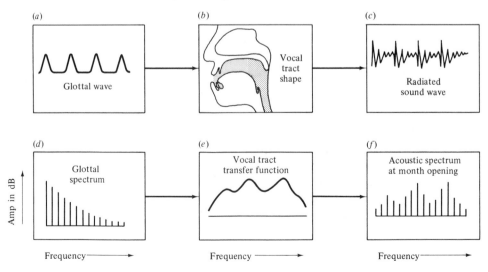

Simple resonators

Just as an expert in optical physics could mathematically calculate the filtration properties of a pair of sunglasses prior to exposing them to light, an acoustical physicist could calculate the natural filtering properties of a vocal tract configuration prior to energizing the system with a sound source. As a beginning student you need not comprehend the mathematical properties of the acoustical filtering which takes place in the vocal tract. However, the general concepts which relate the shape of the vocal tract to the "shape" of the sound spectrum at the mouth opening are important to your understanding.

Let us examine the way a simple acoustical filter works. In Chapter 2 you read about a single Helmholtz resonator, and learned that the natural resonant frequency of that tube, closed at one end, is directly proportional to the area of neck opening (A) and inversely proportional to the length of neck opening (le) and the volume of the resonator (V). It is important to note that the size of the volume, the amount of constriction at the opening, and the length of constriction all interact to determine the precise natural resonant frequency of the tube. You can empirically validate these relationships by blowing across various sized resonators (e. g., a lipstick tube, a pop bottle, and a gallon jug). The larger the volume of the resonator, the lower will be its natural resonant frequency. If you partially occlude the neck opening or increase its length, you will lower the natural resonant frequency, etc.

Multiple resonators

The single Helmholtz resonator does not provide a very adequate physical analogy to the vocal tract during vowel production. More typically, the vocal tract looks like the analogy of the double Helmholtz resonator shown in Figure 7-9. V_1 is analogous to the oropharyngeal air volume, le_1 is the length of the constriction between the tongue and the palate, A_1 is the degree of constriction of air column between tongue and palate, V_2 is the oral cavity volume or volume in front of the tongue-palate constriction, le_2 is the length of the lip protrusion, and A_2 is the area at the lip opening. In such a complex tube, simultaneous multiple resonances are possible. The first resonant frequency should be determined by the formula:

$$F_1 = \frac{c}{2\pi} \sqrt{\frac{1}{V_1}\left(\frac{A_1}{le_1} + \frac{A_2}{le_2}\right)}$$

where c equals the transmission velocity of sound. Similarly, other resonances could be calculated. The frequency location of each resonance depends on the size and shape of the resonance tube (vocal tract). In the human vocal tract, six or more resonances may occur simultaneously, as during the production of vowel sounds. The relative frequency locations of the first three (lowest)

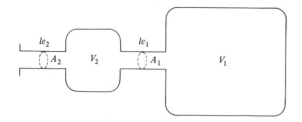

Figure 7-9 Double Helmholtz re-sonator. [*After G. Fant,* Acoustic Theory of Speech Production (*The Hague: Mouton & Co., Publishers, 1970). p. 282. Reprinted by permission of the author and the publisher.*]

resonances appear to be the most important cues for the perception of vowels. Fant (1960) presents data which indicate that the first three resonances within the vocal tract are dependent upon the geometry of the pharyngeal and oral cavities. Since these cavities may be markedly altered when shifting from one vowel to another, the locations along the frequency spectrum at which the first three resonances occur will also be altered. By comparison, Fant (1960) has shown that the resonances 4, 5, and 6 usually emanate from laryngeal cavities which are not as susceptible to variation as are the pharynx and oral cavity. As a result, the resonances 4–6 occur at relatively fixed frequency locations in the output spectrum of the vocal tract even during production of grossly different vowel sounds.

The locations along the frequency spectrum where resonances occur are the regions which provide the greatest transfer of energy from the glottal spectrum to the mouth opening. Energies in frequency regions distant from these natural resonance frequencies will be attenuated. As a result, in the sound spectrum at the mouth opening there are selected frequency regions of relatively strong concentrations of sound energy (called formants) which are related to peaks in the acoustic transfer characteristic (natural resonances) of the vocal tract.

Because the vocal tract produces multiple resonances during vowel production, the acoustic spectrum at the mouth opening at any one moment in time will have several formants. These formants in the output spectrum are directly related to the natural resonances within the vocal tract. The

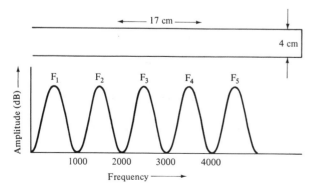

Figure 7-10 Resonance characteristics of a tube 17 cm in length and 4 cm in diameter.

lowest resonance frequency region is called formant 1; the second lowest frequency region, formant 2; etc. In addition to specifying the formants by their location along the frequency spectrum (formant frequencies), they may also be identified by their amplitude and by the steepness of the resonance curve (formant bandwidth). All of these factors may serve as useful cues to the listener in vowel identification.

During the production of a wide-open vowel like /æ/ by an adult male speaker, the vocal tract is similar in shape to a cylinder closed at one end, 17 cm in length and 4 cm in diameter. Such a tube will have natural resonances at 500, 1,500, 2,500, and 3,500 Hz (see Figure 7-10).

Vocal tract resonances (formants)

While the resonances within the vocal tract are determined by the three-dimensional geometry of the entire vocal tube, it is sometimes appealing to simplify this relationship by describing the influences of three major factors: the place of major constriction within the vocal tract, the degree of constriction at that point, and the area and length of the lip constriction. Using these variables, it is possible to show that any time the vocal tube is constricted (perturbed), an alteration of the natural resonance patterns of the unconstricted tube results. Stevens and House (1958) have shown that a reasonable first order approximation of the shape of the vocal tract may be obtained by specifying these parameters as: d_0, the distance from the glottis to the point of major vocal tract constriction; r_0, the radius of the constriction at point d_0; and A/l, the conductivity index at the open end of the vocal tract (in man the conductivity index is dependent upon the area of lip opening divided by by the length of lip protrusion). They assume that the geometry of the vocal airway is primarily affected by the tongue, the curvature of which is parabolic, constrained only at the point of major constriction of the airway and at the tongue root.

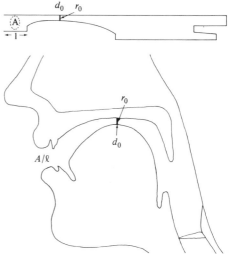

Figure 7-11 Simulated vocal tract shape determined by specification of three parameters: d_0, the distance from the glottis to the point of major constriction within the vocal tract; r_0, the radius of constriction at point d_0; and $A/1$, which is the conductivity index calculated by dividing the area of lip opening by the length of lip opening.

Place of constriction. Although the entire vocal tract participates in the determination of each formant frequency, it is tempting (and not too misleading) to assign primary contributions for each formant to specific regions of the tract.

Moving the place of constriction within the vocal tract alters the volumetric relationships between the front and back cavities. The front cavity is the vocal tract volume anterior to the point of major constriction of the vocal tract. The back cavity is the volume posterior to the constriction. The first formant (F_1) is primarily dependent upon the largest of these cavities, usually the pharyngeal volume. As the place of major constriction is moved toward the front of the mouth, the back cavity enlarges and the first formant gradually decreases in frequency. Since F_2 is primarily determined by the second largest volume, usually the front cavity, moving the place of constriction toward the front of the mouth increases the frequency of F_2. Formant three (F_3) is usually determined by interactions of volumes along the length of the vocal tract and higher order resonances. Hence the physical resonator analogies are not easily specified.

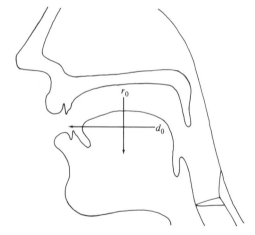

Figure 7-12   Schematic view of the vocal tract to show directional changes in place of articulation and degree of constriction.

Degree of constriction. When d_0 is near the front of the mouth, a tight constriction (small r_0) serves to additionally decrease F_1. As in the simple Helmholtz resonator, a tight constriction on a resonator volume will decrease its resonance frequency. Hence as r_0 decreases, F_1 decreases. However, F_2 increases because the small value of r_0 occurs when the mandible and tongue tip are raised to allow the tongue tip to approximate the alveolar ridge. This tends to decrease the size of the front volume, thereby increasing its natural resonance. Thus, changes in the degree of constriction (r_0) by elevating and lowering the tongue tip will influence the frequency locations of both F_1 and

F_2, because such changes affect the volumetric relationships between the front and back cavities as well as the degree of acoustic coupling between the cavities.

Degree of lip rounding. During the production of front vowels, the influence of lip rounding is minimal insofar as the location of major formants are concerned. For front vowels, place of constriction and degree of constriction are the primary determinants of the formant frequency locations. For the back vowels, lip rounding becomes an important determiner of the location of both F_1 and F_2. When the tongue position is altered from the position for /ɑ/ to that for /u/, the degree of lip rounding increases. Lip rounding constricts the vocal tract at the mouth opening, which serves to decrease both F_1 and F_2.

As the dorsum of the tongue elevates toward the velum when changing the vowel from /ɑ/ to /u/ the tongue root also moves forward (see Figure 7-13). This complex gesture serves to increase the size of the pharyngeal volume during /u/ which results in a lower first resonance for /u/ than for /ɑ/. However, the increased front volume on /ɑ/ as compared to /u/ should result in a lower F_2 on /ɑ/ than /u/, if F_2 were entirely dependent upon volume. Just the opposite occurs due to the increased degree of lip rounding on /u/. That is, the effect of marked lip rounding is to override the expected resonance characteristics due to volume change. This argument suggests that the amount of lip rounding is a most important factor in tuning the entire vocal tract resonator during the production of back vowels in English.

Other factors also contribute to the resonance patterns within the vocal tract. For example, Hudgins and Stetson (1935) and Stetson (1951) have observed that the larynx elevates with an increase in fundamental frequency. Obviously laryngeal height will affect both the length and volume of the vocal tract. Minifie et al. (1970) have shown that the lateral pharyngeal

Figure 7-13 Tracings of lateral head X-rays showing the vocal tract configurations during the production of /ɑ/ and /u/.

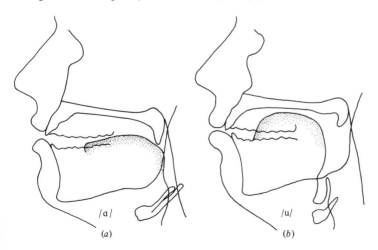

/ɑ/

(a)

/u/

(b)

walls move more inwardly on low vowels than on high vowels. If F_1 is primarily controlled by the pharyngeal volume, such displacements of the lateral pharynx are consistent with, and contribute to, the acoustical changes resulting from tongue movements. That is, high vowels are produced with larger pharyngeal air spaces than are low vowels due to forward movement of the tongue on high vowels. In addition, there is less pharyngeal constriction on high vowels than low vowels. The pharyngeal air space during vowel production is jointly controlled by movements of the tongue and pharyngeal constrictors. The logic of this argument may be extended to reason that the complex acoustical resonance patterns which result during vowel production are related to the concerted movements of several articulators. The precise resonance pattern which results is dependent upon the net three-dimensional geometry of the vocal tract, as influenced by the various articulators.

In conclusion, the modification of the glottal spectrum by the vocal tract during vowel production is lawfully related to the complex physiological gestures within the vocal tract. Although the entire vocal tract contributes to the total acoustical filter function, the primary factors which determine the resonance patterns are: the place of major constriction within the vocal tract, the degree of constriction at that point, and the degree of lip rounding (Figure 7-14). Interactions among these three physiological variables determine the precise acoustical resonances during vowel production.

Figure 7-14 Formant 1 and formant 2 resonances for selected vowel sounds. The arrows at the bottom of the figure depict the influences of place of constriction, degree of constriction, and the degree of lip rounding on vowel resonance patterns.

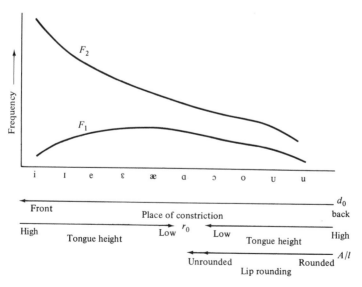

The foregoing argument has been presented as if the articulators involved actually achieve their ideal target positions during each sound produced. Many times, this is not the case. Rather, speakers have a remarkable ability to compensate for physiological constraints imposed on particular articulators (due to phonetic context, pathology, etc.) by adjusting other articulatory maneuvers in order to achieve a desired acoustical end product. It is the interplay among the various articulators which allows the speaker to approximate the desired sound, even under "difficult" speaking situations. For example, gross compensatory adjustments by persons with open cleft palates or surgically removed tongues often cause speech pathologists to be amazed at how "normal" the speech sounds in light of presumed anatomical incompetency.

Table 7-1 Averages of fundamental frequencies and the first three formant frequencies of vowels produced by seventy-six speakers: thirty-three men, twenty-eight women, fifteen children. [*Table from* Handbook of Speech Pathology, *edited by Lee Edward Travis. Copyright* © *1957. By permission of Appleton-Century-Crofts, Educational Division, Meredith Corporation.*]

		i	ɪ	ɛ	æ	ɑ	ɔ	ʊ	u	ʌ	ɝ
Fundamental	M	136	135	130	127	124	129	137	141	130	133
Frequencies	W	235	232	223	210	212	216	232	231	221	218
(Hz)	Ch	272	269	260	251	256	263	276	274	261	261
Formant Frequencies (Hz)											
F_1	M	270	390	530	660	730	570	440	300	640	490
	W	310	430	610	860	850	590	470	370	760	500
	Ch	370	530	690	1010	1030	680	560	430	850	560
F_2	M	2290	1990	1840	1720	1090	840	1020	870	1190	1350
	W	2790	2480	2330	2050	1220	920	1160	950	1400	1640
	Ch	3200	2730	2610	2320	1370	1060	1410	1170	1590	1820
F_3	M	3010	2550	2480	2410	2440	2410	2240	2240	2390	1690
	W	3310	3070	2990	2850	2810	2710	2680	2670	2780	1960
	Ch	3730	3600	3570	3320	3170	3180	3310	3260	3360	2160
F_1/F_2	M	.118	.196	.288	.384	.657	.679	.431	.345	.538	.363
	W	.111	.173	.261	.420	.697	.640	.405	.390	.542	.305
	Ch	.099	.194	.264	.435	.751	.670	.397	.366	.534	.308
F_2/F_3	M	.761	.780	.742	.710	.446	.347	.455	.388	.498	.799
	W	.843	.808	.779	.719	.433	.340	.433	.355	.504	.837
	Ch	.858	.758	.731	.699	.432	.333	.425	.358	.473	.843
F_1/F_3	M	.090	.153	.214	.272	.300	.236	.197	.134	.268	.290
	W	.093	.140	.205	.301	.301	.217	.176	.138	.274	.255
	Ch	.099	.147	.193	.305	.325	.214	.169	.132	.252	.259

Acoustical Cues for Vowel Perception

Even though many formants may be produced during vowel production, only the first three formants appear to be used by listeners in differentiating vowel sounds. In Table 7-1 are the acoustical data on vowels obtained by Petersen and Barney (1952). The F_1/F_2, F_2/F_3, F_1/F_3 ratios were calculated from their data and inserted into the table by the present author.

Observe that the absolute formant frequencies for each vowel differ among men, women, and children. Naturally, differences in overall vocal tract size give rise to different "sized" acoustical filters. Large vocal tracts in adult males generally have lower resonances than do the smaller vocal tracts in women and children. However, it appears reasonable to assume that similar physiological gestures in different sized vocal tracts would yield proportional resonance patterns. Table 7-1 shows that even though the absolute frequencies of the first two formants differ when comparing the same vowel produced by men, women, and children, the ratio relationships among the formant frequencies are very similar. This point can be seen graphically in Figure 7-15.

Most phoneticians agree that vowels are differentiated from one another primarily on the basis of formant frequency information available to the listener. The data just presented suggest that vowels are differentiated by listeners, not on the basis of the absolute formant frequencies involved in the sound elements, but rather by the ratio relationships among the formant frequencies. Of secondary importance to the accurate perception of vowel qualities are such variables as the fundamental frequency, formant amplitudes, formant bandwidths, overall sound pressure level, and vowel duration. If the listener is unable to determine which vowel quality was produced on the basis of formant frequency information, he then has to rely upon these secondary cues.

Formant amplitudes are lawfully related to one another, and depend on the amplitude of the glottal wave, the complex interactions of the amplitude of formant 1, the separation of formants, etc., as described by Stevens and House (1961). Formant bandwidths are dependent upon the acoustical damping characteristics of the oral cavity. Generally speaking, the half power bandwidth increases with increasing formant number. Vowel duration has been observed by many investigators to vary systematically with phonetic context. House (1961) has shown that these variations are partially dependent upon physiological constraints during vowel production and partially dependent upon conventions in our phonologic scheme (English). For an example of physiologic constraint, consider that it takes longer to open the vocal tract to say the low vowel /a/ than it does to say the high vowel /i/. Hence /a/ is longer than /i/. Other vowel duration changes appear to be unique to English.

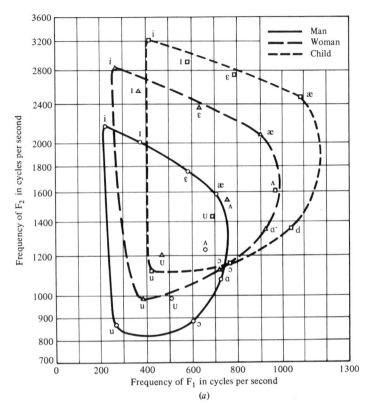

Figure 7-15 (*a*) Absolute frequency distributions of the averaged first formants (F_1) and second formants (F_2) for vowels produced by groups of men, women, and children. [*Figure from* Handbook of Speech Pathology and Audiology, *edited by Lee Edward Travis. Copyright © 1971. By permission of Appleton-Century-Crofts, Educational Division, Meredith Corporation.*] (*b*) A plot of the averaged F_1/F_3, F_1/F_2 data points from vowels produced by men, women, and children. Notice the similarity of the ratios calculated for each speaker group for each vowel, and the relative separation of the ratios from one vowel to another.

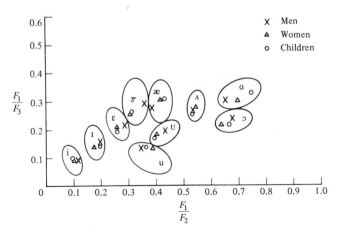

Vowels may be described as continuant sounds in that they may be prolonged without altering their phonemic identification. Although in connected discourse vowel lengths may differ from one vowel to another, duration generally does not affect the perception of the vowel element. Indeed, the duration of a particular vowel may vary from one utterance to the next due to changes in linguistic stress, intonation, etc., without altering the perception of the vowel quality. The vocal tract configurations necessary for the production of individual vowel sounds must be reasonably stable throughout the duration of the vowel. To significantly alter the vocal tract configuration would result in a modification of the output spectrum which would be perceived by listeners as an entirely different vowel sound than the one intended. Minimal vocal tract alterations during vowel production result in allophonic (nonphonemic) variations in vowel quality. Realistically speaking, we have a great deal of pliability in our filter system. We can undergo considerable modification of vocal tract configuration and still produce allophones of an intended vowel. An extrapolation of the logic presented to this point should allow us to appreciate that the modification of the vocal tract that is necessary when moving the articulators from positions required for production of a preceding sound toward the necessary positions for production of a particular vowel, (or away from the vowel position to the required positions for a following sound) will result in dynamically varying vocal tract filter functions immediately preceding (or following) the vowel being produced. If there is vocal fold vibration prior to (or following) the vowel,

Figure 7-16 Spectral changes over time during the production of "buy a pipe."

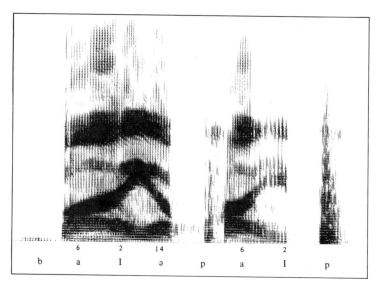

Time ⟶

these dynamic articulatory transitions between speech sounds will regulate the acoustical filtering to provide acoustical transitions between adjacent sounds. These changing formant frequencies during transitions appear to be important cues for speech sound perception. For example, very gradual changes in vocal tract configuration when changing from one vowel to another will result in the perception of a diphthong; very rapid formant transitions occur when changing from a stop consonant sound to a vowel (see Figure 7-16).

Vowel Summary

To summarize at this point, the source-filter theory of sound production has been presented and the logic of this theory applied to vowel production. The relationship between vocal fold vibration and the generation of a complex periodic sound of triangular waveform has been described. The harmonic spectrum of that waveform has been shown to serve as the excitation spectrum to the vocal tract during normal vowel production. The three-dimensional geometry of the vocal tract during the production of a particular vowel sound determines the unique acoustic filtering of the vocal tract. The spectrum of the sound source is modified by this acoustic filter which selectively attenuates the harmonic energies. Thus, the acoustic signal at the mouth opening is a complex periodic signal with the same fundamental frequency as the source tone. The amplitudes of the harmonic energies at the mouth opening are determined by the filter within the vocal tract. Peaks in the output spectrum (known as formants) are determined by the resonances of the vocal tract. The perception of vowel quality is primarily dependent upon the ratio relationships among the formant peaks in the output spectrum.

CONSONANT SOUNDS

Consonant sounds differ from vowels in that the vocal tract is relatively more constricted during consonant production and may be entirely occluded. During vowel production, the vocal tract is relatively open.

In the preceding section on vowels an acoustical theory of vowel production was presented which described the nature of the laryngeal sound source and the acoustical filtering properties of the vocal tract. A similar source-filter approach is useful in the acoustical description of consonant sounds.

Consonant sounds may be described as voiced or voiceless. Those sounds produced with vocal fold vibration are called *voiced* sounds. Thus, the sound source is at the larynx. Sounds with no vocal fold vibration are termed *voiceless*. Voiceless sounds usually have a single sound source—that at the point of major vocal tract constriction where air turbulence is created (noise is produced). Some sounds have more than a single sound source—one at the level of the glottis (voicing), and the other(s) at the point(s) of major vocal tract constriction. The voiced fricative /z/ is a good example of a sound with two sound sources.

Fricatives

Fricative sound sources

As seen in Chapter 6, whenever a mechanical resistance is placed within the vocal tract during speech production (resistance typically being in the form of articulator movement causing a constriction of the airway), an air pressure drop is created across the constriction. The pressure difference across the constriction causes air to flow from the area of higher pressure (oral cavity) to the area of lower pressure (atmosphere at mouth opening). If the respiratory mechanism continues to resupply air behind the constriction, it is possible to maintain a relatively large pressure difference during sustained sound production.

During fricative sound production the degree of vocal tract constriction is quite marked, allowing only a small orifice through which air can flow. When air particles are forced through a narrow opening, the speed with which each particle moves is increased as the particle moves through the orifice. With a small opening, there is greater likelihood that the particles will collide with one another. As the particles are slowed down when they contact one another they begin to follow irregular eddy patterns rather than to flow smoothly in straight lines. This turbulent streaming of air particles causes a nearly random variation of air pressure within the orifice which serves as an aperiodic sound source. If the aperiodic sound (noise) is sustained sufficiently long, it will be perceived as a fricative sound. Thus we may define *fricatives* as sounds produced with very narrow vocal tract constrictions which cause the airflow to be consistently turbulent (Petersen and Shoup, 1966).

Fant (1960) has described the importance of the Reynolds' number in understanding turbulent streaming and noise generation in fricatives. The Reynolds' number is a "dimensionless parameter proportional to the particle velocity v cm/sec and to the effective width h cm of the passage. The

$$\mathrm{Re} = \frac{vh}{\nu}$$

constant $\nu = 0.15$ cm²/sec is the kinematic coefficient of viscosity defined by the ratio of the viscosity coefficient and the density of the gas. Depending on the particular geometry and surface properties of the passage, there is a critical Reynolds' number above which turbulence sets in" (Fant, 1960, p. 273). Since the pressure drop across such constriction will be proportional to the particle velocity, the sound pressure of the generated noise will be related to the magnitude of the pressure drop (beyond a threshold value) and to the effective width of the constriction. It has been empirically determined that circular-shaped orifices provide the most efficient conversion of particle velocity into sound pressure. That is, noise generation is more efficient in circular orifices than in eliptically-shaped orifices of the same cross-sectional area. For example, the large width-to-height ratio of the slit could be one of the factors responsible for the weak intensity of the interdental fricative $/\theta/$ (Fant, 1960, p. 275). The intensity of the $/s/$ sound may be proportionally larger, due in part to the more circular nature of the orifice at the constriction. Quite obviously, the speed of articulatory movements regulating the constriction of the vocal tract at the onset and cessation of fricatives, as well as the duration of the constriction, will markedly affect the intensity of the noise produced (Meyer-Eppler, 1953).

From the foregoing discussion, one may assume that the spectral characteristics of the turbulent sources in fricative sound production are dependent upon the place of articulation (constriction) within the vocal tract, the shape of the orifice at the constriction, and the pressure drop across the constriction. Furthermore, whenever sufficient pressure exists to cause turbulent streaming for a given orifice shape, the spectral characteristics of the sound produced will be similar. For example, the spectral characteristics of the turbulent sound sources for voiced and voiceless fricatives will be considered similar. Quite obviously, the pressure drop at the glottis will reduce the intraoral pressure on voiced fricatives as compared to voiceless fricatives. If, however, sufficient intraoral pressure exists during voiced fricatives to create turbulence at the major oral port constriction, then the spectral characteristics of the turbulent source will be similar, though reduced in amplitude, to the spectral characteristics of the source turbulence on their voiceless cognates. Since similar vocal tract shapes will similarly filter the acoustic sources, one may assume the characteristics of the output spectra of voiced and voiceless fricatives to be similar. However, the voiced fricatives will obviously include a complex periodic wave (voice source) superimposed on the aperiodic noise source. In addition, the voiceless fricatives will differ in amplitude (usually larger) from their voiced cognates.

Fricative resonances

For ease of identification of the place of vocal tract constriction phoneticians label the structures involved in the vocal tract constriction. For example, $/f/$ is a voiceless labiodental fricative; meaning the constriction occurs between

Table 7-2   Classification of English fricatives.

| | Examples—key words | |
Place of constriction	Voiced	Voiceless
labiodental	/v/as in vase	/f/as in farm
linguadental (interdental)	/ð/as in that	/θ/as in thin
lingua alveolar (narrow air channel)	/z/as in zoo	/s/as in save
linguapalatal (wide air channel)	/ʒ/as in measure	/ʃ/as in shoe
linguavelar (lip rounded)		/hw/as in white
glottal		/h/as in hat

the lips and the teeth. Table 7-2 provides a descriptive list of the fricative elements of English.

During fricative production, the closer the sound source is to the lip opening, the higher will be the natural resonant frequency of the vocal tract (acoustic filter). That is, the smaller the volume of air space anterior to the source, the higher will be its natural resonant frequency. This principle helps to explain why the /s/ sound appears higher in "pitch" than the /ʃ/ (sh) sound. During /ʃ/ the lips are protruded and the lip opening is constricted, due to lip rounding. The effect of lip rounding is to lengthen the vocal tube anterior to the source, thereby causing a lower natural resonant frequency for /ʃ/ than for /s/. Similarly, as the place of constriction is moved from the /f/ and /θ/ positions (sound sources near the lip opening with high frequency resonance) to /s/, /ʃ/ and then to /h/, the length of the tube anterior to the source is gradually increased, thereby reducing the natural resonant frequency of the tube anterior to the source. Hence, we get lower "pitched" fricatives as we move from constrictions near the lips to constrictions farther back in the vocal tract. Similar logic could be applied to the understanding of acoustical filtering of the noise sources during the production of voiced fricatives. However, the pitch of voiced fricatives is dependent upon the fundamental frequency of vocal fold motion which determines the fundamental period of the voiced source.

English fricatives

Fricatives are continuant sounds which may be altered in duration (over a reasonably wide range of durations) without significantly affecting their phonemic identification. The following table provides a comprehensive summary of the physiology of production, the spectral characteristics of the sound sources, and the output spectra for the fricatives of English. The primary reference materials from which the information in this table was extracted include Fant, 1960, Strevens, 1960, and Heinz and Stevens, 1961.

Table 7-3 Acoustical properties of English fricatives.

Physiological description	Source spectrum	Output spectrum
Interdental		
/θ/ and /ð/ are produced with the tip of the tongue close to, or touching, the inner edge of the upper incisors. Air is forced through a narrow slit between the bottom of the upper teeth and the top surface of the tongue. The broad width to height nature of the orifice shape yields a low intensity level, broad bandwidth of noise.	Flat noise spectrum from about 1,000 Hz to 10,000 Hz. Energy may drop off at about 3 dB/octave.	Strevens observes that /θ/ has low intensity noise with the highest center of gravity in the frequency domain of any English fricative. Largest amplitudes of energy are from 7,000 to 8,000 Hz. Heinz and Stevens found that listeners identified wide band noises with resonances from 6,500 to 8,000 Hz as either /f/ or /θ/.
Labiodental		
(f) and (v) are produced with the upper teeth close to the inner surface of lower lip. The air stream passes between the teeth and the lower lip, and also through some of the interstices between the upper teeth. The broad width and low height to the elliptical orifice offers a large resistance to the outward flow of air, as well as causing a low intensity, wide band noise to be produced. The noise source is relatively unmodified by the vocal tract since the noise source is located near the output of the resonance tube.	A low intensity noise band from 800 to 10,000 Hz. Amplitude of noise drops approximately 3 dB/ to 6 dB/ Octave.	Low-intensity noise ranging from approximately 1,500 Hz to 7,500 Hz or 8,000 Hz. Strevens has identified low level resonances at 1,900, 4,000, and 5,000 Hz. Fant suggests the major resonance will occur at 6,000–7,000 Hz and is dependent on the resonance of the air column in the constriction and shallow cavity formed by the lips in front of the upper incisors. Fant suggests that this high frequency resonance will be very low in amplitude and that the /f/ sound is perhaps better described by a broad band noise with no observable resonances.
Lingua-Alveolar		
/s/ and /z/ are produced with the tongue tip or tongue blade raised to approximate the alveolar ridge. The tongue is grooved forming a narrow air channel down the center of the tongue. The closer approximation to a circular orifice provides a more efficient conversion of aerodynamic power to acoustic power than does the wide but low elliptical orifice required for /f/ and /θ/. Turbulence is generated at the constriction and also at the cutting edge of the upper incisor teeth.	The sound source spectrum is flat from 300–4,000 Hz followed by a 6 dB/octave drop above 4,000 Hz.	Due to an antiresonance around 3,500 Hz, very little energy is observed in the output spectrum below 4,000 Hz. No characteristic resonance pattern but usually a major energy peak between 4,000 and 7,000 Hz.

Table 7-3   (cont.)

Lingua-Palatal

/ʃ/ and /ʒ/ are produced with the blade of the tongue, or the tip and blade approaching the palate approximately where the alveolar ridge joins the hard palate. They require the tongue to be only slightly grooved, providing a larger area for turbulence. The air stream is set into turbulence in the constriction and possibly at the teeth.	Approximately a flat source spectrum (0 dB/octave) from 300–6,000 Hz.	Lowest output energies around 1,600–2,500 Hz. Very sharp cut-off of high frequency energies around 7,000 Hz. Most of the fricative energy is in the lower frequencies. Strevens and Heinz and Stevens show the first two resonances occurring at about 2,500 and 5,000 Hz, respectively.

Glottal

/h/ is produced by increasing the airflow through the larynx and creating turbulence within a partially constricted glottis.	Broad spectrum noise.	The output spectrum ranges from about 400 Hz to 6,500 Hz. Several peaks occur in the output spectrum for /h/, one around 1,000 Hz and another around 1,700 Hz. Since the whole vocal tract resonates during /h/, lower frequency energies are resonated than for fricatives with more forward places of articulation. There are no physiological constraints placed on the tongue during /h/, providing maximal coarticulation with the following vowel. Hence, the resonances for /h/ may closely approximate those for the following vowel.

Figure 7-17 shows the spectral distributions for all of the fricatives of English, as produced by a single talker.

As with vowel productions, the acoustical resonances during fricative production are dependent upon the place of major vocal tract constriction, the degree of constriction, and the degree of lip rounding. These physiological variables interact to determine the precise acoustical filtering properties of the vocal tract. Stevens (1969) has speculated on the relative contribution to the total resonance pattern of the vocal tract volumes in front of, and behind, the point of major vocal tract constriction during fricative production. For the velar, palatal, and alveolar places of articulation, he demonstrates that it is possible to have, in the front and back cavities, resonances that are coincident in frequency and remarkably overlapping. Such resonance char-

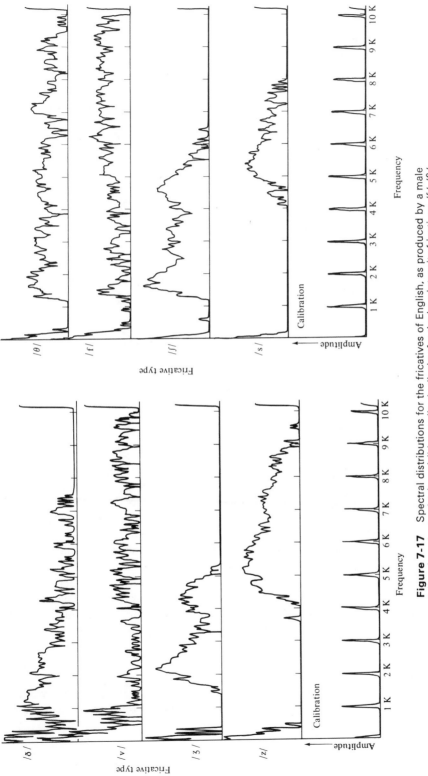

Figure 7-17 Spectral distributions for the fricatives of English, as produced by a male talker. In order to obtain a visible amplitude display for the low intensity fricatives /f/ /θ/ /V/ /ð/, their amplitudes were increased 22 dB more than were the other fricatives.

acteristics would naturally enhance the acoustic output at the resonance frequency. Since such acoustical overlapping is not possible during interdental and labiodental articulations, due to the small volumes anterior to the source, it is interesting to speculate on the role of the front and back cavities during fricative production. It is known that the greatest amplitudes of energy arise from the front cavity resonances. These energies could be enhanced by frequency-overlapping resonances in the cavity behind the constriction.

Harris (1958), has shown that some fricatives (/s/ and /ʃ/, /z/ and /ʒ/) can be differentiated by adult listeners solely on the basis of the spectral properties of the noises produced. That is, the overall spectral characteristics (including intensity, duration, voicing, and spectrum) of /s/ and /ʃ/ and /z/ and /ʒ/ are sufficiently different to allow listeners to discriminate their respective phonemic qualities. However, the fricative pairs /f/ and /θ/, and /v/ and /ð/ are similar enough in place and manner of production to defy consistent phonemic identification on the basis of their overall spectral characteristics. Harris found that listeners relied on the changing formant structures in adjacent vowels to determine whether they heard /f/ or /θ/. Recall that the second formant in vowel production is largely determined by tongue placement. If the tongue is moving toward an interdental /θ/, the vocalic transition is determined by different physiological constraints than are those associated with the labiodental /f/ where the tongue is free to move toward the following sound. The slight changes in the vocalic transitions which result provide sufficient cues to allow the listener to discriminate /f/ from /θ/ or /v/ from /ð/. The fricative noises cue manner of production, while the vocalic transitions and the presence or absence of voicing cue phoneme identification.

Abbs and Minifie (1969), have shown that five-year-old children can easily discriminate among fricative pairs. Children find it easiest to discriminate fricatives that differ in both voicing and spectrum. Fricatives that differ only in spectrum or voicing are more difficult to discriminate. Fricatives that are similar in both spectrum and voicing are the most difficult to differentiate.

The preceding discussion suggests that the acoustical properties of fricatives are dependent upon the physiological aspects of production. Perception of these elements is tied to their acoustical properties. It should be clear from the discussion of coarticulation in Chapter 5 that changes in the precise place of articulation or timing of articulatory movements will have an effect on the acoustical properties of fricatives.

Stops

Some consonant sounds are produced with the vocal tract entirely occluded. When both the oral and nasal cavities are occluded, stop sounds are produced.

There are six stop consonants in English, three are voiced (b, d, g) and three are voiceless (p, t, k). In addition to voicing, stop consonant sounds may differ in the place of articulation: /p/ and /b/ are called bilabial stops because the vocal tract is occluded at the lips; /t/ and /d/ are called alveolar stops because the vocal tract is occluded when the tongue tip and blade contact the alveolar ridge and upper teeth respectively; and /k/ and /g/ are called velar stops because the vocal tract is occluded when the dorsum of the tongue contacts the velum (soft palate and uvula).

Oropharyngeal air pressure

When the vocal tract is occluded at some point within the oral cavity the air escaping from the lungs is trapped behind the constriction (in the oral and pharyngeal air spaces), thereby causing a build-up of oropharyngeal air pressure. When the occlusion is removed by movement of the blocking articulators, the airway becomes open again and air can flow. The air release will be controlled jointly by the pressure drop across the constriction and the size and shape of the orifice at the constriction. Recall from the preceding discussion of fricative sounds that any time the pressure drop across a narrow orifice is sufficiently large, turbulence will be created in the air stream (acoustic noise is generated). Such is the case at the moment of occlusion release. The large pressure drop across the narrow orifice causes rapid particle streaming which becomes turbulent. As the opening is enlarged, the pressure difference across the constriction is reduced and the flow is less turbulent. When the orifice is sufficiently large and the pressure drop sufficiently small, turbulence ceases. Thus, a stoppage of the air stream causes a build-up of oropharyngeal air pressure, which in turn acts as a driving pressure upon the opening of the vocal tract at the constriction, which produces a noise at the point of constriction due to turbulent particle streaming. The duration and intensity of the noise is dependent upon the time-varying size of the orifice (which controls the pressure discharge) and the rate at which the lung resupplies air to the oropharyngeal region.

The oropharyngeal air pressure will be markedly influenced by the duration of vocal tract occlusion and the presence or absence of voicing. If it is assumed that a constant volume-rate of air flow escapes from the lung throughout the duration of a stop sound, then increasing the duration of occlusion would increase the amount of oropharyngeal air pressure.[7] Arkebauer et al. (1967) have shown that peak intraoral air pressure during voiceless stop consonants

---

[7] Obviously there are finite limits to the amount of time the vocal tract may be occluded and retain a constant volume rate of air flow. In the extreme case, when oropharyngeal air pressure equals intrapulmonic pressure, air flow ceases. For the relatively short closure durations during stop consonant production, the assumption of a constant volume flow rate seems reasonable.

is consistently greater than that for voiced stop consonants. Sharf (1962) has shown that the closure durations of voiceless stop sounds are typically greater than for their voiced cognates. He also found that the alveolar stop sounds had shorter closure durations than did the bilabial and velar stop gestures.

It is safe to conclude that closure duration influences the build-up of oropharyngeal air pressure during the production of stop consonant sounds. Additionally, the pressure differences may stem from net differences in the overall size of the vocal tract. Slis and Cohen (1969), Slis (1970), Rothenberg (1968), and Chomsky and Halle (1968) all have speculated that differential constriction of the pharyngeal constrictor muscles could result in smaller pharyngeal air spaces during voiceless than voiced stop productions. If a larger pharyngeal air space existed, they reasoned, it would take a longer period of time to reduce the transglottal pressure drop to a point where voicing would be impossible. Forward movement of the tongue root (Kent and Moll, 1969, Hudgins and Stetson, 1935, Perkell, 1968) and the elevation and lowering of the larynx are physiological determinants of differential oral pressure differences coincident with cognate stop consonant productions. The net effect of increasing the closure duration during voiceless stop sounds, of movement of the tongue root and larynx, and of permitting a larger percentage of the respiratory driving force to work against the constriction, is to provide a greater oropharyngeal air pressure during voiceless stop sound production than during voiced stops. As far as producing acoustic energy is concerned, the most important physiological variable is the amount of oropharyngeal air pressure at the moment of occlusion release.

Transient sound source

The sound source for stop sounds is essentially transient (short-lived), resulting from the turbulence created by the pressure discharge during the occlusion release. Thus, those stop sounds with greater pressure drops across the occlusion will result in noise bursts of longer duration and greater intensity than will stop sounds with smaller pressure drops. This is the reason that voiceless stop sounds are produced with greater duration noise bursts and higher sound energies than are their voiced cognates.

If the impounded air pressure in the portion of vocal tract behind the constriction is released through the oral cavity and lips, the stop sound is called an *explosive* or *plosive*. However, if the release of air pressure is achieved by lowering the velum and allowing air to flow through the nasal cavity, the stop sound is called an *implosive*. Compare the production of the /t/ sound in the word short /ʃɔrt/ with the /t/ sound in the word "shortening" /ʃɔrtnɪŋ/. In the latter example, the /t/ is imploded, while in the former example, it is exploded. It is not required that a nasal sound follow the stop sound in order for it to be imploded. For example, the final sound in the sentence "Put the ball on top," is typically imploded.

Aspirated vs unaspirated stops

The amount of air which is exploded during consonant production will vary from one phonetic context to another. Phoneticians have come to refer to exploded consonant sounds as *aspirated* or *unaspirated*, depending on the amount of air exploded. Technically, aspiration refers to the supplementation of the transient noise burst of an exploded stop consonant by glottal frication (the /h/ sound). For example, the initial sound in the word *pot* /pʰɑt/ is aspirated, while the same sound in the word "spot" /spɑt/ is unaspirated. In both words the sound is identified as a voiceless bilabial stop sound that is exploded. In the first example, the transient noise release is supplemented by glottal frication. In the second example no glottal frication occurs.

In many languages the amount of aspiration which occurs during the production of a stop sound will determine its phonemic identification. For example, in Korean an unaspirated /t/ sound is a different sound than an aspirated /t/ sound. In stressed syllables English speakers tend to give additional emphasis to stop sounds by supplementing the transient release with a glottal fricative /h/. Indeed, many phoneticians transcribe aspirated consonant sounds with an /h/ superscript, as in the transcription for the word curling /kʰɝlɪŋ/. In English, the presence or absence of aspiration on stop sounds is not crucial to the categorical perception of phonemic quality. Rather, aspiration represents an allophonic variation.

The physiological aspects of production and phonetic context play important roles in determining whether or not a stop sound will be aspirated. For example, in those phonetic contexts with successive stop sounds where the first stop sound is produced with a more posterior place of articulation than the second, the release of pressure behind the first constriction (posterior constriction) simply adds to the pressure being built up behind the second constriction (anterior constriction), so that no noise burst will occur in the first stop sound. In the word "actor" /æktɚ/ or the word "footplate" /fʊtpleɪt/ the first of two successive stops is imploded while the second is exploded and aspirated. In the opposite situation, where the first of two successive stops is produced with a more anterior place of articulation, both of the stop sounds will be exploded. In this case, however, the initial sound usually is produced with less plosion than is the second. The initial sound is produced with the driving pressure between two constrictions, while the second is produced with the pressure behind the posterior constriction supplemented by the glottal fricative. This difference can be appreciated by comparing the amounts of aspiration on the adjacent stops sounds in the word "cupcake" /kʌpkeɪk/.

Source spectrum

The spectral characteristics at the mouth opening of stop sounds are dependent upon the acoustical properties of the sound source(s) and the time-varying changes in the three-dimensional geometry of the vocal tract, primarily those portions of the vocal tract anterior to the turbulent source(s). Fant (1960) suggests that a broad band noise spectrum which decreases in amplitude at about 6 dB/octave is an appropriate first order approximation of the turbulent source spectrum during stop sound production. This argument suggests that the noise sources for all stop sounds are similar, no matter whether those noises are produced bilabially, alveolarly, or velarly. In all cases the noise source is a broad band noise with a little more energy available at lower frequencies than at higher frequencies. The 6 dB/octave slope is characteristic of impulse excitations where volume flow rate increases from zero to a large value almost instantaneously. Ideally, an impulse is of infinitely short duration which yields an energy distribution of infinite bandwidth. That is to say, that energy is organized in the time domain, but not in the frequency domain (Halle et al., 1957). The effects of occlusion release during stop sound production cause rapid changes in vocal tract shape, thereby rapidly changing the acoustical filter functions over time. The acoustical result is that concentrations of noise energy in the frequency domain (which depend on the resonating characteristics of the vocal tract) will vary as a function of time. One must conclude, therefore, that for the noise bursts during stop consonants, a modicum of organization exists in both the frequency and time domains.

Output spectrum of noise burst

The filter function of the vocal tract during the noise burst of stop sounds is dependent upon the volumes within the vocal tract which participate in resonation of the source energies. These volumes are largely determined by the place of vocal tract occlusion. Halle et al., (1957) have shown the concentration of output energies during /k/ and /g/ to be in the intermediate frequency regions of 1,500 to 4,000 Hz, whereas the major energies on /t/ and |d| usually fall above 4,000 Hz with the exception of a lesser concentration of energy around 500 Hz. The major resonances associated with these stops are related to the length of vocal tract anterior to the noise source location. The velar or palatal points of constriction for /k/ or /g/ provide a reasonably long tube anterior to the source, which yields lower frequency resonances than occur for /t/ and /d/ which are produced with an alveolar place of constriction. The smaller tube length anterior to the alveolar ridge produces natural resonances at higher frequencies. As a result the noise bursts for alveolar stops have predominate energy distributions at higher frequencies than do velar stops. Hence, alveolar stops sound higher in "pitch" than do velar stops.

The noise bursts associated with bilabial stops have been shown to have the primary concentration of energy in the lower frequency regions (500 to 1,500 Hz). Since there is essentially no vocal tract anterior to the lips that can provide such low frequency resonances, one must postulate a different resonance system. The best theory appears to be one which argues that the impulse excitation from rapid lip opening causes the entire vocal tract to resonate, which accounts for the lower frequency concentrations of noise energy. The initial impulse excitation from the noise burst created by the rapid discharge of pressure at the lips is, of course, immediately supplemented by glottal frication to provide for the 20 to 80 msec noise burst on the voiceless bilabial stop /p/.

The spectral characteristics of bilabial stop sounds raise the question as to the acoustical contribution of those portions of the vocal tract behind the constrictions during the production of alveolar and velar stop sounds. Certainly those portions of the vocal tract can resonate during stop sound production since sound travels in all directions from a source. It is assumed that the amplitudes of those resonances will be small at the mouth opening, since the amount of acoustical resistance between those "back" cavities and the mouth opening is large during stop sounds. As the degree of constriction is lessened upon occlusion release, the back cavities could play a more important role; partly because of the smaller acoustical resistances between those cavities and the mouth opening and partly because of the presence of glottal frication.

The very rapid changes in vocal tract shape upon occlusion release cause concomitant changes in the acoustical filtering. Therefore, the precise acoustical nature of the noise bursts is dependent upon the place of articulation and the speed and extent of occlusion release.

In Chapter 5 the concept of coarticulation was developed in some detail. It should, therefore, not be difficult to understand that phonetic context will markedly alter the precise place of articulation during stop sound production. The contrast between the place of constriction during the production of /g/ in the words "geese" and "gone", demonstrates the palatal and velar places of articulation for that sound. Since the place of articulation is the physiological determinant of the filter length during turbulent sound production, dynamic changes in the place of articulation will cause dynamic changes in the acoustical spectrum at the mouth opening (Fischer-Jorgenson, 1954, Halle et al., 1957).

Vocalic transitions

It is not reasonable to talk about stop consonants as if they existed in isolation. Usually they appear in a phonetic context adjacent to vowel sounds. The acoustical result of moving from a vocal tract position required for vowel production to a vocal tract position for stop consonant production is the occurrence of vocalic transitions. These are changing bands of formant energies which result as a consequence of maintaining voicing during changes in vocal tract shape. Thus, any time the speaker moves his articulators from a vowel position to a consonant position or from a consonant position to a vowel position, vocalic transitions occur. The direction and extent of formant frequency change during vocalic transitions is dependent upon the location of the articulators prior to movement and the distance to be traveled. Vocalic transitions are very rapid adjacent to stop sounds because the movements toward and away from stop sound articulations are very rapid. However, vocalic transitions from one vowel sound to another (as in diphthongs) are relatively slow. Many investigators have shown that vocalic transitions are important cues to the perception of stop consonants. The rate (speed) of vocalic transition tells the listener whether he hears a stop sound, a semi-vowel, or a diphthong (Liberman et al., 1956). The direction of transition (rising or falling), the extent of transition, and the frequencies within the transitional formants are important perceptual cues which stem from changes in the place of articulation (DeLattre, et al., 1955, Öhman, 1966).

Voice onset time

In Chapter 5 we described the differences which can occur in phoneme production from one phonetic context to another. This phenomenon is well illustrated by comparing a voiced stop consonant sound which appears in an initial position with the same sound appearing in the middle of a word. In the word-initial position both "voiced" and "voiceless' stops are produced with a silent closure duration. In the word-middle position, the closure durations are indeed voiced or voiceless. This variance in the "voicing" properties of voiced stop sounds has caused many linguists to avoid using the voiced-voiceless distinction for describing differences among stop consonants. Rather, they use a tense-lax (fortis-lenis) distinction. One of the primary attributes of the tense stop consonant sound is the build-up of intraoral air pressure which causes longer noise bursts than for lax stop sounds. In addition, the glottis is active sooner on lax stop sounds than on tense stops. For example, the longer duration noise burst on tense stops requires that the turbulent pressure discharge from the oral cavity be supplemented by glottal frication. The physiological requirements for creating turbulence at the glottis effectively constrains the vocal folds from initiating periodic vibration. Thus, the onset of voicing is delayed in such instances. During the production of lax stop consonants, where the presence of turbulence is not crucial, the larynx is not thusly constrained and is free to begin periodic vibration (voicing) sooner than during tense stops. Lisker and Abramson (1965) have shown that for word-initial English stop consonants, the voice onset time for lax stops (voiced stops) precedes occlusion release by 35 to 195 msec. For unaspirated tense stops (unaspirated voiceless stops) the voice onset time occurs from 0 to 50 msec after occlusion release; while aspirated tense stops have ranges of voice onset time from 35 to 135 msec after the occlusion release. The perceptual significance of these data lies in an understanding of the importance of voice onset time rather than the presence or absence of voicing in the determination of whether the element was "voiced" or "voiceless."

Summary of perceptual cues for stops

The following acoustical parameters appear to be important cues to the listener in identifying stop consonants in vowel-consonant-vowel environments:

(1) Rate, degree and extent of vocalic transition from V to C

(2) Duration of the closed phase (stop phase)

(3) Presence or absence of voicing during the closed phase

(4) Voice onset time

(5) Duration of the noise burst

(6) Spectral characteristics of the noise burst

(7) Rate, degree and extent of vocalic transition from C to V

Figure 7-18 taken from Slis and Cohen (1969) provides a schematic representation of the temporal and spatial distribution (frequency domain) of the acoustical cues associated with stop consonants. It is curiously interesting to speculate why the overall durations of voiced and voiceless stop

Figure 7-18 Temporal-spatial patterns of voiced and voiceless stops. [After I. H. Slis and A. Cohen, "On the complex regulating the voiced-voiceless distinction II," Lang. and Speech, 11 (1969), Fig. 15. Reprinted by permission of the authors and the publisher.]

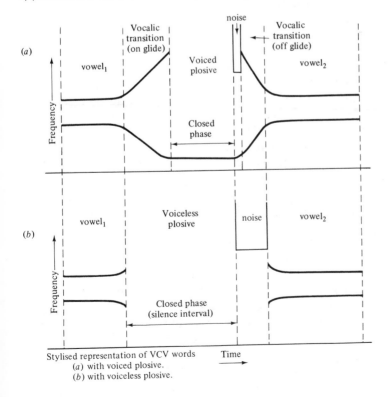

Stylised representation of VCV words   Time
(a) with voiced plosive.
(b) with voiceless plosive.

sounds are similar, whereas the durations of the individual subphonemic segments are dissimilar. The multiplicity of cues which may be used in phoneme identification during stop consonants raises the question of the relative contribution of each cue in consonant perception. As yet we do not know which cues are the most important to listeners. Suffice it to say at this point that listeners use whatever cues are available in a given situation. Since any one of the cues might be sufficient for proper phoneme identification, the presence of multiple cues provides sufficient phonetic redundancy to enable listeners to optimally identify phonemes even in difficult listening situations such as in the presence of noise.

Affricates

Two consonant sounds in English are produced with an occlusion of the vocal tract, which, upon release, is immediately followed by a sustained turbulent sound. These sounds are produced in such a way as to combine the elements of a stop sound with the elements of a fricative. These sounds, called *affricates*, are produced with the major vocal tract constriction at the posterior border of the alveolar ridge. The voiceless affricate /t∫/, as in *church* /t∫ɜt∫/, is produced as a combination of the voiceless alveolar stop sound /t/ and the voiceless linguapalatal fricative /∫/. The voiced affricate /dʒ/, as in *judge* /dʒʌdʒ/, is produced as a combination of the voiced alveolar stop /d/ linguapalatal fricative /ʒ/. The occlusion of the vocal tract at the alveolar ridge during the initial portion of the affricate causes a build-up of air pressure within the oropharyngeal cavity. Upon the release of the occlusion, the escaping air pressure creates a turbulence in the air stream at the point of constriction (alveolar ridge), which produces a noisy sound. If the turbulent sound were solely related to the discharge of a pent-up air pressure resulting from the short duration stoppage of air flow during the initial phase of the element, then a stop consonant would be produced, since stop consonants are characterized by a short duration stoppage followed by a short duration noise burst. However, during the production of affricates, the overpressure within the oropharyngeal cavity is sustained for a longer period of time by resupplying the air which escapes from the oral cavity with more air from the lung. The resulting sound is composed of a short duration closed period (stoppage of air flow) followed by a moderately long period of frication.

The characteristics of the noise sources for affricate sounds and the nature of the acoustical filtering are similar to those discussed previously for fricative and stop sounds. The logic of those arguments can be reasonably extended to accommodate the production of affricate sounds. It is important to realize that for stop sounds and affricate sounds the temporal patterning of articulatory events is highly constrained. Even slight variations in the temporal patterning of the resulting acoustical events will result in misperceptions by listeners. Therefore, the durational patterns of stops and affricates are less variant than are the durational patterns of continuant sounds such as vowels and fricatives, where perception is not as dependent upon durational cues as is the case for stops and affricates.

Non-nasal Semi-vowels

All semi-vowels are produced with vibration of the vocal folds and, hence, are voiced sounds. They are continuant sounds since there is no momentary stoppage of the air stream as in stops or affricates. They are called consonants because there is a greater degree of vocal tract constriction than for vowel elements. They are called semi-vowels because the constriction is not as great as that for other consonant elements. They could as validly be called semi-consonants. Occasionally these sounds are called glides, since their production requires the tongue to move from one position within the vocal tract to another.[8] The four non-nasal semi-vowels are:

/j/, as in *y*ellow /jɛlo/, a palatal semi-vowel

/w/, as in *w*eigh /weɪ/, a lip-rounded velar semi-vowel

/r/, as in *r*ed /rɛd/, a lip-rounded retroflex palatal semi-vowel

/l/, as in *l*ull /lʌl/, a lateral alveolar semi-vowel.

/r/ and /l/

The semi-vowels /r/ and /l/ are dependent upon speed of vocal tract change for proper production. The /r/ sound is usually produced with some degree of lip rounding. The position of the tongue varies considerably with phonetic context. The /r/ in *r*abbit is a palatal retroflex, the /r/ being produced with the tongue tip curled up and back within the oral cavity. The /r/ in any /kr/, /gr/, /rk/, or /rg/ combination is coarticulated in such a way that the major vocal tract constriction during the /r/ sound is a velar constriction. The /r/ in any /tr/, /dr/, /rt/, or /rd/ context is coarticulated with the alveolar stop and results in the /r/ being produced with the major constriction near the alveolar ridge.

The /l/ sound is the only lateral sound in English. The tongue tip is in contact with the alveolar ridge and the air is allowed to pass on both sides of the tongue. The exact position of the constriction is dependent upon phonetic context. When the /l/ sound occurs adjacent to a back vowel, the tongue tip is placed against the hard palate, producing what is called a "dark /l/." When the /l/ sound is adjacent to a front vowel the place of articulation for the /l/

---

[8] The exception to this statement is /l/ which is not technically a glide, being produced with the tongue held in position on the alveolar ridge.

is on the anterior portion of the alveolar ridge, near the upper incisors. The sound produced with an alveolar place of articulation is called a "light /l/." The distinction between the light /l/ and the dark /l/ can be appreciated by comparing the sound qualities of the /l/s in the word *lily* and the word *lawyer*. As with vowel sounds, semi-vowels are produced by acoustically filtering the spectral characteristics of the glottal sound source. Therefore, if the three-dimensional shape of the mechanical acoustical filter (vocal tract) is altered dynamically during the production of these elements, then the spectral characteristics of the acoustical signal at the mouth opening will vary as a function of time.

Fant (1970) presents X-ray tracings of the vocal tract configurations during the steady-state portions of the /r/ and /l/ sounds produced both as palatalized and non-palatalized sounds (see Figure 7-19). The resonances associated with these vocal tract configurations are shown in Table 7-4.

Table 7-4 Formant patterns for /l/ and /r/.

		Non-palatalized	Palatalized
/l/	F_1	350	230
	F_2	750	1,600
	F_3	2,000	2,300
/r/	F_1	500	400
	F_2	1,000	1,500
	F_3	1,800	2,200

Examination of the X-rays shown in Figure 7-19 reveals that the articulatory constriction for the /l/ sound is slightly more forward than for the /r/ sound. Thus, the first major resonance, which is largely determined by the volume behind the constriction, is lower for /l/ than /r/. In addition, the forward movement of the tongue root during the production of the palatalized versions of these sounds causes the pharyngeal volume to increase, thereby decreasing the frequency of F_1 from that obtained in the non-palatalized version. Fant describes F_2 as a half-wavelength resonance of the interior cavities (primarily controlled by the tongue position) and F_3 as substantially dependent upon resonances in the anterior mouth cavity (in front of the alveolar constriction and therefore largely controlled by the lip configuration).

Figure 7-20 shows the schematic representations of the dynamically changing formant frequency patterns which were most often identified by listeners as specific semi-vowels plus a vowel. The semi-vowels are represented by a short duration steady-state portion and a medium duration transition period. The vowels are represented by the relatively long steady-state portion at the end of each utterance. Listeners require the steady-state portions of the

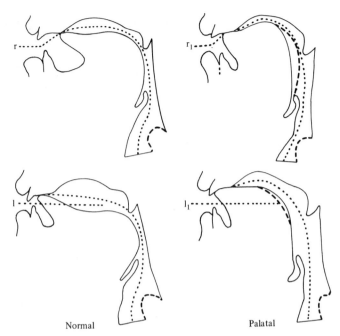

Normal   Palatal

Figure 7-19 Tracings of lateral head X-rays during alveolar and palatal articulations for /r/ and /l/. [*After G. Fant,* Acoustic Theory of Speech Production (*The Hague: Mouton & Co., Publishers, 1970*), *p. 163. Reprinted by permission of the author and the publisher.*]

Figure 7-20 Simulated spectra for the semivowels /r/, l, j, w/. [*After J. D. O'Connor et al., "Acoustic cues for the perception of initial /w, j, r, l/ in English."* Word, *13 (1957), 24-43, Fig. 1.*]

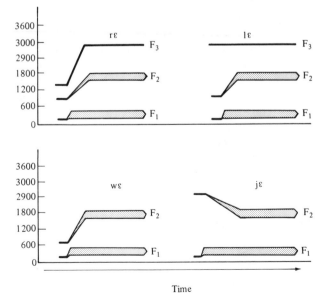

Time

/l/ and /r/ sounds to be of approximately 50 msec duration if appropriate identifications of these elements are to be made (O'Conner et al., 1957, and Lisker, 1957). Shorter durations of the steady-state portion resulted in the simulated utterances being perceived as a stop consonant plus a semi-vowel.

The spectral distribution of energies in the steady-state portions of the semi-vowels (initial portions) is dependent upon the cavity configurations as described above. As the articulators move from the positions required during the steady-state portions of the semi-vowels to the positions required for the following vowels, the filter functions of the vocal tract change in dynamic fashion. Therefore, changes in the frequency of the first formant are the result of a complex interaction of changes in laryngeal height, place of articulation, degree of vocal tract constriction, changes in pharyngeal volume, lip rounding, etc. The determinants of F_1 are thus very similar to those described when changing from one vowel to another. Changes in F_2 appear to be largely controlled by changes in the place and degree of vocal tract constriction. F_3 appears to be primarily related to the degree of lip rounding. O'Conner et al. (1957) suggest that proper identification of differences between /l/ and /r/ requires information from the first three formants. Changes in the first two formants are somewhat similar for /l/ and /r/. However, formant three undergoes a marked upward shift in frequency during /r/, but remains relatively constant during the production of /l/. The reason for this difference appears to be related to the fact that the /r/ sound is begun with lip rounding while the /l/ sound is usually produced with the lips spread (except when coarticulated with a following lip-rounded vowel). The effect of lip rounding has been described in greater detail earlier in this chapter as causing a decrease in the natural resonant frequencies of the vocal tract. During the production of semi-vowels, a low resonance frequency for F_3 is associated with lip rounding. Therefore, as the lips move from the lip-rounded configuration of /r/ to the lip-spread configuration of the following vowel which has a lip-spread configuration, a marked increase in the frequency of the third formant occurs. Since /l/ is produced with the lips in a spread position, little change will occur in F_3 when moving from /l/ to an unrounded vowel. The presence of change in the third formant appears to be an important perceptual cue to listeners in differentiating /l/ from /r/ (see Figure 7-20). One might expect quite the opposite effect if comparing the utterances /ru/ and /lu/. Thus, the acoustical variations during the production of semi-vowels are influenced profoundly by physiological coarticulation phenomena which vary with phonetic context. That is, the phonetic environment will determine the requirements for sequential alteration of vocal tract shape.

In addition, the duration of the transition appears to be systematically longer for the /r/ than for /l/. The transition durations for /l/ appear to range from about 70 to 100 msec. The transitions for /r/ can be as long as 300 msec. before significantly altering the perception of /r/ (O'Conner et al., 1957).

/j/ and /w/

The /j/ is produced with a high front tongue position very similar to that used for the production of the vowel /i/ as in *e*ach. The /j/ is produced by moving rapidly from the /i/ tongue position to the articulatory position of another vowel. For example, in the phrase "I am what I am," a slow tongue movement from the final articulatory position during the diphthong /aɪ/ to the articulatory position for /æ/ yields an acoustical signal which is perceived as /aɪ æm wɑt aɪ æm/ whereas a rapid tongue movement will yield an acoustical signal perceived as /aɪ jæm wɑt aɪ jæm/ which would sound like Popeye saying "I yam what I yam." The difference between the semi-vowel /j/ and a diphthong with an initial /i/ or /ɪ/ element is primarily related to the temporal sequencing of muscular events regulating the speed of changing vocal tract shape. A more rapidly changing shape will produce a semi-vowel, whereas a more slowly changing shape will produce a diphthong.

The production of the semi-vowel /w/ is likewise similar to the production of a diphthong with an initial /u/ element. The shape of the vocal tract for /w/ is very similar to that for /u/: a high back elevation of the dorsum of the tongue toward the velum with a marked concomitant lip rounding. With the /u/, that vocal tract configuration is sustained for a relatively long period of time. During /w/ the vocal tract shape is rapidly altered toward the position required for an adjacent following vowel. If the change takes place slowly, the sounds are perceived as a diphthong (u + vowel). Again the temporal sequencing of events distinguishes between the semi-vowel /w/ plus a vowel and the diphthongization of (u + v).

The high degree of constriction within the vocal tract during the initial, short duration, steady-state portion of the semi-vowels /w/ and /j/ yield low F_1 values similar to those obtained during the production of the vowels /u/ and /i/, respectively. The low resonances are related to the marked degree of vocal tract constriction, and the relatively large pharyngeal air spaces.

The first formant for both /w/ and /j/ is about 240 Hz. Since O'Conner et al., (1957) have shown that listeners are able to perceptually differentiate /w/ and /j/ from each other and from other sounds in English when presented with only the first two formants, this discussion will be restricted to the acoustical regulation of F_1 and F_2 for these sounds.

The duration of transition is approximately 100 msec for both /w/ and /j/. The frequency for the second formant transition for /j/ must be above 2,300 Hz for proper perception by listeners. O'Conner et al., (1957) have shown that context dependent transitions from 2,280 to 3,600 Hz were all adequately perceived as /j/. The starting frequency of the second formant transition is usually below 600 Hz when producing /w/. During the formant transitional phase of these sounds, the direction and extent of transition is dependent upon the phonetic context. As seen in Figure 7-20, the transition from /w/ to /ɛ/ is greater in extent than the transition from /j/ to /ɛ/ since the articulatory position of the tongue for the /j/ is more similar to that for /ɛ/ than is the the articulatory position for /w/.

Nasal Semi-vowels

Three semi-vowels of English are produced with complete occlusion of the oral cavity. They are /m/, /n/ and /ŋ/, voiced continuants produced with an open velopharyngeal port which provides a communicating airway from the pharynx through the nasal cavities. Since they are produced with an open port, there is relatively little constriction of the airway from the glottis to the nares. Because the length of the air tube is longer from the glottis to the nares than from the glottis to the lips, lower resonances occur during the production of nasal sounds than during vowel sounds. The soft linings of the nasal cavities cause increased damping of the acoustic signal. Therefore, the amplitudes of the resonances (formant amplitudes) will be smaller and the bandwidths of the resonance curves will be broader (formant bandwidths) for nasal semi-vowels than for vowels. The overall intensity of nasal sounds is less than the intensity of non-nasal vowels. This reduction in intensity has caused many linguists to refer to these sounds as possessing a "nasal murmur." The classification of nasal semi-vowels is according to the place of oral cavity constriction:

/m/ as in mummy /mʌmɪ/, is a bilabial nasal semi-vowel

/n/ as in Nancy /nænsɪ/, is an alveolar nasal semi-vowel

/ŋ/ as in uncle /ʌŋkl/, is a velar nasal semi-vowel.

The place of constriction within the oral cavity determines the size of the oral cul-de-sac which will function as an acoustic resonator during the production of nasal semi-vowels.

When the oral constriction is near the velum as in /ŋ/, very little oral cul-de-sac is present and the resonance tube consists of the pharyngeal and nasal cavities, providing resonance characteristics similar to those during normal vowel production (i. e., a communicating airway from the glottal sound source to the opening of the resonance tube, with relatively little constriction along the length of the tube. Fant (1970) has shown that the fixed formants of the pharyngeal and nasal cavities occur at approximately 250, 1,000, 2,000, 3,000 and 4,000 Hz, with the lowest formant having the dominant intensity.

For both /m/ and /n/ the size of the oral cavity behind the constriction is substantial enough to have a significant effect on the nasal resonances. Since the primary cavity affected by the oral "side branch" is the pharyngeal airspace, the major acoustic effect is a lowering of F_1 due to the increased volume of the pharynx. During nasals, F_1 is usually below 250 Hz. In addition, antiresonances are present which affect the acoustic signal. The location of these antiresonances in the frequency domain is determined jointly by the place of oral cavity constriction and the amount of velopharyngeal opening. Antiresonances serve to decrease the spectral energies at specific frequency locations, which cumulatively have the effect of reducing the total amplitude of the sound generated.

The antiresonances during nasal sound production have the effect of reducing and sometimes eliminating from the acoustic signal some of the low intensity formants described above. That is, a major resonance and an antiresonance can occur at the same frequency, which has the effect of cancelling the resonance. Hattori, Yamamoto, and Fujimura (1958) have shown that nasal vowels are characterized by an increase in energy below 300 Hz, an antiresonance around 500 Hz, and a decrease in interformant fill from 1,000 to 2,500 Hz. The predominant effect of nasalization is a reduction in overall amplitude of the vowel sounds. Similar results have been shown by Curtis, (1942), Joos (1948), and House (1957).

Cooper (1952), Malecot (1956), and House (1957) have shown that the formant transitions adjacent to nasal sounds provide significant auditory cues for differentiating among the nasal consonants. The presence of a "nasal murmur" may tell the listener he hears a nasal sound, but the formant transitions preceding and following the murmur tell him which nasal he hears. The bilabial nasal is produced with no encumbrance on the tongue, so the tongue is free to maximally coarticulate during the production of adjacent phonemes. The alveolar and velar nasals require involvement of the apical and dorsal tongue articulators, respectively, thereby inhibiting their freedom to coarticulate during the production of adjacent phonemes. The physiological constraints placed on these articulators during the production of nasal sounds have an effect on the filter functions of the vocal tract preceding or following the production of the nasal. The movement toward a place of occlusion (or away from a place of occlusion) by an articulator results in a changing formant frequency pattern. The specific frequencies of the formants, and their direction and extent of change over time are acoustic cues used by listeners to identify the place of vocal tract constriction. Thus, the formant patterns in the surrounding acoustic environment plus the presence of a nasal murmur appear to be important cues to the perception of nasals.

During the production of vowel sounds in nasal environments, the effects of coarticulation will cause the vowels to be nasalized. The velum simply does not have enough time to open and close the velopharyngeal port for each phoneme in a string. Therefore, in words like mint, man, moon, and monsoon, the vocalic elements are nasalized. The degree of nasalization is dependent upon the relative amounts of acoustical impedence in the oral and nasal cavities, (determined by degrees of opening in the oral port and nasal port). Low vowels have little oral cavity acoustical impedance, therefore the amount of velopharyngeal opening must be large before these sounds are perceived as excessively nasal. High vowels are produced with larger amounts of oral acoustical impedance, therefore smaller velopharyngeal port openings will result in these sounds being perceived as nasal vowels (Lintz and Sherman, 1961).

IMPACT OF COARTICULATION ON SPEECH ACOUSTICS

To this point, most of the arguments presented in this chapter have been based on the assumption that it is possible to provide acoustical descriptions of individual speech sounds. Only casually have we implied that context-dependent variations in articulatory positioning (and the consequent temporal regulation of articulatory movement) will exert significant influences on the acoustical output associated with each speech sound. As a reader, you need only to review the comprehensive discussion of physiological coarticulation in Chapter 5, and apply that information to the logic of the source-filter theory of speech acoustics presented in this chapter to appreciate that dynamic speech production involves the production of several phones on the same articulatory gestures. Since the particular gestures involved in the production of any given phone will vary slightly from one phonetic context to another, it is not surprising that the absolute acoustical characteristics of the sound produced will also vary. In point of fact, context-dependent variations in articulatory behavior, constrained by the rules of our phonology and the mechanics of our articulatory mechanisms, allow substantial variations in acoustical output to occur—and yet, these variant signals evoke similar perceptual responses. Although it is not the purpose of this chapter to do so, it is provocative to speculate on how much acoustical variance can occur during any given phone, and still result in perceptual invariance. That is, how much does a given phone have to vary in terms of formant frequencies, formant amplitudes, formant bandwidths, overall intensity, fundamental frequency, duration, etc., before it is perceived as a different sound?

You are cautioned as a reader not to apply the information presented in this chapter as the ultimate truth about acoustical phonetics. The information we have provided is intended to be used as a guideline to give you a way of thinking about the relationships between speech physiology and speech acoustics. Obviously, the acoustical descriptions which we have provided must be modified to accommodate the impact of coarticulation during dynamic utterance.

SUPRASEGMENTAL ASPECTS OF SPEECH PRODUCTION

Changes in the intonational patterns of the voice (melody of the voice), changes in linguistic stress (relative emphasis given to syllable within an utterance), and changes in the durational characteristics of utterances (including pausal patterns, tempo and rate of syllable utterance) all assist in providing vocal variety and contribute to the meaningfulness of the message generated. These changes occur at the suprasegmental level, that is, they occur across a number of phonemes. The regulation of the rate of utterance is primarily controlled by the number and extent of the pauses distributed throughout the discourse. Only limited variations in the rate of utterance may be achieved by altering the durational characteristics of the speech sounds themselves. Durationally, the pauses are the most free to vary. When changing the emotionality of the message, changes in all of the suprasegmental parameters interplay to provide the proper emotional "tone" for the message.

Even though a number of investigations have attempted to specify the precise roles played by each of the suprasegmental parameters in oral communication, there is yet little definitive information to that end. For example, differences in type of sentence uttered (interrogative, declarative, exclamative) are encoded within the suprasegmental characteristics of the utterance. It is difficult to consistently specify what these changes will be, since individual speakers tend to individually regulate these parameters when changing the meaning of a sentence spoken aloud. Even so, within broad limits these parameters can be specified for various grammatical configurations (Lieberman, 1967).

The regulation of these suprasegmental parameters provides the variation within the acoustical signal which allows the listener to extract the proper semantic intent of the message. Vanderslice (1968) has suggested that the potential meanings in an ambiguous sentence such as "My English history teacher was pretty" can be sorted out by the listener from changes in the intonation, stress, and durational variations in the utterance.

A CAUTION

Although it is tempting in a chapter such as this to speculate on the perceptual importance of specific acoustic attributes of the speech signal (both segmental and suprasegmental) which might be used by the listener as "cues" for speech perception, one must be cautioned not to do so. The reason for such caution is that the speech signal at the mouth opening is not what is responded to by the listener in speech perception. Quite obviously, the acoustical nature of the speech sounds at the mouth opening of the vocalizer will be modified by the resonating characteristics of the conductive mechanism of the ear of the listener (external auditory meatus, tympanic membrane, ossicular chain and cochlear fluids) prior to being transduced into neural events by the listener. Within the ear, harmonic distortion, difference tones, combination tones, and combination noise bands may be introduced, due to the mechanics of cochlear function, to alter the "raw material" within the speech wave prior to its being neurally encoded for perceptual identification. Since it is the vibratory patterns within the cochlea that are the raw material for neural encoding, one must raise the question of how much influence the distortion products within the conductive mechanism of the ear have on speech perception. Is it possible that we use some of the distortion products as significant cues for the perception of certain speech sounds?

A POINT OF VIEW

There is much within the acoustical signal at the phonemic level (segmental level) and suprasegmental level which assists the listener in decoding the meaning of an intended message. Quite obviously, proper interpretation of a message is partially dependent upon what is brought to the listener by the acoustical signal. However, it is also important that the listener brings an adequate linguistic competence to the listening situation so that he can understand the message. That is, unless the listener understands the rules of the language spoken by the talker, and has had some experience in using the language, it is unlikely that he will be able to interpret correctly the meaning of the utterance. Thus, speech perception is partially dependent upon the acoustical signal and partially dependent upon the language experience of the listener. These concepts will be expanded upon in the following chapters.

REFERENCES

ABBS, M. S. and MINIFIE, F. D. 1969. Effect of acoustic cues in fricatives on perceptual confusions in preschool children. *J. Acoust. Soc. Amer.* 46: 1535–42.

ARKEBAUER, J. H., HIXON, T. J. and HARDY, J. C. 1967. Peak intraoral air pressure during speech. *J. Speech Hear. Research.* 10: 196–208.

CHOMSKY, N. and HALLE, M. 1968. *The Sound Pattern of English.* New York: Harper & Row, Publishers, Inc.

COOPER, F. S., DeLATTRE, P. C., LIBERMAN, A. M. BORST, J. M. and GERSTMAN, L. J. 1952. Some experiments on the perception of synthetic speech sounds. *J. Acoust. Soc. Amer.* 24: 597–606.

CURTIS, J. F. 1942. An experimental study of the wave-composition of nasal voice quality. Ph.D. Thesis. Univ. Iowa.

DELATTRE, P. C., LIBERMAN, A. M. and COOPER, F. S. 1955. Acoustic loci and transitional cues for consonants. *J. Acoust. Soc. Amer.* 27: 769–73.

FISCHER-JORGENSEN, ELI. 1954. Acoustic analysis of stop consonants. *Miscellanea Phonetica.* 11: 42–59.

FANT, G. 1960. *Acoustic Theory of Speech Production.* The Hague: Mouton.

FLANAGAN, J. L. 1958. Some properties of the glottal sound source. *J. Speech Hear. Research.* 1: 99–116.

HALLE, M., HUGHES, G. W. and RADLEY, J. P. A. 1957. Acoustic properties of stop consonants. *J. Acoust. Soc. Amer.* 29: 107–16.

HARRIS, K. S. 1958. Cues for the discrimination of American English fricatives in spoken syllables. *Lang. and Speech.* 1: 1–7.

HATTORI, S., YAMAMOTO, K. and FUJIMURA, O. 1958. Nasalization of vowels in relation to nasals. *J. Acoust. Soc. Amer.* 30: 267–74.

HEINZ, J. M. and STEVENS, K. N. 1961. On the properties of voiceless fricative consonants. *J. Acoust. Soc. Amer.* 33: 589–96.

HOUSE, A. S. 1957. Analog studies of nasal consonants. *J. Speech Hear. Dis.* 22: 190–204.

HOUSE, A. S. 1961. On vowel duration in English. *J. Acoust. Soc. Amer.* 33: 1174–78.

HUDGINS, C. V. and STETSON, R. H. 1935. Voicing of consonants by depression of larynx. *Arch. Neerlandaises Phonet. Exp.* 11: 1–28.

JOOS, M. 1948. Acoustic phonetics. *Suppl. Lang.* 24: 1–136.

KENT, R. D. and MOLL, K. L. 1969. Vocal-tract characteristics of the stop cognates. *J. Acoust. Soc. Amer.* 46: 1549–55.

LIBERMAN, A. M. DELATTRE, P. C., GERSTMAN, L. J. and COOPER, F. S. 1956. Tempo of frequency change as a cue for distinguishing classes of speech sounds. *J. Exp. Psychol.* 52: 127–37.

LIEBERMAN, P. 1967. *Intonation, perception and language.* Res. Monogr. No. 38. Cambridge, Mass.: MIT Press.

LINTZ, L. B. and SHERMAN, D. 1961. Phonetic elements and perception of nasality. *J. Speech Hear. Research.* 4: 381–96.

LISKER, L. 1957. Closure duration and the intervocalic voiced-voiceless distinction in English. *Lang.* 33: 42–49.

LISKER, L. 1957. Minimal cues for separating /w r l y/ in intervocalic position. *Word.* 13: 256–67.

LISKER, L. and ABRAMSON, A. 1965. Voice onset time in the production and perception of English stops. *Status Rep. Speech Res.* New York: Haskins Labs. No. 1, 3.1.

MEYER-EPPLER, W. 1953. Zum erzeugungsmechanismus der geräuschlaute. *Z. Phonetik.* 7: 196–212.

O'Connor, J. D., Gerstman, L. J., Liberman, A. M., DeLattre, P. C. and Cooper, F. S. 1957. Acoustic cues for the perception of initial /w, j, r, l/ in English. *Word*. 13: 24–43.

Öhman, S. E. G. 1966. Coarticulation in VCV utterances: spectrographic measurements. *J. Acoust. Soc. Amer.* 39: 151–68.

Perkell, J. S. 1966. *Physiology of speech production: Results and implications of quantitative cineradiographic study.* Cambridge, Mass.: MIT Press.

Petersen, G. E. 1957. Acoustical properties of speech waves. Part II of Chapter 5 of *Handbook of Speech Pathology* (Edited by Travis, L. E.) New York: Appleton-Century-Crofts, Inc.

Petersen, G. E. 1959. Vowel formant measures. *J. Speech Hear. Research.* 2: 173–83.

Peterson, G. E. and Barney, H. L. 1952. Control methods used in the study of vowels. *J. Acoust. Soc. Amer.* 24: 175–84.

Peterson, G. E. and Shoup, J. E. 1966. The elements of an acoustic phonetic theory. *J. Speech Hear. Research.* 9: 68–99.

Rothenberg, M. 1968. The breath-stream dynamics of simple-released-plosive production. *Bibl. Phonet.* No. 6.

Sharf, D. J. 1962. Duration of post-stress intervocalic stops preceding vowels. *Lang. and Speech.* 5: 26–30.

Slis, I. H. 1970. Articulatory measurements on voiced, voiceless and nasal consonants. *Phonet.* 21: 193–210.

Slis, I. H. and Cohen, A. 1969. On the complex regulating the voiced-voiceless distinction, I and II. *Lang. and Speech.* 11: 80–102, 137–55.

Stetson, R. H. 1951. *Motor Phonetics.* Amsterdam: North-Holland Publishing.

Stevens, K. N. 1969. Acoustical aspects of speech production, pp. 347–55 in *Handbook of Physiology.* Washington D.C.: American Physiological Society.

Stevens, K. N. and House, A. S. 1955. Development of a quantitative description of vowel articulation. *J. Acoust. Soc. Amer.* 27: 484–93.

Stevens, K. N. and House, A. S. 1961. An acoustical theory of vowel production and some of its implications. *J. Speech Hear. Research.*

Strevens, P. 1960. Spectra of fricative noise in human speech. *Lang. and Speech.* 3: 32–49.

Timcke, R., von Leden, H., and Moore, P. 1958. Laryngeal vibrations: Measurements of the glottic wave. Part 1. The normal vibratory cycle. *Arch. Otolaryngol.* 68: 1–19.

Vanderslice, R. 1968. The prosodic component: Lacuna in transformational theory. Oral presentation at a seminar in Computational Linguistics. Rand Corp.

8

ELEMENTS OF
AUDITORY PHYSIOLOGY

Theodore J. Glattke

INTRODUCTION

The auditory system presents a multi-faceted system to the physiologists
who would study it. A complex mechanical link couples air-borne sound to
the sensory receptors for hearing. These are located in a fluid-filled enclosure.
Once stimulated, the receptors may give rise to excitation of several hundred
thousand neural "units" through chemical and/or electrical mediation. Each
advancement in observation techniques has provided new clues as to the
means by which we experience the sensation of hearing, but we are a long
way from a unified concept regarding the mechanisms responsible for pitch,
loudness, and speech perception.

The point of departure for this chapter coincides with Békésy's observations of the ear, beginning in the 1920s. There is a rich history preceding
Békésy, however, and there are a number of excellent reference sources

Much of the form of this review has evolved from discussions with F. B. Simmons,
E. D. Schubert, J. H. Dewson, III, A. Starr, and J. H. Winstead. If the chapter has merit,
much is due to these discussions, though the author alone assumes responsibility for errors
which may be contained herein.

which will provide the student with historical perspective. These include Bast and Anson (1949), Wever (1949), Fletcher (1953), Wever and Lawrence (1954), Békésy (1960), and Zemlin (1968). The present chapter will review briefly the structure and mode of response of the principal elements in the auditory system.

THE EXTERNAL AND MIDDLE EAR STRUCTURES

The *pinna* is the outermost portion of the ear. It is composed of cartilage and ligaments, and is held in position by a number of ligaments and muscles. The cartilage forms several landmarks in the skin covering the pinna. These are identified in Figure 8-1. In humans, the musculature is not of functional advantage. Extrinsic muscles couple the pinna with portions of the *temporal bone* of the skull, and some persons can move their pinnae voluntarily. By contrast, however, the horse uses some ten muscle groups to control orientation of its pinnae, and can move them through wide arcs without changing its head position (Vallancien, 1963).

The largest depression in the pinna, the *concha* (i. e., shell), forms the entrance to the *external auditory meatus*. The foundation for the meatus is cartilage for the outer one-third of its length, and is a hard bony channel for the medial two-thirds. In man, its length is approximately 2.5 cm, and its diameter is about 0.7 cm. The walls of the meatus are slightly concave, with the smallest lumen occurring near the border of the bony and cartilagenous portions. The meatus curves slightly downward, and it contains a number of hair follicles and cells which secrete *cerumen*, a wax-like substance which serves to moisten the skin of the meatus and reduce the possibility of foreign body intrusion.

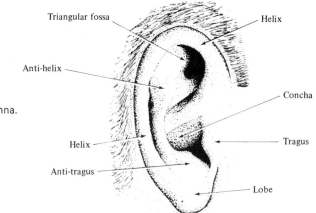

Figure 8-1   The human pinna.

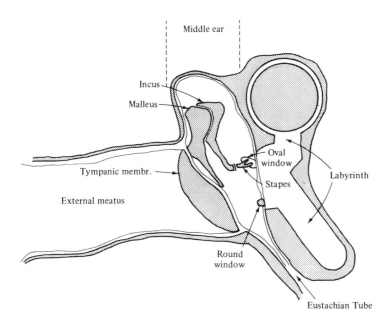

Labels on figure: Middle ear, Incus, Malleus, Tympanic membr., External meatus, Oval window, Stapes, Labyrinth, Round window, Eustachian Tube

Figure 8-2 A schematic drawing of the air conduction apparatus and the fluid-filled labyrinth. Three semicircular canals have been represented as a single canal, and the cochlear portion of the labyrinth is shown as a straight tube in this schematic. [*After G. von Békésy and W. A. Rosenblith, "Mechanical properties of the ear," in S. S. Stevens (ed.), Handbook of Experimental Physiology (New York: John Wiley & Sons, Inc., 1951), pp. 1075–115.*]

Figure 8-2 shows a schematic representation of the components of the outer and middle ear, and their anatomical relation to each other and the inner ear. It may provide a useful reference for the discussion which follows.

The external auditory meatus terminates at the *tympanic membrane.* The membrane is formed of three layers of tissue. The outer layer is a delicate continuation of the skin of the meatus. The middle layer is fibrous, and the inner layer is continuous with the moist lining of the middle ear space. When viewed from the external meatus, the tympanic membrane appears translucent, like a piece of ground glass. A perspective on the tympanic membrane as viewed from the entrance to the external auditory meatus is shown in Figure 8-3. The fibrous middle layer of the membrane may give the impression that a grid of lines runs through the membrane. The membrane is concave inward, and the point of maximum depression is the *umbo.* This is the point of attachment of the tip of the *manubrium* (handle) of the *malleus,* one of the three bones in the middle ear space. This attachment is secured by means of fibrous tissue. The membrane is held in place at the medial end of the meatus by a ligamentous ring. A portion of the tympanic membrane is termed the *pars flaccida.* This portion is free of the fibrous tissue found elsewhere in the membrane.

287

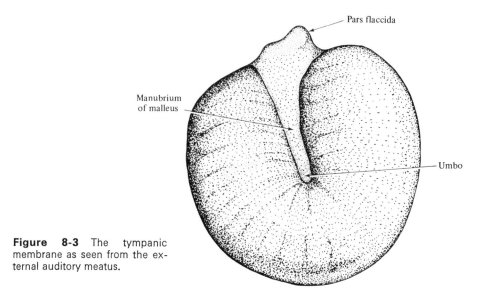

Pars flaccida

Manubrium
of malleus

Umbo

Figure 8-3 The tympanic membrane as seen from the external auditory meatus.

The space on the medial side of the tympanic membrane is air-filled, and is normally vented by the *eustachian tube*, which communicates with the nasopharynx. This middle ear space also contains three small bones, the ligaments which support them, and the ligaments from two muscles which attach to two of the bones.

The three bones, called the *ossicles*, connect the tympanic membrane to the inner ear space. The first of these, the malleus, is named for its mallet-like appearance. The malleus articulates with a second, slightly larger ossicle, the *incus*, which appears somewhat like an anvil when viewed from some perspectives. The third ossicle, connecting the incus with the inner ear, is stirrup-shaped, and termed the *stapes*. The malleus has already been described as being firmly attached over much of the length of the manubrium to the tympanic membrane. The stapes seats into an opening which has the oval shape of its *footplate* (or bottom of the stirrup), the *oval window*. The attachment to the oval window is insured by an *annular ligament* around the circumference of the footplate. The ossicles' attachments to each other are maintained by capsules of ligamentous material surrounding each joint. Figure 8-4 shows several views of human ossicles dissected from the middle ear space.

Additional ligaments aid in suspending the ossicular chain, and these attach between the ossicles and the walls and *attic* (i. e., top) of the middle ear space. The ligaments of the *tensor tympani* and *stapedius* muscles also intrude into the middle ear space.

Figure 8-4 Human ossicles dissected from the middle ear. The malleus is about 5·5 mm in length; the stapes footplate measures about 3·2 mm by 1·4 mm. (*Békésy and Rosenblith, 1951*).

Malleus

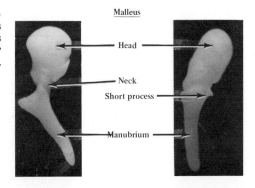

Head

Neck

Short process

Manubrium

Incus

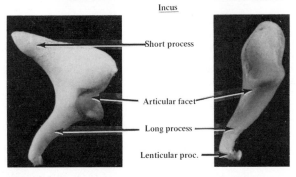

Short process

Articular facet

Long process

Lenticular proc.

Stapes and the 3 ossicles

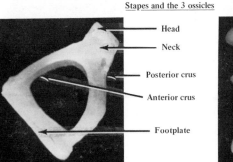

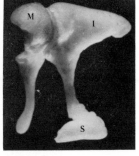

Head

Neck

Posterior crus

Anterior crus

Footplate

The ligament of the stapedius muscle emerges from a bony pyramid inferior and posterior to the stapes to attach to the *posterior crus* (arm). The muscle is enclosed in a cavity inferior to the pyramid, and the nerve supply to the muscle is from a portion of the VIIth cranial nerve (facial). The ligament of the tensor tympani appears superficially on the medial anterior wall of the middle ear cavity and crosses the space to attach to the malleus near the short anterior process. The muscle is encapsulated adjacent to the eustachian tube.

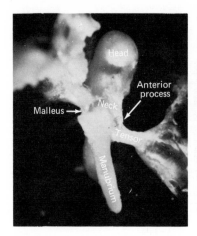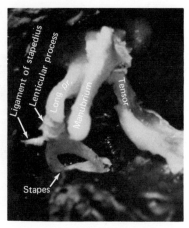

Figure 8-5 Human ossicles suspended in the middle ear space. The tympanic membrane has been removed, and the left part of the figure shows the attachment of the ligament of the tensor tympani muscle to the malleus. The view in the left portion of the figure is taken from a perspective anterior to the middle ear cavity along an axis above and roughly parallel to that of the eustachian tube. The photograph at right shows the attachment of the tendon of the stapedius muscle to the posterior crus of the stapes. The view is anterior to and approximately parallel with the axis of the external auditory meatus.

The tensor tympani is innervated by a portion of the Vth cranial nerve (trigeminal). Figure 8-5 shows views of the suspended ossicles and the attachments of the ligaments of these two muscles.

In addition to all of these components associated with hearing, a portion of the VIIth cranial nerve, the *corda tympani,* courses through the middle ear space to the innervate anterior taste buds of the tongue.

External and Middle Ear Action

The pinna is essentially a sound collector, but it is a poor one in humans. It appears transparent to much sound energy (i. e., low frequencies), and it is not free to move independently of the head. There has been some suggestion that the convolutions of the pinna may assist in sound discrimination by providing for reinforcement of sound frequencies having wavelengths proportional to the distances between the convolutions (Batteau, 1968). Most authors relegate the human pinna to the position of an earring holder, and little else.

The external auditory meatus is not a dynamically responsive portion of the ear. Its length does influence the sound reaching the tympanic membrane, however. The meatus behaves like a broadly-tuned resonator in the manner of a glass bottle. Sound frequencies with wavelengths approximating four times the length of the meatus are selectively reinforced. If the length of the meatus is about 2.5 cm, wavelengths of 10 cm should be reinforced. At sea level and room temperature, this would correspond to a frequency of about 3,500 Hz. These approximations have been made by several authors, and a resonance effect has been shown to occur in the predicted frequency region (Wiener and Ross, 1946). For example, Shaw (1966) shows this resonance to be in the region of 2,400 Hz, in agreement with Békésy's (1960) computations.

Practically, this means that sound energy provided in a free field (no echoes) with uniform representation at all frequencies will arrive at the tympanic membrane with an enhancement of those frequencies in the resonance region. Predictably, this region varies slightly from person to person and grossly from species to species, depending on the size and shape of the external meatus. The pinna may also affect this resonance (Flynn and Elliott, 1965).

Transformer Action of the Middle Ear

The sensory apparatus of the inner ear is located in a fluid-filled chamber. When sound energy crosses the boundary between two media, such as air and the fluid of the inner ear, the efficiency of transfer is affected by the physical characteristics of the media. The mass and stiffness of the media determine their reluctance to be compressed by the pressure variations which comprise sound. This reluctance is manifested in a frictional component, offering simple *resistance*, and a so-called *reactive* component. The resistive component is independent of the driving frequency imposed on the medium. The reactive component is a direct manifestation of the mass and stiffness effects at a given frequency. Resistive and reactive components sum in a complex fashion to result in an *acoustic impedance*.

If sound energy attempts to cross the boundary between a medium of low impedance (one which may be disturbed easily by sound energy) to one of high impedance, some of the energy will not cross. Rather, it will be reflected back toward the source of the sound. The amount of energy reflected back will be due in part to the ratio of the acoustic impedances of the two media.

For the fluid in the inner ear, approximate calculations indicate that 99.9% of the energy striking the air/fluid boundary would be reflected back toward the source (Wever and Lawrence, 1954, p. 72). Thus, only 1/1,000th of the incident energy would cross the boundary, and a 30 dB loss would occur in sound pressure.[1] These approximate calculations assume that the

---

[1] This can be shown as follows: The pressure ratio, p/p_0 is equal to $\sqrt{E/E_0}$, the square root of the energy ratio.

$$N \text{ dB} = 20 \log \sqrt{1000/1}$$
$$N \text{ dB} = 20 \log 31.62$$
$$N \text{ dB} = 20 \times 1.4996$$
$$N \text{ dB} = 29.99$$

sound energy arriving at the inner ear is transmitted through the fluid of the inner ear in the form of an acoustical pressure wave, i. e., that the molecules of the fluid are alternately in a state of compression or rarefaction (Wever and Lawrence, 1954).

An alternate view is that sound energy reaching the stapes is expended simply in pushing the fluid of the inner ear to and fro, and that the inner ear fluid is probably not compressed (Fletcher, 1953). The significance of this alternate view is that the approximate calculations of the inner ear impedance may be inappropriate. Both viewpoints help to set the stage for describing the function of parts of the middle ear apparatus. The middle ear functions in part to increase the efficiency of transfer of sound energy to the inner ear. Two of its physical properties appear to assist in this function, *the ratio of the areas of the tympanic membrane and stapes,* and *a lever action brought on by the differences in length of the malleus and incus.*

Area ratio hypothesis

The area of the tympanic membrane has been estimated at 85 mm². Békésy (1960) has studied the vibration patterns of the tympanic membrane under conditions of sound stimulation and has noted that a portion of the membrane is fixed rigidly around its circumference, and only about two-thirds moves freely. He has estimated this *effective area* at 55 mm². Improved observation techniques making use of laser optical systems (Tonndorf and Khanna, 1968) are now making available more detailed descriptions of the mode of tympanic membrane displacement, but the reduced effective area concept has not changed.

If the effective area of the tympanic membrane is 55 mm², and the area of the stapes footplate is 3.2 mm² (Békésy, 1960), the ratio of the areas is about 17/1. When attached to each other with a single ossicle, like the columnella found in the frog, this physical characteristic in itself affords the tympanic membrane/stapes footplate combination an opportunity to raise pressure by a factor of seventeen.

The middle ear mechanism does this like the example shown in Figure 8-6. A thumbtack can be pushed into a piece of wood with ease. Without great force, an attempt to push a piece of doweling having the same diameter as the head of the tack would be unsuccessful. The doweling or tack represents a transformer between a low impedance medium (one's thumb) and a high-impedance medium (the block of wood). Since the areas of both ends of the doweling are equivalent, it provides no enhancement of the pressure applied by one's thumb. The tack does provide for a pressure enhancement, however. The force distributed over the head of the tack is brought to bear on the point, and the force per unit area is markedly increased. The extent of increase is directly proportional to the ratio of the area of the head of the tack to the

A thumbtack provides a pressure gain

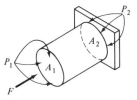

$$P_1 = \frac{F}{A_1} \quad P_2 = \frac{F}{A_2}$$

$$\frac{P_2}{P_1} = \frac{F}{A_2} \div \frac{F}{A_1} = \frac{A_1}{A_2}$$

$$P_2 = P_1 \frac{A_1}{A_2}$$

But $A_2 = A_1$

$$P_2 = P_1$$

$$P_1 = \frac{F}{A_1} \quad P_2 = \frac{F}{A_2}$$

$$\frac{P_2}{P_1} = \frac{F}{A_2} \div \frac{F}{A_1} = \frac{A_1}{A_2}$$

$$P_2 = P_1 \frac{A_1}{A_2}$$

But $A_2 < A_1$

$$P_2 > P_1$$

The middle ear does the same

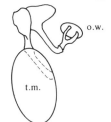

o.w.

t.m.

$$P_1 = \frac{F}{\text{Area of t.m.}}$$

$$P_2 = \frac{F}{\text{Area of o.w.}}$$

$$P_2 = P_1 \frac{\text{Area of t.m.}}{\text{Area of o.w.}}$$

$$P_2 > P_1$$

Figure 8-6 Illustration of the effects of the area ratio of the tympanic membrane and stapes footplate. As in the case of a thumbtack, the pressure applied at the stapedial footplate is increased in proportion to the ratio of the areas of the footplate (or point of the tack) and the tympanic membrane (or head of the tack).

area of the point of the tack. Thus, in the case of the tympanic membrane and stapes footplate, the pressure increase is about seventeen times. In terms of decibels, this increase is about 24.6 dB.

Lever hypothesis

The second mechanism by which the middle ear may enhance the transfer of energy from the atmosphere to the inner ear is its lever action. The ossicles are arranged to function as a Class II lever. The fulcrum (pivot) is placed at one end of the lever, the applied force at the other; and the load between the

Figure 8-7 Illustration of the effects of the lever action of the malleus and incus. The malleus and incus function much like a crowbar, and the resulting force applied to the incudostapedial joint increases proportionately with the ratio of the lengths of the long processes of the malleus and incus. The actual ratio in humans is about 1.3 to 1.

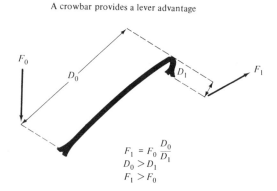

A crowbar provides a lever advantage

$$F_1 = F_0 \frac{D_0}{D_1}$$
$$D_0 > D_1$$
$$F_1 > F_0$$

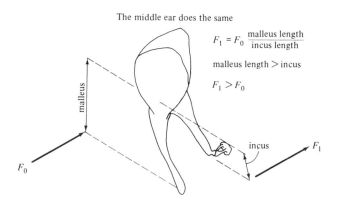

The middle ear does the same

$$F_1 = F_0 \frac{\text{malleus length}}{\text{incus length}}$$

malleus length > incus

$$F_1 > F_0$$

fulcrum and applied force. The resulting force is increased proportionately with the ratio of the distance between the load and the fulcrum. This effect is illustrated in Figure 8-7. The analogy shown in Figure 8-7 is of a crowbar. If a bar is placed on a pivot point, it can be used to pry nails or large masses loose from their resting place. The increase in effective driving force is offset by a loss in displacement. Thus, depending on the placement of the fulcrum, one might swing the end of the crowbar several feet to provide a few inches of displacement at the other end.

This analogy between the crowbar and the ossicles assumes, of course, that the malleo-incudal joint slippage is minimal, else a hinged crowbar would be required for the model. The analogy ends at the incudostapedial joint.

Measures of the lengths of the ossicles and the ratio of the stapes displacement vs malleus displacement suggest that the lever ratio formed by the malleus and incus is about 1.3:1 (Wever and Lawrence, 1954; Fischler et al., 1967).

The product of the enhancement of the lever and area ratio mechanisms of the middle ear transformer system should give a net increase in pressure of about twenty-two times the sound pressure presented to the tympanic membrane. This gain corresponds to approximately 26.8 dB. Békésy (1960) has reported measures of the actual pressure-transformation ratio of the middle ear apparatus. As observed in human cadaver material, the actual increase in pressure between the tympanic membrane and stapes was in the range of 20 to 24 dB below about 2500 Hz, which is in the range of the prediction based upon the anatomical configuration of the middle ear. In addition, persons who have lost their middle ear structures show a loss in sensitivity in the range of 20 to 30 dB, though exceptions have been noted.

The fine aspects of motion of the tympanic membrane and ossicles have also been the object of scrutiny. Békésy's (1960) ingenious experiments were first reported in the 1930s and 1940s. He found that the tympanic membrane displacement was in the form of a rotation about an axis (or "hinge") located on the superior margin of the membrane. Thus, it "swings" in and out of the middle ear space, its inferior portion traversing a greater distance than the superior portion. Above 2,400 Hz, its displacement patterns become complex, and it vibrates segmentally (Békésy, 1960; Tonndorf and Khanna, 1968).

Three modes of stapedial motion have been described. Békésy (1960) observed that the stapes swings in and out of the vestibular space much like a gate, with its axis of rotation (or hinge) located near the posterior edge. Guinan and Peake (1967) have reported a piston-like action, in which the entire footplate moves in and out of the vestibule. At very high intensities (140 dB) the stapes appears to rotate or "rock" about an axis which coincides with the footplate's long axis. Thus, the superior portion of the stapes footplate "tips" into the vestibule while the inferior portion is displaced toward the middle ear space (Békésy, 1960).

Parenthetically, it should be noted that the actual displacement amplitudes observed for the stapes are minute. Most observations can be made only at high intensities because of the sensitivity of the electronic apparatus or the resolution of the optical systems which have been used to obtain the measures. For stimuli in the region of 75 dB SPL (Sound Pressure Level), Békésy (1960) reported stapes displacement of 20 Å with a 400 Hz stimulus. (Å, an angstrom, is 10^{-8} centimeters.) He also showed that stapes displacement decreased when stimulus frequency increased and SPL was held constant. Thus, his results agree well with Rubinstein et al. (1966), who reported about 10 Å displacement for 1,000 Hz in the region of 75 dB SPL. Rubinstein et al. (1966) have extrapolated from their (high intensity) data to suggest that stapedial displacement at threshold for 1,000 Hz is 1.5×10^{-3} Å.

To close the discussion of the transformer action of the middle ear it might be well to consider the impedance of the ear as a whole, i. e., as observed

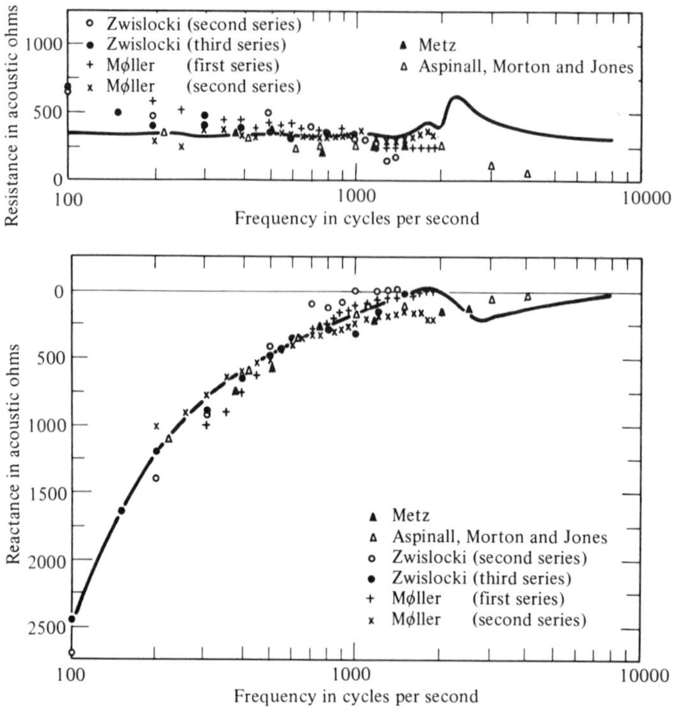

Figure 8-8   Impedance of the human ear as measured at the tympanic membrane. The overall impedance consists of a resistive component, shown in the top of the figure, and a reactive component, in this case stiffness. The resistive component is independent of stimulus frequency, except over the range from 1,800–3,000 Hz. The stiffness component causes increased impedance at low frequencies, and becomes negligible at high frequencies. Data from various investigators are shown in the figure. (See Zwislocki, 1962, 1963, 1963 a, 1970.) [*After J. S. Zwislocki, "Acoustics of the middle ear," Middle Ear Function Seminar (Fort Knox: U.S. Army Medical Research Laboratory, 1963).*]

from the tympanic membrane. Recall that impedance has a resistive (energy-consuming) and a reactive component. Measures of whole-ear impedance require that the sound pressure created in the external meatus by a known source be compared with the sound pressure produced by the same source in an acoustic network with known, variable acoustic reactance and resistance.[2] The results of many investigators, using various techniques, are shown in Figure 8-8. The data show the general tendency of the entire system to have reduced reactance from low to midrange frequencies.

[2] See Figure 2-27 in A. M. Small's chapter on acoustics for examples of acoustic elements which may produce reactive and resistive effects.

The measurement innovations of Zwislocki (1962, 1963a, b, 1970) and others have provided a relatively easy means of obtaining these measures, and they provide a convenient means of detection of a malady of the conduction system. For example, an interruption in the ossicular chain which would effectively uncouple the tympanic membrane from the cochlea would be reflected in an impedance measurement showing decreased stiffness and resistance. Fluid in the middle ear, or stapes fixation due to otosclerosis would tend to result in an increased stiffness and resistance.

In addition to the study of the normal and pathological ear, the measures of impedance offer a means of indirectly assessing the action of the middle ear muscles. When the muscles contract the tympanic membrane is pulled medially, adding to the concavity of the tympanic membrane. The stapes is pulled laterally, or retracted slightly from its normal resting position. This provides for an added stiffness component, and the added component will increase the overall impedance of the ear for lower frequency stimuli.

The muscles contract reflexively in awake subjects, and an obvious conclusion is that they function to provide a measure of protection by increasing the impedance of the middle ear system and attenuating the sound energy reaching the inner ear. If this were true, it should be possible to show a change in auditory threshold produced by contraction of the muscles of the middle ear. Jepsen (1963) has reviewed this problem, and offers evidence from other investigators showing that a threshold change does indeed occur during contraction of the muscles. For example, Reger (1960) reported average threshold shifts of about 30 dB for low-frequency stimuli for subjects who could voluntarily contract their middle ear muscles.

Another line of thought suggests that the muscles may contribute to particular desirable changes in sensitivity or "tuning" for certain stimuli.

Figure 8-9 EMG activity recorded from the stapedius muscle in the cat. The figure shows the electrical activity (EMG) of the stapedius muscle of one ear of a cat prior to and during the presentation of a 1,000 Hz tone to the opposite ear. The reflex may be evoked for both ears by a stimulus presented monaurally. Generally, the threshold for the reflex is related to the sensation level of the stimulus, and the reflex contraction may be maintained for periods of relatively long duration. [*These data are reproduced from F. Blair Simmons, "An analysis of the middle-ear-muscle acoustic reflex of the cat," Middle Ear Function Seminar (Fort Knox: U.S. Army Medical Research Laboratory, 1963).*]

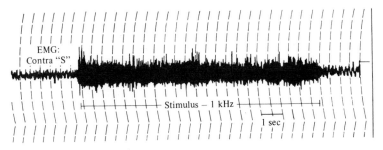

In either case, their contribution for impulsive stimuli, such as a gunshot, would be limited, for they exhibit a response latency of about 10 msec (Galambos and Rupert, 1959). Direct recordings of the EMG activity of the muscles have also demonstrated the reflex, and an example of the activity from the stapedius muscle of a cat is shown in Figure 8-9. The thresholds for the reflex are related to the *sensation level* of the stimulus, and estimates range from 60 to 100 dB, SL in normals (Jepsen, 1963).

THE INNER EAR STRUCTURE

The oval window leads to a space, the *vestibule*, which is continuous with the bony labyrinth of the *semicircular canals* and the *cochlea*. The canals, each of which completes an arc out of and back to the vestibule, are oriented in three planes. They contain part of the sensory apparatus for the balance system. The vestibule itself contains other elements of this system, the *utricle* and *saccule*. The labyrinth forming the cochlea coils like a snail's shell. Reference is conveniently made to its *base* and *apex* because each of its two and one-half turns has a progressively smaller radius. The relationship of the bony cochlear coils to the semicircular canals and vestibule is schematized in Figure 8-10(*a*). It is important to note that a person examining a dried specimen of the temporal bone would not find a bony snail shell-like object but a series of canals etched there.

In life, the bony labyrinth encapsulates the membraneous labyrinth. The so-called *vestibular labyrinth* includes the utricle, saccule and membraneous semicircular canals, including their sensory apparatus, the *ampulae*. This portion of the membraneous labyrinth communicates with the cochlear portion via the *ductus reuniens*, and with the *subarachnoid space* in the skull via the *endolymphatic duct*. The membraneous portion of the labyrinth is shown in Figure 8-10(*b*). The fluid medium in which the membraneous labyrinth resides is called *peri*lymph, and that enclosed within the membraneous portion is *endo*lymph. (The prefixes, *peri-* and *endo-*, signify fluid *out*side and *in*side of the membraneous system.)

The cochlear portion of the membraneous labyrinth does not float in the perilymph, but is attached to the bony portion broadly on two sides. This effectively divides the cochlear labyrinth into three channels, or *scalae*. That which is continuous with the vestibule is the *scala vestibuli*. The scala terminating at the round window is the *scala tympani*. The membraneous labyrinth between them is the *scala media*. The scala vestibuli and scala tympani are continuous with each other at the apex of the cochlea, and this point is the *helicotrema*.

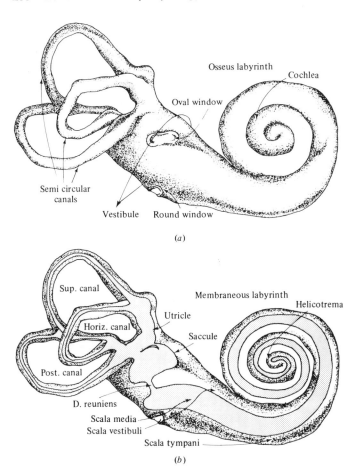

Figure 8-10 (a)

(b)

Figure 8-10 Schematic drawings of the bony and membraneous labyrinths. (*a*) The outline of the labyrinth in the temporal bone of the skull. (*b*) The relationship of the membraneous portion of the labyrinth to the bony canals. The membraneous labyrinth contains endolymph, and it may be thought of as being suspended in the perilymph. [*Courtesy P. Kaizawa.*]

The nature of the attachment of the scala media to the walls of the cochlea is shown in Figure 8-11(*a*). The bony canal is not circular, but is punctuated on one side by the *bony spiral lamina* (shelf) and the limbus. (Many elements in the cochlea will have the term "spiral" included in their names, reflecting that the element is present through much of the spiraling length of the cochlea.) The lamina coils with the length of the cochlea, and the nerve fibers which innervate the cochlea find their entrance through holes along the

A section through the cochlea shows...

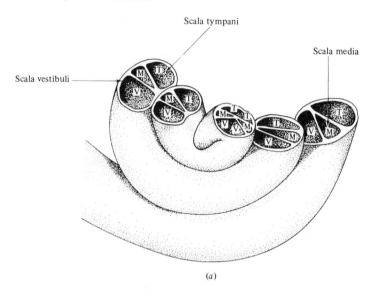

Scala tympani

Scala media

Scala vestibuli

(a)

Figure 8-11 Schematic drawings of the cochlea. (a) The perspective obtained when the cochlea is opened along a line across its widest point; (b) The structures in a section of a single turn; (c) The structure of the organ of Corti, which is contained within the scala media.

A magnified view of one turn shows...

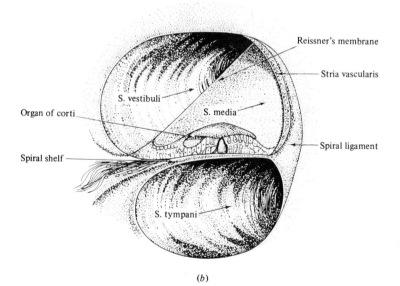

Reissner's membrane

Stria vascularis

S. vestibuli

Organ of corti

S. media

Spiral ligament

Spiral shelf

S. tympani

(b)

margin of the shelf. This series of openings is the *habenula perforata. Reissner's membrane* extends from the limbus, forming the margin between the scala media and scala vestibuli. The boundary between the scala media and the scala tympani is formed by the *basilar membrane.*

The basilar and Reissner's membranes are continuous with the *spiral ligament* on the wall of the cochlea opposite the spiral lamina. Several perspectives of the cochlea are shown in Figure 8-11(*a*).

Figure 8-11(*b*) shows a cross-section of a single cochlear turn, and the elements contained in the scala media are identified. The aggregate of supporting cells, the tectorial membrane, and hair cells form the actual receptor organ for hearing, the *organ of Corti* (Figure 8-11(*c*) below). The fibers of the VIIIth Cranial (auditory) nerve terminate on the *inner* and *outer hair cells.* Their name is taken from the ciliary projections from each cell.

The cilia are arranged in a "W"-like configuration, and when viewed from the top of the organ of Corti, the open portion of the "W" is oriented toward the tunnel of Corti. The cilia are in intimate contact with the tectorial membrane, but it does not appear certain that they are actually deeply imbedded in the membrane (Spoendlin, 1968). The tectorial membrane appears to be attached medial to the inner hair cells by fiber-like trabeculae (Lim and Lane, 1969a).

The principal parts of the Organ of Corti are. . .

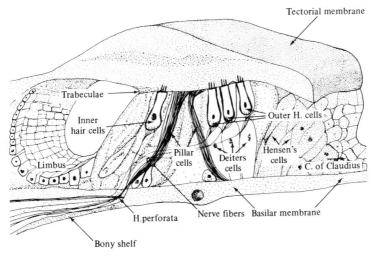

(*c*)

Figure 8-12 provides a view of a surface preparation of the organ of Corti of the Guinea pig as obtained by electron microscopy. Inner (IH) and three rows of outer (A, B, C) hair cells are apparent, along with Hensen's (H) and pillar (OP, IP) cells. The tectorial membrane has been removed to obtain this view.

Figure 8-12 A scanning electron micrograph illustrating a surface view of the organ of Corti (Guinea pig). The cilia of the inner hair cells (IH), and the cilia and cell bodies (1, 2, 3, and A, B, C) of the outer hair cells; Hensen's (H), outer and inner pillar cells may be observed (OP, IP). An unmyelinated nerve fiber (N) may be seen crossing the tunnel of Corti. [*This figure was provided through the courtesy of Dr. David J. Lim.*]

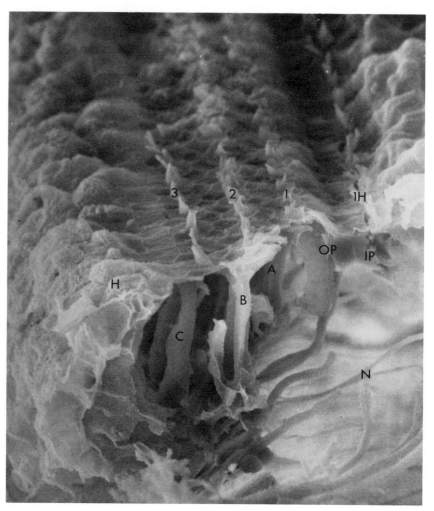

MECHANICAL ACTION IN THE COCHLEA

To this point, discussion of the action of the ear has led to the description of the transformer action of the membranes and ossicles of the middle ear, and the delivery of acoustic energy to the inner ear in the form of displacement of the stapes. If a simple impulsive stimulus (a "click") is used to stimulate the ear, the stapes rocks in and out of the vestibular space. The stapes movement should cause a momentary displacement of the fluid, and the scala media will be first depressed toward the scala tympani, then elevated toward the scala vestibuli. This pattern of displacement appears first at the basal end of the scala media, and then traverses the length of the cochlea. Békésy (1960) made the first observations of this phenomenon, and termed it the *traveling wave*.

A detailed analysis of the action of the scala media in response to displacement of the stapes (Békésy, 1960) has revealed that the physical characteristics of the basilar membrane determines the nature of the action. The membrane is about 35 mm in length, 0.04 mm wide at the base of the cochlea, and 0.5 mm wide at the apex, and there is a continuous gradation in width along its length (Békésy and Rosenblith, 1951). A gradient of elasticity corresponds to this change in width, and the membrane is stiffer by a factor of about 100 at the base than at the apex. Other factors aside, a relatively stiff element responds preferentially to high frequency stimulation. Thus, a crystal glass will "ring" at a high frequency when struck. Compare this effect with the slow undulations of a mound of gelatin. The transient stimulus mentioned earlier contains energy from a broad range of frequencies. The traveling wave produced by a transient stimulus appears to cause relatively rapid undulations near the base of the cochlea, and progressively slower-developing wave patterns toward the apex. The mechanical action thus reflects the presence of high frequency energy at the base and low frequency energy toward the apex. It is providing a *spatial display* of the stimulus frequencies contained in the impulsive stimulus.

When a stimulus consisting of only one frequency is used, the displacement pattern of the scala media grows to a maximum amplitude as it travels along the membrane. Just beyond the point at which the maximum amplitude is reached, the displacement amplitude diminishes quickly. Fletcher's (1953) and later investigators' mathematical models of cochlear action have provided detailed illustrations of the pattern of basilar membrane motion at several points in time during stimulus presentation. Figure 8-13 shows the growth and decay of a traveling wave for a 200 Hz stimulus at six points in time. The location of the maximum amplitude at 28.5 mm from the basal end is not at all arbitrary as Békésy's studies indicated the basilar membrane does indeed provide a preferential response for each frequency, and the location of the maximum displacement is predictable by the membrane's physical character.

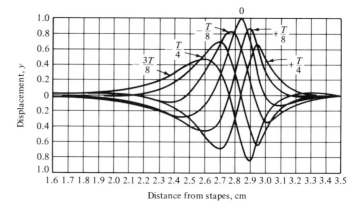

Figure 8-13 Displacement patterns of the basilar membrane for a simple 200 Hz stimulus. The appearance of the basilar membrane (scala media) is illustrated at six points in time spaced at 0.625 msec intervals. Each interval corresponds to 1/8th of the period of the stimulus. Note the relatively slow growth of the displacement pattern from the basal end, and rapid decrement toward the apex. [*From* Speech and Hearing in Communication, *by Harvey Fletcher. Copyright © 1953 by Litton Educational Publishing, Inc., by permission of Van Nostrand Reinhold Company.*]

Figure 8-14 Relative displacement amplitudes and phases of the basilar membrane for various frequencies. To arrive at these figures, the "envelope" of the traveling wave was determined on one side of the basilar membrane. The envelope shows only the maximum amplitude of displacement along the basilar membrane. The actual shape of the displacement pattern at each instance in time is not shown by the envelope representation. The data points shown by the triangles, squares, and circles are the result of Békésy's observations of the scala media. The phase data in each part of the figure show the time lag of the development of the traveling wave for each frequency. In general, the development of the wave from the point of first measurable displacement to the maximum requires a time interval equal to about half of the period of the stimulus frequency. For 1,000 Hz, this would be about 0.5 msec; for 200 Hz, about 2.5 msec, etc. The decay of the envelope requires about one-half the time necessary for its growth to a maximum. [*From* Speech and Hearing in Communication, *by Harvey Fletcher. Copyright © 1953 by Litton Educational Publishing, Inc., by permission of Van Nostrand Reinhold Company.*]

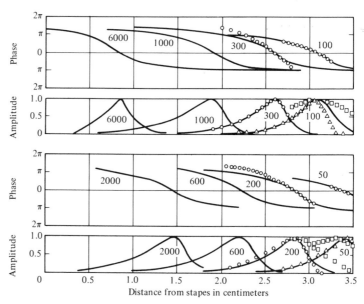

The most straightforward way to test for this effect would be to stimulate the cochlea with simple tones, one at a time, and determine the location of the displacement maximum caused by each tone. The illustrations in Figure 8-14 show the results of a number of observations and estimations of the location of traveling wave maxima for various stimulus frequencies. The envelope of each traveling wave, showing only the maximum displacement at several points along the basilar membrane, is represented. The data points shown by circles, squares, and triangles are the results of Békésy's observations of cochlear function, and the solid curves represent the results of Fletcher's calculations.

It is often helpful to think of the membrane as functioning as a filter. A given point on the membrane is responsive to all frequencies below a certain frequency, and filters out frequencies above this point. This seems to follow because low frequencies cause disturbances which traverse the entire membrane, and the activity due to high frequencies is limited to the more basal sections of the cochlea.

The movement of the basilar membrane is thought to be translated into effective stimulation for the nervous system through the interaction of the hair cells and tectorial membrane. The medial attachment of the membrane is to the fixed bony spiral lamina, and the outer attachment is to the more flexible spiral ligament. When the wave passes through a point on the membrane, its resulting movement is swing-like, with a hinge located in the bony spiral lamina. The tectorial membrane also pivots on a "hinge," but this hinge is located in a plane above that of the basilar membrane. At the point of contact between the cilia of the hair cells and the tectorial membrane, some relative lateral or "shearing" movement occurs. This effect is illustrated in Figure 8-15. This shearing action is thought to be the effective stimulus for auditory sensation. The shear is maximum in the lateral (across the scala) direction at the point of maximum amplitude of the traveling wave. It is greatest in the longitudinal direction along the steepest portion of the traveling wave envelope, which is the "low frequency" or apex side of the envelope maximum.

Figure 8-15 Shearing action in the cochlea. When the basilar membrane is displaced due to stimulation, the resulting action on the cilia of the hair cells is a lateral shear. This is due to the interaction of the relative displacements of the tectorial and basilar membranes.

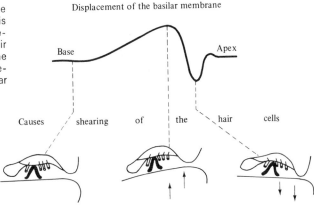

Displacement of the basilar membrane

Base   Apex

Causes   shearing   of   the   hair   cells

Within limits, the actual amplitude of the traveling wave is directly proportional to the stimulus intensity. Thus, the points on the membrane experiencing maximum stimulation will be determined by the frequency selectivity of the membrane, and the actual amplitude of the shear will be determined by the effective amplitude of the stimulus. The points adjacent to those experiencing maximum stimulation will experience stimulation which is determined by the gradient of tuning of the membrane.

The preceding discussion of the mechanical action of the ear has described the results of so-called "air conduction" stimulation. That is, an apparent traveling wave is produced in the inner ear by virtue of sound energy conducted to the inner ear from the air via the ossicles. Another route of stimulation is known to be functional, however, and is considered in the next section.

Bone-Conduction Stimulation of the Cochlea

The bones of the skull carry sound energy just as air and fluid, or wood and steel. It is thus possible to stimulate the ear by placing a vibrator on the skull, even though this energy may not arrive at the inner ear via the external meatus and middle ear apparatus. An important key to understanding how this form of stimulation may work was provided by Békésy (1960). His studies on cochlear models showed that the "stapes" of the inner ear may be located anywhere in the inner ear space and still produce a traveling wave which progresses from the base to the apex of the cochlea. That is, a pressure differential may be created across the scala media anywhere in the cochlea and still produce a rather normal sequence of mechanical activity leading to shearing action of the hair cells.

For bone conduction stimulation of the cochlea, the exact means by which sound energy is delivered to the fluid remains to be elucidated, but there are at least three avenues of thought which seem appealing.

The first is the *inertial* bone conduction theory (Barany, 1938). This theory suggests that, for low frequency stimulation, the portion of the skull containing the cochlea vibrates as a whole, and thus the whole cochlea is made to move slightly. The stapes, because of its attachment to the other ossicles and its flexible attachment to the temporal bone at the oval window, also moves, but its motion may lag behind the movement of the skull. The inertia of the middle ear conduction apparatus is what contributes to this lag in the movement of the stapes. The net result of this action is an apparent movement of the stapes in and out of the oval window. Thus the bone-conducted stimulus appears at the cochlea just as if it were borne by the normal air conduction route.

For higher frequency stimulation, *compressional* bone conduction may be the means by which the cochlea is stimulated. The theory of compressional bone conduction holds that the bony labyrinth may compress slightly in response to the pressure variations caused by sound. If the bony labyrinth compresses, the oval and round windows must flex because the fluid is relatively incompressible. The round window should flex to a greater extent than the oval window, because the oval window is stiffer than the round window and is attached to the ossicular chain (Kirikae, 1960). Because there would be more resulting "give" in the scala tympani than in the scala vestibuli, a momentary pressure difference may occur across the scala media, and result in the production of a traveling wave.

Another suggestion is the *osseotympanic* theory (Békésy, 1960). This theory suggests that the movement of the mandible simply lags behind the movement of the skull, or the mandible does not move at all. Its flexible attachment to the skull lies just beneath the skin of the soft cartilagenous portion of the external meatus. The relative movement of the skull with respect to the mandible, the theory holds, actually sets up pressure variations in the air present in the external meatus. The result is that sound is produced and carried to the inner ear via the ossicles.

All of these theories suggest that the windows of the cochlea must be *free to move*, and they imply that the middle ear apparatus should be at least partly functional. The experiments of Tonndorf (1966) and others have demonstrated that both windows may be sealed, and that bone-conducted stimuli can still evoke an indication of a response from the ear. These observations have prompted the suggestion that the cochlear and/or vestibular ducts, providing connection of the fluid spaces of the ear to the subarachnoid space in the skull, may serve as a "third window" (Tonndorf, 1966; Naunton, 1963).

To close this discussion on action of the middle and inner ear apparatus, it might be useful to describe one additional means of assessing the function of the inner ear. The technique involves the observation of some of the electrical activity of the cochlea.

The Cochlear Microphonic

In 1930 Wever and Bray reported that electrical activity recorded from the auditory nerve in the vicinity of the cochlea (of a cat) mirrored the waveform of the sound stimulus. Practically what this means is that the recorded activity could be played through an audio amplifier and loudspeaker, and that it would sound like the stimulus which had been presented to the animal's ear. This Wever-Bray effect apparently contained a number of different types of responses, but the most prominent element in their recording was probably the *cochlear microphonic*. This electrical potential may be recorded within or near the cochlea. It is a large electrical potential by physiological standards,

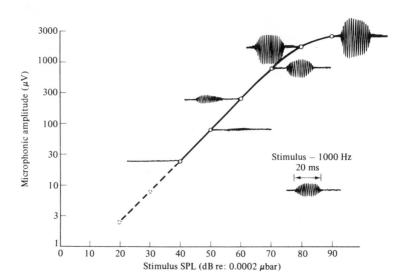

Figure 8-16 Cochlear microphonics recorded from the round window of a cat. The figure shows the peak-to-peak amplitude of the cochlear microphonic, and some examples of the waveform of the response to a 1,000 Hz stimulus. Over the linear portion of the curve, a 10 dB increase in stimulus SPL was met with an increase of the cochlear microphonic amplitude of about 3 to 1, or a corresponding 10 dB increase. At about 70 dB SPL, the microphonic response fails to grow in a one-to-one proportion with the stimulus, and in some cases the microphonic amplitude may actually decrease with further increments in stimulus intensity. These data were taken from a cat which had been implanted for over three years prior to the date of the recording. [*The data are provided courtesy of F. Blair Simmons and John H. Winstead.*]

and it faithfully mirrors the stimulus waveform configuration over a very large range of variation of stimulus parameters.

A popular location for a recording electrode designed to pick up the cochlear microphonic is the round window. A ball-tipped or looped piece of wire serves the purpose, and may be left in place against the window for long periods of time (years, actually) apparently without causing significant damage. An example of a round-window record of the cochlear microphonic to a 1,000 Hz stimulus tone is shown in Figure 8-16. The salient features of the cochlear microphonic seem to be these:

(1) It is stable for constant moderate stimulus input during long periods of time (Simmons and Beatty, 1962).

(2) It grows linearly with the stimulus intensity over a range of approximately 60 dB (Wever and Lawrence, 1954).

(3) It is without a "threshold" but simply appears to grow out of the noise in the recording whenever a stimulus of sufficient

intensity is applied (Wever, 1966). A one microvolt or 10 microvolt amplitude is often used as a laboratory "standard," however.

(4) It is usually resistant to insult provided by changes in the physiological state of the animal, and may persist for up to 30 min after death (Békésy, 1960).

(5) Its existence appears to depend on the presence of normal hair cells (Butler et al., 1962).

Aside from providing a general means of estimating the integrity of the cochlea and related structures, the cochlear microphonic has been a useful tool in the study of the action of the cochlea. The cochlea of the Guinea pig, for example, is covered by a very thin bone, and is oriented so that all of its turns may be viewed from the bulla, a large air-filled cavity located next to the middle-ear space in those animals. Taking advantage of this anatomical configuration, Tasaki, et al. (1952) placed recording electrodes in each of the turns of the cochlea, and reported what they termed the "space-time" pattern of the microphonic. Essentially, they found that the microphonic developed along the turns of the cochlea in the manner predicted by the theories and observations of Békésy regarding the traveling wave. An example of recordings of this type is shown in Figure 8-17. The records were taken from the first and third turns of the cochlea of a Guinea pig. Clearly, the turn III responses for low frequency stimuli were of greater amplitude than those of turn I. The reverse was true for high frequency stimuli. In addition, the microphonic developed in the turn III recordings somewhat later in time than in those from turn I, reflecting the travel time of the traveling wave.

The microphonic has been a useful tool in studying cochlear responses to stimuli more complex than simple tones (Boer and Six, 1956; Deatherage et al., 1957; Glattke, 1968; Dallos, 1969a, 1969b). It has been used to investigate responses of the cochlea to stimuli which may demonstrate inherent nonlinear effects in the cochlea (see Figure 8-16) (Dallos, 1969,

Figure 8-17 Cochlear microphonics obtained from two points in the cochlea of guinea pig. These data show the cochlear microphonic recorded from the basal and apical turns of the cochlea of a guinea pig for stimuli of various frequencies, and they demonstrate in a crude fashion the frequency selective response of the cochlea. [*The data are provided through the courtesy of the Division of Otolaryngology, Stanford Univ., School of Medicine.*]

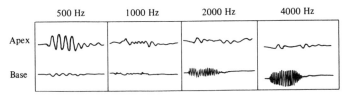

1969a; Worthington and Dallos, 1971), and to study the subtle phase relationships of the traveling wave (Tasaki et al., 1952; Tonndorf, 1958; Teas et al., 1962; Nordmark et al., 1969; Dallos et al., 1971).

Another series of investigations concerning the cochlear microphonic origin have been especially valuable. It should be recalled that Békésy's observations and reasoning have led to the shearing action model of hair cell stimulation. (See Figure 8-15.) During one phase of his investigations, he developed a moving probe; one that could be used to stimulate small portions of the organ of Corti while simultaneously recording the cochlear microphonic resulting from that stimulation. He was able to displace the hair cells in the radial direction predicted by the shearing principle, and found that the microphonic response produced by this type of displacement was greater than that produced by displacement along other axes.

The overview of cochlear function which all of these observations support seems to be as follows: The physical characteristics of the basilar membrane dictate its preferential "tuning" to stimuli of various frequencies. The traveling wave therefore reaches a maximum amplitude at some point determined by the stimulus frequency. At this point of maximum amplitude, shearing action in a radial direction is maximal for the hair cells. Radial shearing action also appears to yield the greatest cochlear microphonic potential, a potential presumably generated by the hair cells. Since the fibers of the auditory nerve terminate on the hair cells, it seems reasonable to suggest that the cochlear microphonic may reflect some type of action by which the hair cells stimulate the fibers of the auditory nerve. All of this reasoning leads to a theory that stimuli of different frequencies must stimulate different nerve fibers, and that this spatial array of stimulation is established in the cochlea.

The coding of auditory stimuli in the nervous system beyond the cochlea has been studied largely by an examination of the electrical properties of the cells which make up that system. Before proceeding with a presentation of the various modes of response of the auditory nervous system, it would be well to pause and consider some aspects of the basis for these electrical recordings and the innervation patterns of the auditory system.

SOME MORPHOLOGICAL AND ELECTRICAL CHARACTERISTICS OF NEURONS

A generalized drawing of a simple neuron is shown in Figure 8-18. Neurons consist of a *cell body* and its associated projections, *dendrites,* and a morphologically distinct projection, an *axon.* Axonal arborizations, shown as collaterals, and dendrites terminate in a variety of end-branchings. The

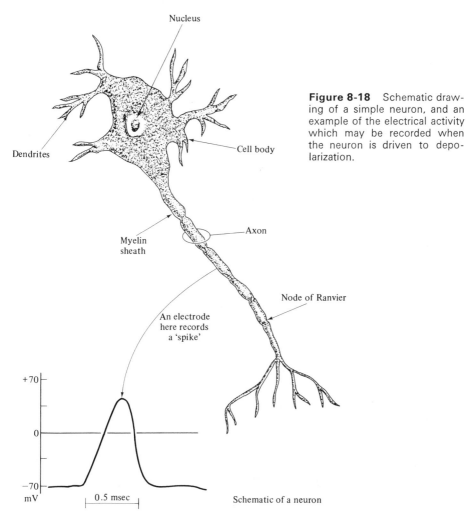

Nucleus

Dendrites

Cell body

Myelin
sheath

Axon

Node of Ranvier

An electrode
here records
a 'spike'

+70

0

−70
mV

| 0.5 msec |

Schematic of a neuron

Figure 8-18 Schematic drawing of a simple neuron, and an example of the electrical activity which may be recorded when the neuron is driven to depolarization.

dendrites may be thought of as carrying information to the cell body; the axon as carrying information away from the cell body, presumably to the next neuron in the chain.

The most peripheral neurons ("first-order") in the auditory-vestibular system have two axonal processes, and are called bipolar neurons. One axon terminates on the sensory cells in the cochlea, and the other forms a functional connection with the next neuron in the chain. The junction between neurons is known as a *synapse*.

Many varieties of electrical potentials are produced in the nervous system. They range from steady differences in potential measured across a cell membrane through very rapid changes in potentials ("spikes") which have a time course measured in fractions of milliseconds. Recordings of the electrical activity of single neurons or of large areas of nerve tissue (such as with scalp-EEG electrodes) provide the most convenient means of determining their reaction to stimulation. If a small electrical conductor (an electrode) is pushed into a single axon and used to measure the electrical potential of that location relative to the outside of the cell membrane, it will generally be found to have a "resting" potential of 70 millivolts negative with respect to the outside. When the neuron is driven to excitation, the resting potential suddenly changes to about +40 millivolts relative to the outside and is then restored to its resting value. This process of depolarization and re-polarization ordinarily is completed within about 0.5 milliseconds.

This electrical "spike" is a manifestation of a transient, reversible change in the physical character of the neuron. The change involves the controlled release of potential energy which has been stored in the form of a concentration gradient for small *cations*[3] across the cell membrane.

The means by which this event occurs remains to be elucidated completely. Hodgkin and Huxley (1952) have provided a working hypothesis commonly referred to as the "sodium-pump" hypothesis. Some of the features of this hypothesis are disputed (Tasaki, 1968), but the ionic basis for observed action potentials described by Hodgkin and Huxley has survived repeated scrutiny.

As summarized by Huxley (1954), the concentration of sodium (Na^+) inside the giant squid axon is about one-tenth that found outside the cell membrane. The potassium (K^+) concentration is about forty times that found outside the cell. The process of excitation results in momentary rapid diffusion of Na^+ and K^+ through the cell membrane which is followed by restoration of their original concentrations. The "sodium-pump" restores and maintains the concentration gradient. The Na^+ and K^+ diffusion is known to occur over slightly different time courses, and the sodium theory falls short in explaining how given "channels" in the nerve membrane may be ion selective once they are open (Baker, 1968). With the hindsight afforded by Tasaki's (1968) experiments, the sodium theory also fails to provide a distinct role for calcium (Ca^{++}). Tasaki's hypothesis argues that the condition for excitation is displacement of divalent cations (Ca^{++}) from binding sites in the membrane by monovalent cations (K^+). The change in membrane conductivity is not interpreted in terms of ion-selective impedance changes, and this feature of Tasaki's concepts makes them more acceptable than the early Hodgkin-Huxley hypothesis.

The nerve fibers themselves appear to discharge in an "all-or-none" fashion. That is, spike discharges are very consistent in their waveshape, amplitude, and duration. Single neurons may respond with bursts of spikes

---

[3] Positively charged ions.

at rates between 1,000 and 2,000 spikes per second for sustained periods of time. The spike potentials are very *local* potentials, however, and cannot be recorded when an electrode is more than a few microns away from the source. Microelectrodes, with tip diameters measured in fractions of microns, may be used to record these potentials for hours (Frank and Becker, 1964; Frank, 1959). When electrode tips exceed about 20 microns, it is usually impossible to isolate the electrical activity from single units in the auditory portion of the nervous system, though exceptions to this have been reported (Simmons and Linehan, 1968). Rather than a burst of spike activity, a so-called slow-wave evoked response may be observed with larger electrodes. The slow-wave potential is multiphasic, with negative and positive components distributed over several milliseconds. Figure 8-19 shows examples of slow-wave response to a "click" stimulus. The recordings were taken from three anatomically defined structures in the brain stem which are known to be primarily associated with the auditory pathway.[4] The electrodes had been in place for over a year prior to the time these recordings were made. The long time period over which these "chronic" recordings can be maintained permits their observation during a large variety of stimulus conditions.

The relation between spike and slow-wave responses has not been defined completely. In some cases, the shape of the slow-wave has been shown to be correlated with the probability of the occurrence of a single unit discharge (Fox and O'Brien, 1965). The slow-waves grow in amplitude in response to stimulus frequency and intensity changes. This growth may reflect the fact that more single neurons are participating in the response, or it may mean that those which are responding are discharging in better synchrony with each other.

Specific aspects of the conduction of nerve impulses along individual neurons and across synapses will not be covered here. Generally, Frank (1959) and other chapters of the *Handbook of Physiology* and Eccles (1964) will be useful foundations for the interested student. Otherwise, it should be borne in mind that the conduction velocity ranges from 0.5 to more than 100 meters per second, depending on the diameter of the neuron and whether or not it has a myelin sheath (Grundfest, 1940). The delays in transmission across synaptic junctions have been estimated to range from "vanishingly small" to about 0.9 milliseconds, with a modal value of about 0.3 msec (Eccles, 1964). With these approximations in mind, notice should be taken of the time delays between the evoked responses shown in Figure 8-19, particularly between the cochlear nucleus and the inferior colliculus. The approximately 2.5 msec time delay between response onset for these two structures is a reflection of the distance between them and the fact that one

---

[4] The cochlear nucleus, inferior colliculus, and medial geniculate will be described more completely in the next section.

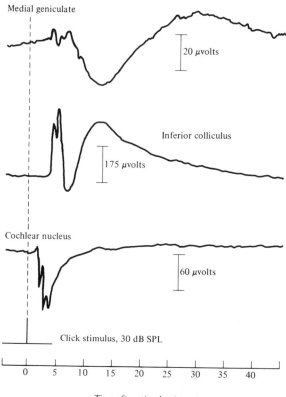

Three examples of auditory-evoked response

Medial geniculate

20 μvolts

Inferior colliculus

175 μvolts

Cochlear nucleus

60 μvolts

Click stimulus, 30 dB SPL

| 0 | 5 | 10 | 15 | 20 | 25 | 30 | 35 | 40 |

Time after stimulus (msec)

Figure 8-19 Examples of auditory-evoked slow-wave responses from three locations in the auditory nervous system. These data show the responses evoked by a single transient (click) stimulus at a level approximately 20 dB above threshold. Positive-going voltage changes are shown plotted in an upward direction. The data show changes in latency of onset of response corresponding to travel time of the neural impulses and delays imposed by synaptic transmission. The very early response recorded from the electrodes located in the medial geniculate may be due to activity present at a great distance from the electrodes, rather than activity evoked from the medial geniculate itself. [*The data are provided courtesy of the Division of Otolaryngology, Stanford Univ. School of Medicine.*]

or two synaptic boundaries are crossed by the pathways leading between them.

The innervation patterns of the auditory pathways are very complex, and there is not total agreement among investigators. Part of the disagreement comes with each new advance in observation technique rather than from "errors" in previous experiments. The electron microscope, for example, has been applied very successfully by Lim and Lane (1969a) (1969b) in the study of the topography of the structures of the ear.

Generally, the auditory portion of the central nervous system consists of neurons which lead away from the cochlea and toward the auditory cortex, and neurons which lead away from the cortex and toward the cochlea. (None have been shown to traverse the entire distance, and many synapses intervene between the cortex and cochlea.) The neurons leading away from the cochlea are "ascending" or *afferent* neurons. The neurons leading toward the cochlea are "descending" or *efferent* neurons. The afferent neurons may be thought of as carrying incoming information to the central nervous system. Efferent neurons provide for the flow of information back toward the periphery, and may regulate the activity of afferent neurons and the receptor organ. Some of the details of these two systems are described in the next section.

INNERVATION PATTERNS OF THE AUDITORY SYSTEM

A schematic drawing of four major innervation patterns of the auditory nerve in the cochlea is shown in Figure 8-20. The short *radial fibers* terminating on the inner hair cells are thought to be afferent fibers (Fernandez, 1951; Davis, 1962; Spoendlin, 1968). Some *radial* fibers cross the tunnel of Corti to provide efferent innervation for the outer hair cells (Spoendlin, 1968). *Spiral tracts*, running for an average 0.6 mm length provide afferent innervation for the outer hair cells (Smith, 1961; Davis, 1962; Spoendlin, 1968). The *internal spiral* bundle fibers may terminate on the afferent neurons of the inner hair cells to provide efferent control (Fex, 1968; Spoendlin, 1968). The intraganglionic spiral bundle is not shown in the figure. It courses within the modiolus (a hollow core surrounded by the cochlear turns) and gives off collaterals to inner and outer hair cells, perhaps providing afferent and efferent innervation. (See Fernandez, 1951, and Spoendlin, 1968).

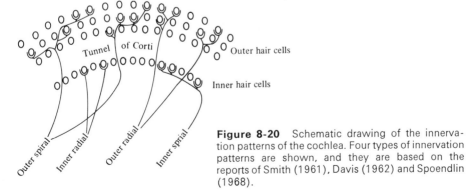

Figure 8-20 Schematic drawing of the innervation patterns of the cochlea. Four types of innervation patterns are shown, and they are based on the reports of Smith (1961), Davis (1962) and Spoendlin (1968).

Cochlear innervation (schematic)

The fibers leaving the organ of Corti do not acquire their myelin sheaths until they pass through the *habenula perforata*. Just beyond this point, their cell bodies form the *spiral ganglion*. Their axons then twist into concentric coils and join with the vestibular branch of the nerve to pass into the brain stem at the border of the pons and medulla. There appear to be about 20,000 to 30,000 hair cells in the organ of Corti, about 30,000 afferent fibers leaving the ear, and about 500 efferent fibers.

Virtually all of the afferent fibers synapse with the cell bodies of the second neurons in the ascending system when they arrive at the brain stem. The aggregate of cell bodies, dendrites, and collaterals forms the *cochlear nucleus*. Microscopic studies of the cochlear nucleus have shown that there may be as many as thirteen anatomical divisions receiving fibers from all parts of the cochlea (Lorente de No, 1933). On the basis of gross structure, the nucleus may be divided into three principal parts, however. These are the dorsal, posterior-ventral, and anterior-ventral nuclei (Rose et al., 1959).

As shown in Figure 8-21, most fibers leaving the cochlear nucleus cross to the other side of the brain stem. They may pass via three major tracts. Those fibers from the dorsal cochlear nucleus form the *stria* (line) of *Monakow* and the *stria of Held*, and pass to the contralateral superior olivary complex. The fibers from the anterior portion of the cochlear nucleus join with fibers of the *trapezoid body* and pass into the superior olivary complex bilaterally. The superior olivary complex appears to be the first in the ascending system to receive a major number of fibers from both ears.

Figure 8-21   Schematic drawing of the major auditory tracts in the brain stem. The portion of the figure on the left shows the tracts superimposed on a surface drawing of the brain stem viewed from the dorsal aspect, and the other portion shows the tracts grossly represented in sections of the brain stem taken at four levels. [*Courtesy P. Kaizawa.*]

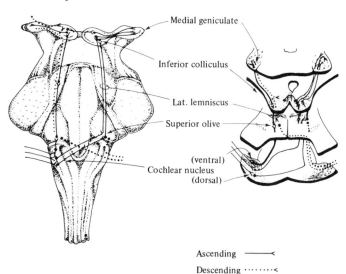

Medial geniculate

Inferior colliculus

Lat. lemniscus

Superior olive

(ventral)
Cochlear nucleus
(dorsal)

Ascending ———<
Descending ·······<

The major ascending tract from the superior olivary complex is the *lateral lemniscus*. Some fibers in this tract may form synapses with higher-ordered fibers in the nucleus of the lateral lemniscus. The greater number of fibers appear to pass directly to the *inferior colliculus*. At this level the fibers may synapse and/or cross to the contralateral inferior colliculus via the *commissure* of the inferior colliculus. Most fibers form a synapse with neurons which pass via the *brachium* of the inferior colliculus to the *ipsilateral medial geniculate*. After forming synapses in the medial geniculate, elements of the ascending system radiate in a diffuse fashion. Reaching the cortex, they project to the *transverse temporal gyri* and *insular cortex*.

The illustration in Figure 8-21 gives the impression that the ascending neurons are arranged in discrete tracts consisting of four or five neurons. The point-to-point representation in the illustration is a gross simplification of the actual configuration of the neurons. The arborizations of the axon leading from each cell body are very diffuse, and they may form synaptic connections with several neurons. Thus, the number of neurons exiting each nucleus exceeds the number of neurons leading to the nucleus. As Chow (1951) has suggested, this proliferation results in a dramatic increase in the number of auditory neurons from level to level in the ascending system. Chow indicated that the auditory cortex may contain 100 to 300 times the number of neurons (30,000) in the auditory nerve. The nuclei in the brain stem may have from two to fourteen times the number of cells in the nerve. The representation in Figure 8-21, then, shows only the *minimum* number of synapses which occur between the ear and the auditory cortex, and it falls far short of displaying the actual complexity of the system.

The available data regarding the origin and routing of the efferent pathways are not as complete as the data for the afferent neurons. Some known efferent tracts are illustrated in Figure 8-21, and among these the *olivocochlear bundle* has received the most attention. It originates in the region of the superior olivary complex. The majority of its projections form a stria just below the floor of the IVth ventricle, and these neurons cross the brain stem to reach the organ of Corti of the opposite ear. The descending neurons between the cortex and brain stem nuclei are more diffuse than the olivocochlear bundle, and they have been elusive to investigators (Rose and Woolsey, 1958; Massopust and Ordy, 1962; Nobel and Dewson, 1966).

One further caution should be borne in mind when considering the anatomical material just presented. The data included here were drawn from non-human materials, and investigations such as Chow's (1951) have not been repeated for the human auditory nervous system. Some species differences are known to exist, and generalizations from animal studies to humans may be tenuous. For example, the gross configuration of the superior olivary complex in the cat brain stem is different than the same structure in the brain stem of man.

The same general caution applies to the electrophysiological data which will be described in the next section. Nearly all of the electrical data from neurons have been gathered from animal preparations. (See Suzuki (1969) for a recent review of human-evoked responses.) The data reported here were gathered from cat or monkey preparations, and there may be undiscovered species differences that will change current interpretations of the data over the years.

Frequency Coding in the Auditory System

The earliest theory on the nature of the hearing process were actually theories of pitch perception. Since pitch is intimately related to stimulus frequency, they might also be referred to as theories of frequency coding. Until the past two decades, theories of frequency coding were aligned with either a "place" principle or a "neural-rate" principle. There is much evidence to suggest that both types of coding may be involved in the realm of auditory experience. Some of the evidence supporting each view will be presented in this section.

The place theory of hearing holds that different stimulus frequencies are discriminable from each other because they give rise to excitation patterns in different places in the nervous system. Helmholtz (1877) is credited with articulating this theory as it applies to the cochlea. His anatomical observations led him to conclude that the sensory apparatus consisted of individually tuned elements which vibrated in response to the frequency to which each was tuned. The result was a spatial array, not unlike that provided by the strings of a piano. The traveling-wave concept has replaced this "tuned-resonance" theory, but the spatial analysis that results is common to both views of the function of the inner ear. (The interested reader should refer to Wever (1962) for a concise history of the theories of cochlear function.)

A strict place theory of hearing would require that the spatial array provided by the cochlea be preserved in the nervous system. This effect does seem to occur to a certain extent. The issue may be clouded, however, by a lack of knowledge as to which "level" in the nervous system is responsible for providing a pitch percept. Since it is the "highest" center, the cortex. is prime candidate for the task, but there is no definite proof that it is the only system capable of providing a pitch percept related to simple, unchanging tonal stimuli. With this in mind, what is the evidence which favors a place theory of frequency coding in the nervous system?

The most salient feature of the response of single units in the auditory nervous system is that they are frequency selective. If a unit is going to respond to a simple tonal stimulus (some in the auditory cortex do not), it will do so for a relatively limited range of stimulus frequencies. This effect is often measured by determining the minimum sound pressure level (SPL)

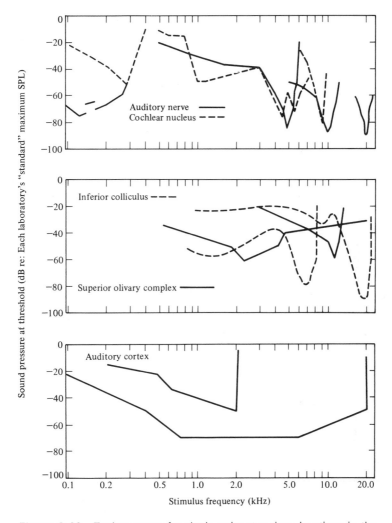

Figure 8-22 Tuning curves for single units at various locations in the auditory nervous system. The data shown here were gathered in five different laboratories and grouped together on similar coordinate systems. They show the minimum sound pressure level necessary to evoke a change in the discharge pattern of the units under study as a function of stimulus frequency. (The "0 dB" reference is about 100 dB SPL.) Note that there is considerable variation in the shape of the tuning curves at each level. The broadest tuning curves have been reported for cortical units, however. [*Auditory nerve data, redrawn from Kiang (1965) with permission of the M.I T. Press. Inferior colliculus data, redrawn by permission from Rose et al.,* J. Neurophysiol., *26 (1963), 294–320. Superior olivary complex data, redrawn by permission from Moushegian et al.,* J. Neurophysiol., *27 (1964), 1174–91. Auditory cortex data, redrawn and reproduced by permission from Y. Katsuki, N. Suga, and Y. Kanno, "Neural mechanisms of the peripheral and central auditory system in monkeys,"* J. Acoust. Soc. Amer., *32 (1962), 1396–1410.*

necessary to evoke a change in the activity pattern of the unit under study. The change may be either an increase or decrease in discharge rates observed in the absence of stimuli, or a subtle reorganization of the pattern of discharges of the unit. The plotted curve relating the threshold SPL to stimulus frequency is the *tuning curve* of the unit under study. The test frequency for which the least SPL is necessary to evoke a change in unit behavior is the *characteristic frequency* (CF) of that unit. Figure 8-22 shows tuning curves collected for units at various levels throughout the auditory nervous system in cat. They illustrate several features. First, the thresholds for single unit CFs recorded in the cat tend to be as low or lower than human listening thresholds for tones of the same frequencies. Also, the units tend to be responsive to a wider frequency range as the stimulus intensity is increased. Finally, the tuning curves obtained from units in the periphery of the nervous system tend to be asymmetrical about the CF of the unit, and they mirror the envelope of the traveling wave, though they often show much sharper tuning than the envelope (Møller, 1969a; Rose et al., 1959).

If a microelectrode is advanced through the cochlear nucleus, it is also possible to find an orderly progression of unit CFs (Rose et al., 1959). Each of the three major divisions of the cochlear nucleus appears to have representation of the entire cochlea, i. e., units which respond to low and high frequencies. Similar findings have been reported for the superior olive, inferior colliculus, and medial geniculate (Thurlow et al., 1951; Katsuki et al., 1962; Ades et al., 1939; Rose et al., 1963). This spatial organization is known as *tonotopic organization*.

Many investigations, reviewed by Woolsey (1960) indicated that the surface of the cortex was organized in a tonotopic fashion. Under certain conditions of stimulation, recording, and anesthesia, it is possible to demonstrate the existence of several cortical areas in the cat in which the spatial array of the cochlea is preserved. However, when the animal is lightly anesthetized the sharp boundaries become somewhat diffuse (see, for example, Gross and Small, 1961). Generally, the studies which demonstrated this surface tonotopic organization were based on surface slow-wave evoked responses. Single unit studies indicate that there is not an orderly progression of unit CFs corresponding with movement of the electrode along the cortical surface (Evans et al., 1965).

The architecture of the cortex is sufficiently different than other levels in the brain as to suggest diffusion. It may be, for example, that the surface recordings are inappropriate for determining tonotopic arrangement, and such organization may be present in intermediate layers or in "columns" of cells lying in from the surface (Evans, 1968; Goldstein et al., 1970). Thus, the place theory should not be considered to have been disproven by these findings. Rather, concepts regarding the organization of the cortex are changing.

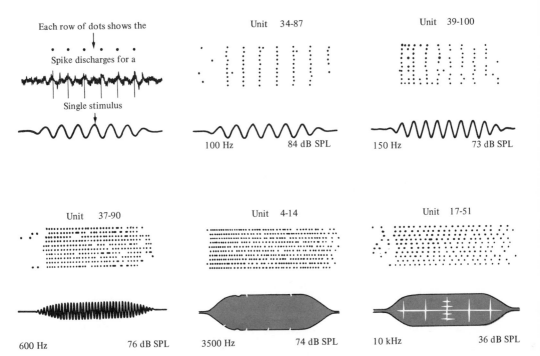

Figure 8-23 Stimulus frequency following behavior by single units in the cochlear nucleus. The figure shows that the "dot" displays are produced so that a row of dots corresponds to the spike discharges from a single unit during presentation of a stimulus. Ten rows of dots grouped together represent the response patterns to ten replications of the stimulus. The data shown for five units indicate that they may respond in exact synchrony with each cycle of low-frequency tones, and at higher frequencies they respond in an orderly manner at some consistent fraction of the stimulus frequency. [*Reproduced courtesy of the Division of Otolaryngology, Stanford Univ. School of Medicine.*]

The most popular alternate theory to explain the coding of frequency information is the neural-rate theory. This theory does not require that the cochlea provide a spatial analysis of the input stimulus according to its frequency components. Rather, the cochlea must simply transmit all of the timing information of the stimulus to the nervous system. The nervous system must somehow provide patterns of discharges which preserve the stimulus frequency, or timing, characteristics. The foundation for the modern theories of the neural-rate type was provided by Wever's (1949) volley theory.

The volley theory acknowledges that it is impossible for single neurons to discharge at rates much greater than 1000 spikes per second for longer than a few milliseconds. The pitch of a stimulus is, nonetheless, coded in the rate of discharge of the units which are responsive to the stimulus. The frequency character of the stimulus is preserved, according to this theory, because the units systematically cycle, or volley, in their response to the stimulus. A given unit may respond only to the first, third, fifth, seventh, etc., cycles of the input stimulus, and another may follow the second, fourth, sixth, eighth, and so on. Some central system is sensitive to all of the units which are responding in this volley fashion, and this central mechanism extracts the appropriate frequency cues from the activity patterns of the units.

There is much evidence to suggest that units in the peripheral portions of the nervous system discharge in a fashion appropriate to this theory (Anderson et al., 1971). Figure 8-23 shows the discharge patterns of several units in the cochlear nucleus. Each discharge from the unit is represented as a dot, and the pattern of dots formed by ten horizontal rows above the stimulus is the response pattern for ten replications of that stimulus. It can be noted that the dots tend to be arranged in orderly vertical columns. This indicates that the units discharged at approximately the same points in time for each stimulus presentation. Further, the time intervals between the dots in each row are consistent, suggesting that they may be related to the stimulus frequency. If the dots did not occur so that there was one for each cycle of the stimulus, they may have occurred with each second or fifth or tenth cycle.

As single unit recordings are taken from levels ranging from the auditory nerve (Kiang, 1965; Rose et al., 1967) through the structures of the brain stem (Halai and Whitfield, 1953; Rose et al., 1963; Evans, 1968) the following of stimulus frequency by discharge rate is less apparent. Discharge patterns from the medial geniculate, for example, rarely show rates of following above a few hundred Hz (Galambos, 1952).

At the cortex, many units do not respond to a simple short tonal stimulus. Rather, they appear to respond only when the stimulus frequency or amplitude is changed. This modulation of the stimulus may produce a few discharges which are synchronized with the rate of modulation, but which are not related to the stimulus frequency. An example of this type of data, gathered by Whitfield and Evans (1965) and reviewed by Evans (1968), is shown in Figure 8-24. The upper trace of (a) and (b) of the figure shows the electrical activity recorded by the electrode. No response is observed for the continuous (nearly one second) stimulus schematized in (a). In (b), the stimulus frequency was moved higher and lower at the rate indicated by the cycles of the stimulus envelope. The few responses which occur do so just prior to the peaks of the cycles. Nelson et al. (1966) and Suga (1965) have shown related findings in the activity patterns of units in the inferior colliculus. The units did respond to continuous tones, but responded to frequency modulated tones differentially. Direction of the frequency change influenced some of the units, and a few responded to frequency-modulated tones at frequencies outside of their tuning curves. As peripheral as the cochlear nucleus, Møller (1969b) has found direction of frequency change to influence unit behavior to a limited extent.

H4$_{12}$

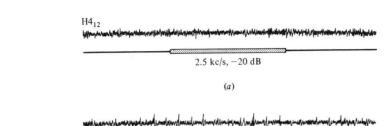

2.5 kc/s, −20 dB

(a)

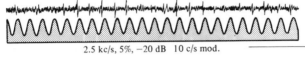

2.5 kc/s, 5%, −20 dB   10 c/s mod.

(b)

Figure 8-24 An example of unit behavior at the level of the auditory cortex. (a) The absence of regular discharges of the unit to a stimulus of approximately 1 second duration. (b) The stimulus frequency was modulated about a center frequency of 2.5 kHz. The unit was observed to respond to the stimulus only on occasions when the frequency was swept from below 2.5 kHz to above 2.5 kHz. Calibration lines in the lower right corner of the figure are for 0.5 second and 0.5 millivolts. [*From I. C. Whitfield and E. F. Evans, "Responses of auditory cortical neurons to stimuli of changing frequency,"* J. Neurophysiol., *28 (1965), 655-72.*]

Data of the type reviewed in this section lead to the following conclusions, among others. First, there is neural behavior which supports both the place and neural-rate theories of frequency coding, and this behavior is evidenced principally in the more peripheral portions of the auditory system. Recordings from the higher centers neither strongly support nor negate either theory. Rather, they suggest that these regions may not have the principal responsibility for relaying "place" or "neural rate" information, and that the hierarchy of the nervous system is arranged such that the phylogenetically newer structures (cortex) are occupied with something other than simple pitch perception.

If the reader has the impression that he has been left hanging by this discussion of possible mechanisms of frequency coding, he is correct. Both types of frequency representation may occur in the nervous system. Wever suggests that the neural-rate theory may be most appropriate for low-frequency stimulation, and that place representation may be the cue for higher frequencies. Licklider (1959, 1962) has developed an elaborate theory incorporating this possible dual representation. He suggests that the cochlear spatial analysis determines which neural elements may be excited in the periphery, and that a temporal analysis of the neural activity patterns may follow the cochlear analysis. The results of this temporal analysis may then be recoded into a place of maximal response through a sophisticated neural correlation device. This general line of thought, though not necessarily the specific model, may be very appropriate for reasoning through the processes of frequency coding.

Intensity Coding in the Auditory System

Increases in stimulus intensity have an obvious effect at the cochlea: they are met with an increase in the amplitude of the traveling wave. The cochlear response, as measured by the cochlear microphonic, appears to grow in direct proportion to the intensity of the stimulus over a range of approximately 60 dB. At least two effects would naturally follow this growth of activity in the cochlea. First, the sensory units normally stimulated by the traveling wave would receive a greater amount of stimulation. Second, more sensory cells might be stimulated by the growth and spread of the traveling wave.

The intensity of a stimulus is, of course, a primary factor in determining the loudness associated with the perception of that stimulus. One might think of loudness as being based in a neural signal which is present against a background of irrelevant neural activity. The irrelevant activity is the "noise" in the system, and is provided by the units which are not receiving stimulation by the input to the ear. "Recruiting" more units to participate in a response by increasing the stimulus intensity would help to improve this neural "signal-to-noise" ratio simply because more units would be participating in the response and there would be less irrelevant activity.

What of the first effect? How does the pattern of unit behavior change when a more intense stimulus is presented to the ear? The answer is not a simple one, for there are many subtle changes which may occur. The unit activity patterns shown in Figure 8-25 provide examples of many of these changes. The first obvious effect is that the discharge rate of a unit may increase with increments of stimulus intensity. The patterns of Unit 37–92 show this effect. This phenomenon was demonstrated when the first single unit recordings were made in the periphery of the auditory system (Galambos and Davis, 1943, 1944). The exact manner in which the rate of discharge may change with stimulus increments is variable from unit to unit. Some investigations have suggested that at least two types of rate growths may occur in the auditory nerve (Nomoto et al., 1964), while others (Kiang, 1965) suggest that it is fruitless to try to classify units in terms of this characteristic.

A second characteristic of the unit responses is that the rate of discharge may not change, but the unit may be able to maintain a high rate of discharge for a longer period of time for stimuli of higher intensity. Thus, the total number of spikes occurring during each stimulus presentation may increase. The discharge patterns of Unit 35–83 illustrate this effect.

The third characteristic is that the pattern of discharges of the unit may change, but the overall rate or total number of discharges which occur during presentation of a stimulus may not be affected. For example, the patterns of Unit 33–83 show the presence of a silent interval after presentation of the stimulus at 65 and 85 dB, but minimal changes can be seen in the

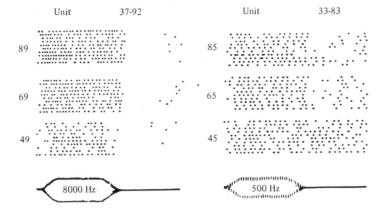

Figure 8-25 Changes of unit discharge patterns with changes in stimulus intensity. The dot patterns show unit responses to ten replications of a stimulus of 50 msec duration at the indicated intensities. Unit 37–92 shows an increase in discharge rate with increments in stimulus intensity. Unit 35–83 shows a relatively fixed rate of discharge, but an increase in the duration of the burst of discharges with increased stimulus intensity. Rather than showing a change in discharge rate, unit 33–83 shows a change in the organization of discharges, with the addition of a short silent interval after stimulus presentation as stimulus intensity is increased. Unit 37–94 shows complete inhibition of discharge after stimulus onset for stimuli of maximal intensity, and a shift in pattern to actual increments in discharge rate as the stimulus intensity is lowered. These patterns, and variations of these patterns, may be found in unit discharge characteristics throughout the nervous system. [*Reproduced courtesy of the Division of Otolaryngology, Stanford Univ. School of Medicine.*]

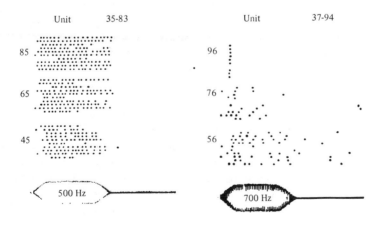

response pattern during the stimulus. This type of pattern change may provide an excellent contrast between a "response" and the succeeding spontaneous activity.

A fourth effect is an extension of the other three. The spontaneous activity of units at levels above the auditory nerve may be inhibited by the presence of a simple tonal stimulus. Activity patterns of Unit 37–94 illustrate this effect. This characteristic of unit behavior may serve to improve the neural "signal-to-noise" ratio because much of the background activity in the nervous system would be inhibited during stimulus presentation. The discharge patterns shown here were obtained from the cochlear nucleus (cat), but are representative of responses obtained throughout the nervous system.

All of these modifications of unit response characteristics may function together to improve the neural representation of a stimulus. The inhibition of units, for example, may provide support for a general "place" principle of hearing. The interconnections of neurons in the nervous system may permit a very active response area to be surrounded by units which are inhibited. Typically, this "inhibitory surround" may be as effective in defining the margins of the active area in the nervous system as a black circle is in defining the margins of a white spot drawn on a white piece of paper. This type of effect has been studied in the visual system, as well, and the "Mach-band" concept has been useful in understanding the ability to distinguish contrasts in illumination patterns. (See, for example, the review of this topic by Carterette et al., 1969.)

The observations of the inhibition of single units in the auditory system that have been made for stimuli delivered monaurally naturally lead this discussion into a description of responses to stimuli delivered to the two ears simultaneously. This is so because the ability to localize sounds in space may depend on the ability of the nervous system to inhibit (or enhance) the activity patterns from one of the two ears which are signalling the presence of a stimulus.

Binaural Effects in the Auditory System

The superior olivary complex has been described as the "lowest" nucleus in the afferent auditory system which receives a great number of fibers from both cochleas. The superior olivary complex and all of the major auditory centers above have units which behave preferentially to stimuli presented to each or both ears simultaneously. Any of the following combinations are possible in the response character of these units:

(1) A unit may be excited by a stimulus delivered to the ipsilateral (i. e., same side) ear, only. (See Galambos et al., 1959).

(2) A unit may be excited by a stimulus delivered to the contralateral (i. e., opposite side) ear, only (Galambos et al., 1959).

(3) A unit may be excited by a stimulus delivered to the ipsilateral ear and inhibited by a stimulus delivered to the contralateral ear (Moushegian, et al., 1964b).

(4) A unit may be inhibited by a stimulus delivered to the ipsilateral ear and excited by a stimulus delivered to the contralateral ear (Hall, 1964, 1965) (Moushegian et al., 1964b).

(5) A unit may respond to simultaneous delivery of stimuli to both ears with an increase or suppression of activity (Moushegian et al., 1964a, b).

(6) Time lags between the delivery of stimuli to both ears may be reflected in discharge patterns marked by corresponding suppression and enhancement of unit activity (Moushegian et al., 1964a).

Gathering all of these effects together, it is possible to build elaborate models of how the nervous system may react to stimuli delivered binaurally, as they are in nature. For example, Bergeijk (1962) has developed a theory which incorporates excitation, inhibition, and latency shifts in unit behavior patterns as they relate to changes in time of arrival and stimulus intensity at the ears. The salient feature of the model is that neural activity from the superior olivary complex and auditory nuclei above this point reflects the presence of a more intense (or earlier) stimulus to the contralateral ear by a graded increase in the probability of occurrence of a discharge. Stimuli at the ear ipsilateral to the complex produce a decrease in the probability of a discharge of the units in that nucleus. Localization of a source thus depends grossly on the amount of activity dispatched from the two superior olivary nuclei. If the left side is more active, then the percept will be localized to the right ear. The reverse would be true for localization to the left. The variety of activity patterns from the units in the superior olivary complex and nuclei above this location certainly supports these notions, as does the anatomy of the system. Deatherage's (1966) review of this topic is most inclusive.

One additional point should be noted here. The small differences in time of arrival which can be detected for stimuli presented independently to the two ears are on the order of microseconds. No single unit can discharge at microsecond intervals, but the small differences in timing can be detected. If such temporal analysis is possible for binaural stimuli, it may be appropriate to consider it possible for simple tones presented monaurally to be analyzed in a similar fashion to provide for stimulus frequency coding (Nordmark, 1963). Licklider's (1959) triplex theory has provided a basis for such a model.

It may appear that, save for some speculation regarding the function of the superior olivary complex, much of the evidence in the area of auditory physiology serves only to eliminate structures from contention as areas which provide specific functions. Such is not the case, however, when the data which have been reviewed are considered in light of consequences of lesions to various parts of the auditory nervous system. The results of the lesion studies have usually prompted ingenious modifications of techniques in the electrophysiological research. Some of these studies will be reviewed in the next section.

SOME BEHAVIORAL CONSEQUENCES
OF LESIONS IN THE AUDITORY SYSTEM

One type of investigation which has been useful in determining the role played by various levels has involved the controlled production of a lesion to known areas, and the subsequent investigation of apparent loss of function due to that lesion. The technique often requires that an experimental animal be trained to perform a task when an appropriate auditory stimulus is presented. This stimulus may be a simple tone, or one of changing frequency, or intensity, or one coming from the right or left. After the performance of the animal has reached a satisfactory competence level (say, 80% correct responses), a surgical lesion is made in the region of the nervous system under study. After recovery from surgery, the animal is placed back into the same testing situation. The experimenter may then observe the number of trials required for the animal to regain his former competence, or whether the animal ever does regain such competence in performing the task at hand. If failure to perform the task is correlated with placement of the lesion, the experimenter may have some basis for suggesting that the damaged structure may have functioned normally to aid in the animal's perception of the stimulus.

Some obvious results include the fact that complete destruction of the labyrinth or auditory nerve results in deafness on the side of the lesion. But what of the deep structures in the central nervous system?

Cortex. Destruction of the known auditory cortex in cat does not impair the animal's threshold for simple tonal stimuli (Kryter and Ades, 1943; Raab and Ades, 1946; and Rosenzweig, 1946). In addition, discrimination of changes in stimulus intensity (Oesterreich and Neff, 1960) and frequency (Neff and Diamond, 1958; and Diamond and Neff, 1957) may be relearned after bilateral cortical ablation (destruction). The series of experiments by Neff and his associates, using cats, has defined two types of deficits associated with bilateral ablation of known auditory cortex: localization of sound in space (see Neff's review, 1968) and *pattern* discrimination involving stimulus frequency changes (Diamond and Neff, 1957; Neff and Diamond, 1958; and Diamond et al., 1962).

Their frequency discrimination experiments usually involved stimuli at 800 and 1,000 Hz. A series of three tones at 800 Hz (symbolized as . . .) followed by a series at 800, 1,000, and 800 Hz (. · .) was differentiated by cats following cortical ablation (Diamond and Neff, 1957). When the patterns were reversed in sequence (. · . . . .), appropriate avoidance behavior was *not* demonstrated after cortical ablation (Diamond et al., 1962). With very extensive lesions, a sequence discrimination (. . . · · . . . vs . · . . · . . ·.) was impaired, where tonal discrimination (. . . vs . ·.) was intact (Diamond and Neff, 1957). Neff (1960) has summarized findings of this type by suggesting that the cortex is essential for differentiation of sequence of stimulation or amount of stimulation per unit time for stimulus patterns involving identical intensities and frequencies (which presumably stimulate the same neural units).

Dewson et al. (1970) have reported a disruption in sequence discrimination (tone-noise vs noise-tone) using primates. Small unilateral lesions were made in auditory "association" cortex. The lesions were adjacent and inferior to the primary cortex of the temporal lobe, and the primary area was spared. The nature of the disruption induced by such lesions was subtle: the temporal ranges at which the animals performed competently (79% correct) were limited. Stimulus durations and silent intervals between the stimuli thus had to be shortened if the animals were to reach the same level of competence evidenced prior to the introduction of the lesion. Among the hypotheses considered by the authors, the one suggesting that auditory short-term memory was influenced by the lesions seems most attractive.

Another series of experiments by Dewson et al., (1969) should be noted here. Monkeys which had experienced bilateral lesions of primary auditory cortex fared well in relearning tone-noise discrimination, but failed to relearn a discrimination task involving two speech sounds, [i] and [u]. When matched for intensity and duration, these two speech sounds pose a discrimination task based on the location of two or three spectral maxima (formants), a task far more complex than the simple discrimination of one tone from another.

Medial geniculate. While destruction of primary auditory cortex is known to cause retrograde degeneration of neurons to portions of the medial geniculate, complete destruction of the geniculate bodies does not occur. Thus, the cortical lesion studies suggest that simple detection and discrimination tasks may be accomplished by the medial geniculate or by regions of the cortex which do not receive projections from the medial geniculate. Sectioning of the brachium of the inferior colliculus, thus cutting off the classical auditory pathway *peripheral to* the medial geniculate, produces behavioral effects which are more devastating than cortical lesions alone. In particular, localization may be impaired to a greater degree (Strominger and Oesterreich, 1970), and sensitivity to changes in stimulus intensity is poorer (by as much as 10 dB) (Oesterreich and Neff, 1960).

Other centers. Only a relatively small amount of data has been gathered regarding specific lesions below the medial geniculate or brachium of the inferior colliculus. As Neff (1968) has reviewed, transection of the trapezoid body produces a localizing deficit, suggesting that the integrity of the input to the superior olivary complex must be preserved.

Studies of human patients have indicated that complex discrimination functions may be impaired by deep central nervous system lesions. Jerger et al., (1969) have described a series of studies on a patient with bilateral temporal lobe damage. The impairments of localization and complex stimulus discrimination (speech) observed in laboratory animals were also observed in this patient. Gershuni (1968) has summarized data from many laboratories with animal and human experience. Much of the data dealt with impairments for transient events and speech. He argues convincingly that the cortical auditory system is a spatial and temporal projection system which is especially important in detection of transitional cues.

If one point be drawn from this section, it is related to complex stimulus discrimination. It should be recalled that unit discharge patterns in the higher nervous system structures rarely follow individual cycles of simple tonal stimuli. Rather, they discharge in bursts which may be unrelated to the frequency of a tonal stimulus. The bursts occur only when a stimulus is changed along one of its dimensions. In view of such data, it is attractive to think of the higher nervous system centers as functioning to render decisions on changes in the acoustic environment of the individual. The lower nuclei may each perform a variety of tasks related to stripping redundancy from the neural events present in each auditory nerve, and excitation of these nuclei may lead to specific, well-defined sensations. Complex sorting and discrimination tasks, according to this line of thought, would be left to the "higher" centers.

One task the higher centers may assume is the governing of the activity patterns of the brain stem nuclei. The appropriate stimulus for activation of such efferent control is not known. Rather, stimuli such as a series of brief shocks are delivered to the tract or nucleus thought to provide this efferent control. The effects of this prior stimulus are observed on a lower center's afferent evoked activity in response to an acoustic input. This type of investigation shall be considered in the next section.

THE EFFERENT AUDITORY SYSTEM

All of the preceding sections on coding of stimulus parameters have implicitly dealt with the ascending, or afferent portion of the nervous system. The efferent system poses special problems to investigators, with its elusive anatomical configuration and adequate stimulus being formidable among these problems. Clues as to the nature of its function come from three general types of studies. The first type involves the study of the effects of direct electrical (shock) stimulation to known efferent neurons.

For example, prior electrical stimulation of certain areas of the auditory cortex may produce subtle effects on the discharge patterns of units in the medial geniculate (Watanabe et al., 1966). The great bulk of data from this type of study deals with the olivocochlear bundle, however. Accessible from the floor of the IVth ventricle, it can be approached for electrical stimulation with relative ease. Galambos (1956) demonstrated that electrical stimulation of this bundle of neurons would cause enhancement of the cochlear microphonic and a decrease in the amplitude of the gross whole nerve response recorded from the same ear. This amplitude decrement presumably is related to an inhibition of the response of the neurons. This same technique has been used in conjunction with recordings made from various other levels in the nervous system, and there has been some suggestion that enhancement, as well as inhibition, of responses may result.

If two transient stimuli are delivered to the ear with a small (say 2 to 5 msec) interstimulus interval, two gross evoked responses are recordable from the auditory nerve. The second response is of smaller amplitude than the first, possibly indicating that some of the neurons which contributed to the first response were incapable of discharging in response to the second stimulus. With prior electrical stimulation of the olivocochlear bundle, the response to the first click is attenuated (like Galambos' results) but the response to the second click is not attenuated to as small a percentage of the amplitude of the first click as before, when no prior electrical stimulus was given (Dewson, 1967). Findings like these suggest that the units which were inhibited by the efferent tract stimulation were placed on "hold" for the period of time occupied by the first acoustic stimulus, and allowed to respond maximally to the second stimulus. It may be most appropriate to think of the efferent system as a *regulatory* system aiding in stimulus sorting, rather than as an inhibitory system which shuts out all auditory input.

Dewson (1968) has pursued this "sorting" hypothesis in another series of studies. Monkeys were trained to discriminate between two English vowels, and their ability to maintain this discrimination while the speech sounds were presented against a controlled background of noise was studied. After experiencing lesions of the olivocochlear bundle, the animals' performances in noise was again evaluated, and found to be poorer than that observed prior to the lesions. They did perform well when no competing noise was present, however. This line of research seems especially promising in determining the role of the efferent system.

Other efforts have gone into investigating the means by which the efferent system acts upon the afferent system. Fex (1962, 1968) has studied efferent action in a wide variety of experiments and suggests, for example, that some regulation may occur at the junction of the hair cells and neurons, and also directly upon afferent neurons. The anatomical relationships among the efferent and afferent systems (Rasmussen, 1964 and Spoendlin, 1968) certainly support such conclusions.

The application of neurochemical blocking or facilitating agents has also been used to define the mechanisms available to the efferent system (Whitfield, 1968). This, too, may provide additional valuable information as to its function. At present, however, its actual mode of operation remains without complete definition.

A SUMMARY

This brief overview of the auditory system has sketched several possible mechanisms for the effective stimulation of the system, and for its reaction to various types of stimulation. The transmission of energy to the inner ear was shown to be facilitated by the action of the middle ear structures. The resultant mechanical activity of the inner ear was described, and emphasis was placed on the shearing forces applied to the hair cells as a means of initiating a response from the auditory nervous system.

The means by which stimulus frequency is coded in the nervous system has not been exactly defined, but it appears that both place of excitation and rate of neural discharge may contribute to the percept associated with a given stimulus frequency. Several factors were also suggested as contributing to the formulation of a neural code for stimulus intensity. Rate and pattern of neural discharge may couple with anatomical arrangement of neurons to effect this code.

Those neural units which react preferentially to changes in the parameters of binaural stimuli were described as possessing a broad galaxy of responses which could all contribute to the laterality of a tonal image. Again, anatomical configuration and rate of neural discharge may combine to provide the appropriate mechanism for two-eared listening.

An extremely brief review of lesion studies was provided. These studies were generated, usually, to determine the effects of disability of anatomically defined structures in the auditory nervous system. The general finding has been that the processing of complex auditory stimuli was dependent upon the integrity of the auditory cortex. Electrophysiological studies have come to use very complex stimuli for the study of unit behavior patterns. This changing feature of these studies is important, because persistence coupled with the appropriate stimulus set may help to define critical aspects of the responses of the auditory nervous system to speech and other complex stimuli.

If this line of thought seems to be based on pure fiction, it may be helpful to recall some of the characteristics of speech signals. From one perspective, speech consists of a sequence of bursts of noise interspersed with silent intervals. The noise bursts may contain spectral maxima at various well-defined frequencies, and these maxima may shift during the production of a given speech segment. This type of stimulus is not unlike the frequency-modulated stimuli used in the study of cortical single neurons described earlier in this chapter. Such stimuli were the only ones effective in evoking a response from many cortical units. Could it be that speech, as one set of gestures which comprise language, is perceived and sorted exactly like all of the other stimuli with which an individual is bombarded? A definite answer is not apparent, but sufficient evidence exists to prompt the question! In addition to the physiological evidence presented previously, consider, also, that speech materials are often used in audiological evaluations to provide cues for the differential diagnosis of disorders of the nervous system.

For example, pure tone thresholds for 500, 1,000, and 2,000 Hz should be a fairly good predictor for the threshold for speech reception, as significant energy in speech is located in these frequency regions. Speech reception is usually measured by requiring the patient to repeat the words he hears and, obviously, requires perceiving the signal well enough to permit reporting it back to the tester. This is, of course, different than detection, as detection of any signal is usually a simpler task than perceiving all of its attributes. A person who shows only minimal loss of threshold sensitivity for pure tones but a markedly greater loss for speech stimuli or an impairment of speech discrimination may be suspect as having a disorder affecting the nervous system as distinct from one involving the cochlea or middle ear apparatus. Perhaps it is being too anthropomorphic to remind the reader of cats who fail to make complex discriminations successfully after removal of cortex, but who show minimal loss of sensitivity for pure tones. Then again, perhaps not.

If this chapter has met its goals, it has provided the introductory student with sufficient information to enable him to comprehend the elegance and complexity of the auditory nervous system. The literature search presented here has not been complete, but it should have provided the student with a few leads into the vast literature in this area, so that he may pursue some specific questions on his own.

REFERENCES

ADES, H. W., METTLER, F. A. and CULLER, E. A. 1939. Effect of lesions in the medial geniculate bodies upon hearing in the cat. *Amer. J. Physiol.* 125: 15–23.

ANDERSON, D. J., ROSE, J. E., HIND, J. E. and BRUGGEE, J. F. 1971. Temporal position of discharges in single auditory nerve fibers within the cycle of a sine wave stimulus: Frequency and intensity effects. *J. Acoust. Soc. Amer.* 49: 1131–39.

BAKER, P. F. 1968. Nervous conduction: Some properties of the ion-selective channels which appear during the action potential. *Brit. Med. Bull.* 24: 179–82.

BARANY, E. 1938. A contribution to the physiology of bone conduction. *Acta Otolaryngol.* Suppl. 26.

BAST, T. H. and ANSON, B. J. 1949. *The Temporal Bone and the Ear.* Springfield, Ill.: Charles C. Thomas, Publisher.

BATTEAU, D. W. 1968. Role of the pinna in localization: Theoretical and physiological consequences, pp. 234–43. *In* A. V. S. De Reuck and J. Knight (eds.), *Hearing Mechanisms in Vertebrates.* Boston: Little, Brown and Company.

BÉKÉSY, G. VON. 1960. *Experiments in Hearing.* New York: McGraw-Hill Book Co., Inc.

BÉKÉSY, G. VON and ROSENBLITH, W. A. 1951. Mechanical properties of the ear. pp. 1075–115. In S. S. Stevens (ed.) *Handbook of Experimental Psychology.* New York: John Wiley and Sons, Inc.

BERGEIJK, W. A. VAN. 1962. Variation on a theme of Békésy: A model of binaural interaction. *J. Acoust. Soc. Amer.* 34: 1431–37.

BOER, E. DE and SIX, P. D. 1960. The cochlear difference tone. *Acta Otolaryngol.* 51: 84–88.

BUTLER, R. A., HONRUBIA, B. M., JOHNSTONE, B. M. and FERNANDEZ, C. 1962. Cochlear function under metabolic impairment. *Ann. Otol. Rhinol., and Laryngol.* 71: 648–56.

CARTERETTE, E. C., FRIEDMAN, M. P. and LOVELL, J. D. 1969. Mach bands in hearing. *J. Acoust. Soc. Amer.* 45: 986–98.

CHOW, K. L. 1951. Numerical estimates of the auditory central nervous system of the Rhesus monkey. *J. Comp. Neurol.* 95: 159–75.

DALLOS, P. 1969a. Comments on the differential electrode technique. *J. Acoust. Soc. Amer.* 45: 999–1007.

DALLOS, P. 1969b. Combination tone $2f_L\text{-}f_h$ in microphonic potentials. *J. Acoust. Soc. Amer.* 46: 1437–44.

DALLOS, P., SCHOENY, Z. G. and CHEATHAM, M. A. 1971. On the limitations of cochlear microphonic measurements. *J. Acoust. Soc. Amer.* 49: 1144–54.

DAVIS, H. 1962. Advances in the neurophysiology and neuroanatomy of the cochlea. *J. Acoust. Soc. Amer.* 34: 1377–85.

DEATHERAGE, B. H. 1966. Examination of binaural interaction. *J. Acoust. Soc. Amer.* 39: 323–49.

DEATHERAGE, B. H., DAVIS J., and ELDREDGE, D. H. 1957. Physiological evidence for the masking of low frequencies by high. *J. Acoust. Soc. Amer.* 29: 132–37.

DEWSON, J. H., III. 1967. Efferent olivocochlear bundle: Some relationships to noise masking and to stimulus attenuation. *J. Neurophysiol.* 30: 817–32.

DEWSON, J. H., III. 1968. Efferent olivocochlear bundle: Some relationships to stimulus discrimination in noise. *J. Neurophysiol.* 31: 122–30.

DEWSON, J. H., III, COWEY, A. and WEISKRANTZ, L. 1970. Disruptions of auditory sequence discrimination by unilateral and bilateral cortical ablations of superior temporal gyrus in the monkey. *Exp. Neurol.* 28: 529–48.

DEWSON, J. H., III, PRIBRAM, K. H. and LYNCH, J. C. 1969. Effects of ablations of temporal cortex upon speech sound discrimination in the monkey. *Exp. Neurol.* 24: 579–91.

DIAMOND, I. T., GOLDBERG, J. M. and NEFF, W. D. 1962. Tonal discrimination after ablation of cortical projection areas of the auditory system. *J. Neurophysiol.* 25: 223–35.

DIAMOND, I. T. and NEFF, W. D. 1957. Ablation of temporal cortex and discrimination of auditory patterns. *J. Neurophysiol.* 20: 300–15.

ECCLES, J. C. 1964. *The Physiology of Synapses.* New York: Springer-Verlag.

EVANS, E. F. 1968. Cortical representation, pp. 234–43. *In* A. V. S. De Reuck and J. Knight. (eds.), *Hearing Mechanisms in Vertebrates.* Boston: Little, Brown and Company.

EVANS, E. F., ROSS H. F. and WHITFIELD I. C. 1965. The spatial distribution of unit characteristic frequency in the primary auditory cortex of the cat. *J. Physiol.* 179: 238–47.

EVANS, E. F. and WHITFIELD, I. C. 1964. Classification of unit responses in the auditory cortex of the unanaesthetized and unrestrained cat. *J. Physiol.* 171: 476–93.

FERNANDEZ, C. 1951. The innervation of the cochlea (Guinea pig). *Laryngoscope* 61: 1152–72.

FEX, J. 1962. Auditory activity in centrifugal and centripetal cochlear fibers in cat. *Acta Physiol. Scand.* Suppl. 189, 1–68.

FEX, J. 1968. Efferent inhibition in the cochlea by the olivocochlear bundle, pp. 169–86. *In* A. V. S. De Reuck and J. Knight (eds.), *Hearing Mechanisms in Vertebrates.* Boston: Little, Brown, and Company.

FISCHLER, H., FREI, E., SPIRA, D. and RUBINSTEIN, M. 1967. Dynamic response of middle ear structures. *J. Acoust. Soc. Amer.* 41: 1220–31.

FLETCHER, H. 1953. *Speech and Hearing in Communication.* Princeton, N.J.: D. Van Nostrand Company, Inc.

FLYNN, WM. E. and ELLIOTT, D. N. 1965. Role of the pinna in hearing. *J. Acoust. Soc. Amer.* 38: 104–105.

FOX, S. S. and O'BRIEN, H. H. 1965. Duplication of evoked potential waveform by curve of probability of firing of a single cell. *Science* 147: 888–90.

FRANK, K. 1959. Identification and analysis of single unit activity in the central nervous system. *In Handbook of Physiology.* Sect. 1, Vol. 1, Neurophysiology. American Physiological Society.

FRANK, K. and BECKER, M. 1964. Microelectrodes for recording and stimulation. *In Physical Techniques in Biological Research.* Vol. V, part A. New York: Academic Press.

GALAMBOS, R. 1952. Microelectrode studies on medial geniculate body of cat. III. Response to pure tones. *J. Neurophysiol.* 15: 381–400.

GALAMBOS, R. 1956. Suppression of auditory nerve activity by stimulation of efferent fibers to the cochlea. *J. Neurophysiol.* 19: 424–37.

GALAMBOS, R. and DAVIS, H. 1943. The response of single auditory nerve fibers to acoustic stimulation. *J. Neurophysiol.* 6: 39–57.

GALAMBOS, R. and DAVIS, J. 1944. Action potentials from single auditory nerve fibers? *Science* 108: 513.

GALAMBOS, R. and RUPERT, A. 1959. Action of the middle ear muscles in normal cats. *J. Acoust. Soc. Amer.* 31: 349–55.

GALAMBOS, R. SCHWARTZKOPFF, J. and RUPERT, A. 1959. Microelectrode study of superior olivary nuclei. *Amer. J. Physiol.* 197: 527–36.

GERSHUNI, G. V., BARU, A. V. and KARASEVA, T. A. 1968. Role of auditory cortex in discrimination of acoustic stimuli. *Neurosci. Transl.* 1: 370–82.

GLATTKE, T. J. 1968. Apical cochlear responses to pulse trains. *J. Acoust. Soc. Amer.* 44: 819–21.

GOLDBERG, J. M. and NEFF, W. D. 1961. Frequency discrimination after bilateral section of the brachium of the inferior colliculus. *J. Comp. Neurol.* 116: 265–90.

GOLDSTEIN, M. H. JR., DALY, R. L., ABELES, M. and McINTOSH, J. 1970. Functional architecture in cat primary auditory cortex: Tonotopic organization. *J. Neurophysiol.* 33: 188-97.

GROSS, N. B. and SMALL, A. M. JR. 1961. Frequency correlates on the auditory cortex of the cat brain. *Exp. Neurol.* 3: 375–87.

GRUNDFEST, H. 1940. Bioelectric potentials. *Amer. Rev. Physiol.* 2: 213–42.

GUINAN, J. J. JR. and PEAKE, W. T. 1967. Middle ear characteristics of anesthetized cats. *J. Acoust. Soc. Amer.* 41: 1237–61.

HALAI, S. and WHITFIELD, I. 1953. Responses of the trapezoid body to acoustic stimulation with pure tones. *J. Physiol.* 122: 158–71.

HALL, J. L. II 1964. Binaural interaction in the accessory superior olivary nucleus of the cat. Cambridge: M.I.T. Technical Report 416.

HALL, J. L. II 1965. Binaural interaction in the accessory superior olivary nucleus of the cat. *J. Acoust. Soc. Amer.* 37: 814–823.

HELMHOLTZ, H. L. F. VON *On the Sensations of Tone as a Physiological Basis for the Theory of Music.* 1877. Trans. and rev. by A. J. Ellis. New York: Dover, 1954.

HODGKIN, A. L. and HUXLEY, A. F. 1952. A quantitative description of membrane current and its application to conduction and excitation in nerve. *J. Physiol.* 117: 500–44.

HUXLEY, A. F. 1954. Electrical processes in nerve conduction, pp. 23–34. *In* H. T. Clarke (ed.), *Ion Transport Across Membranes.* New York: Academic Press.

JEPSEN, O. 1963. Middle-ear muscle reflexes in man, pp. 192–240. *In* J. Jerger (ed.), *Modern Developments in Audiology.* New York: Academic Press.

JERGER, J., WEIKERS, N. J., SHARBROUGH, F. W., III and JERGER, S. 1969. Bilateral lesions of the temporal lobe. *Acta Otolaryngol.* Suppl. 258: 1–51.

KATSUKI, Y., SUGA, N. and KANNO, Y. 1962. Neural mechanisms of the peripheral and central auditory systems in monkeys. *J. Acoust. Soc. Amer.* 24: 1397–410.

KIANG, N. Y.-S. 1965. *Discharge Patterns of Single Fibers in the Cat's Auditory Nerve.* Cambridge: M.I.T. Press.

KIRIKAE, I. 1960. *The Structure and Function of the Middle Ear.* Tokyo: Univ. Tokyo Press.

KOBRAK, H. G. 1959. *The Middle Ear.* Chicago: Univ. Chicago Press.

KRYTER, K. D. and ADES, H. W. 1943. Studies on the function of the higher acoustic nervous centers in the cat. *Amer. J. Psychol.* 56: 501–36.

LICKLIDER, J. C. R. 1959. Three auditory theories. *In* S. Koch (ed.), Vol. 1 *Psychology: A Study of a Science.* New York: McGraw-Hill Book Company.

LICKLIDER, J. C. R. 1962. Periodicity pitch and related auditory process models. *Internat. Audiol.* 1: 11–36.

LIM, D. J. and LANE, W. C. 1969a. Vestibular sensory epithelia. *Arch. Otolaryngol.* 90: 47–56.

LIM, D. J. and LANE, W. C. 1969b. Cochlear sensory epithelium: A scanning electron microscopic observation. *Ann. Otol.* 78: 827–41.

LORENTE DE NO., R. 1933. Anatomy of the eighth nerve. The central projection of the nerve endings of the internal ear. *Laryngoscope* 43: 1–38.

MASSOPUST, L. C. JR. and ORDY, J. M. 1962. Auditory organization of the inferior colliculi in the cat. *Exper. Neurol.* 6: 465–77.

MØLLER, A. R. 1969a. Unit responses in the cochlear nucleus of the rat to pure tones. *Acta Physiol. Scand.* 75: 530–41.

MØLLER, A. R. 1969b. Unit responses in the cochlear nucleus of the rat to sweep tones. *Acta Physiol. Scand.* 76: 503–12.

MOUSHEGIAN, G., RUPERT, A. and WHITCOMB, M. A. 1969a. Brain stem neuronal response patterns to monaural and binaural tones. *J. Neurophysiol.* 27: 1174–91.

MOUSHEGIAN, G., RUPERT, A. and WHITCOMB, M. A. 1969b. Medial superior olivary unit response patterns to monaural and binaural clicks. *J. Acoust. Soc. Amer.* 46: 196–202.

NAUNTON, R. 1963. The measurement of hearing by bone conduction, pp. 1–29. *In* J. Jerger (ed.), *Modern Developments in Audiology.* New York: Academic Press.

NEFF, W. D. 1960. Role of the auditory cortex in sound discrimination, pp. 211–16. *In* G. L. Rasmussen and W. F. Windle (eds.), *Neural Mechanisms of the Auditory and Vestibular Systems.* Springfield Ill.: Charles C. Thomas.

NEFF, W. D. 1968. Localization and lateralization of sound in space, pp. 207–33. *In* A. V. S. De Reuck and J. Knight (eds.), *Hearing Mechanisms in Vertebrates.* Boston: Little, Brown and Company.

NEFF, W. D. and DIAMOND, I. T. 1958. Neural basis of auditory discrimination, pp. 101–26. *In* H. F. Harlow and C. N. Woolsey (eds.), *Biological and Biochemical Bases of Behavior.* Madison: Univ. Wisconsin Press.

NELSON, P. G., ERULKAR, S. D. and BRYON, J. S. 1966. Responses of units of the inferior colliculus to time-varying acoustic stimuli. *J. Neurophysiol.* 29: 834–60.

NOBEL, K. W. and DEWSON, J. H. III 1966. A corticofugal projection from insular and temporal cortex to the homolateral inferior colliculus in cat. *J. Aud. Res.* 6: 67–75.

NOMOTO, M., SUGA, N. and KATSUKI, Y. 1964. Discharge pattern and inhibition of primary auditory fibers in the monkey. *J. Neurophysiol.* 27: 768–87.

NORDMARK, J. O. 1963. Some analogies between pitch and lateralization phenomena. *J. Acoust. Soc. Amer.* 35: 1544–47.

NORDMARK, I., GLATTKE, T. J. and SCHUBERT, E. D. 1969. Waveform preservation in the cochlea. *J. Acoust. Soc. Amer.* 46: 1587–88.

OESTERREICH, R. E. and NEFF, W. D. 1960. Higher auditory centers and the DL for sound intensity. *Fed. Proc.* 19: 301.

RAAB, D. H. and ADES, H. W. 1946. Cortical and midbrain mediation of a conditioned discrimination of acoustic intensities. *Amer. J. Psychol.* 59: 59–83.

RASMUSSEN, G. L. 1964. Anatomic relationships of the ascending and descending auditory systems, pp. 5–19. *In* W. S. Fields and B. R. Alford (eds.), *Neurological Aspects of Auditory and Vestibular Disorders.* Springfield, Ill.: Charles C. Thomas.

REGER, S. N. 1960. Effect of middle ear muscle action on certain psychophysical measurements. *Ann. Otol. Rhinol. Laryngol.* 69: 1179–98.

ROSE, J., BRUGGE, J., ANDERSON, D. and HIND, J. 1967. Phase-locked response to low frequency tones in single auditory nerve fibers of the squirrel monkey. *J. Neurophysiol.* 30: 769–94.

ROSE, J., GALAMBOS, R. and HUGHES, J. 1959. Microelectrode studies of the cochlear nuclei of the cat. *Bull. Johns Hopkins Hosp.* 104: 211–51.

Rose, J., Greenwood, D., Goldberg, J. and Hind, J. 1963. Some discharge characteristics of single neurons in the inferior colliculus of the cat. I. Tonotopical organization, relation of spike counts to tone intensity, and firing patterns of single elements. *J. Neurophysiol.* 26: 294–320.

Rose, J. and Woolsey, C. N. 1958. Cortical connections and functional organization of thalamic auditory system of the cat, pp. 127–50. *In* H. F. Harlow and C. N. Woolsey (eds.), *Biological and Biochemical Bases of Behavior.* Madison: Univ. Wisconsin Press.

Rosenzweig, M. 1946. Discrimination of auditory intensities in the cat. *Amer. J. Psychol.* 59: 127–36.

Rubinstein, M., Feldman, B., Fischler, H., Frei, E. and Spire, D. 1966. Measurement of stapedial-footplate displacements during transmission of sound through the middle ear. *J. Acoust. Soc. Amer.* 40: 1420–26.

Shaw, E. A. G. 1966. Ear canal pressure generated by a free sound field. *J. Acoust. Soc. Amer.* 39: 465–70.

Simmons, F. B. 1963. An analysis of the middle ear muscle acoustic reflex of the cat. *In* J. Fletcher (ed.), *Middle Ear Function Seminar.* Fort Knox: U.S. Army Med. Res. Lab.

Simmons, F. B. and Beatty, D. L. 1962. The significance of round window recorded cochlear potentials in hearing. *Amer. Otol. Soc. Trans.* 95: 182–217.

Simmons, F. B. and Linehan, J. A. 1968. Observations on a single auditory nerve fiber over a six-week period. *J. Neurophysiol.* 31: 799–805.

Smith, C. A. 1961. Innervation pattern of the cochlea. *Amer. Otol. Soc. Trans.* 48: 35–60.

Spoendlin, H. 1968. Ultrastructure and peripheral innervation pattern of the receptor in relation to the first coding of the acoustic message, pp. 89–125. *In* A. V. S. De Reuck and J. Knight (eds.), *Hearing Mechanisms in Vertebrates.* Boston: Little, Brown and Company.

Spoendlin, H. 1969. Innervation patterns in the organ of Corti of the cat. *Acta Otolaryngol.* 67: 239–54.

Strominger, N. L. and Oesterreich, R. E. 1970. Localization of sound after section of the brachium of the inferior colliculus. *J. Comp. Neur.* 138: 1–18.

Suga, N. 1965. Analysis of frequency-modulated sounds by auditory neurons of echo-locating bats. *J. Physiol.* (Lond.) 179: 26–53.

Suzuki, T. (ed.) 1969. Electrophysiological measurements of human auditory function. *Acta Otolaryngol.* Suppl. 252: 1–103.

Tasaki, I. 1968. *Nerve Excitation: A Macromolecular Approach.* Springfield Ill.: Charles C. Thomas.

Tasaki, I., Davis, H. and Legouix, J. P. 1952. The space-time pattern of the cochlear microphonics (Guinea pig) as recorded by differential electrodes. *J. Acoust. Soc. Amer.* 24: 502–19.

TEAS, D. C., ELDREDGE, D. and DAVIS, H. 1962. Cochlear responses to acoustic transients: An interpretation of whole-nerve action potentials. *J. Acoust. Soc. Amer.* 34: 1438–59.

THURLOW, W. R., GROSS, N. B., KEMP, E. H. and LOWY, K. 1951. Microelectrode studies of neural activity of cat. I. Inferior colliculus. *J. Neurophysiol.* 14: 289–304.

TONNDORF, J. 1958. Localization of aural harmonics along the basilar membrane of Guinea pigs. *J. Acoust. Soc. Amer.* 30: 938–43.

TONNDORF, J. 1966. Bone conduction studies in experimental animals. *Acta Otolaryngol.* Suppl. 213: 1–132.

TONNDORF, J. and KHANNA, S. M. 1968. Submicroscopic displacement amplitudes of the tympanic membrane (cat) measured by laser interferometer. *J. Acoust. Soc. Amer.* 44: 1546–54.

VALLANCIEN, B. 1963. Comparative anatomy and physiology of the auditory organ in vertebrates, pp. 522–56. *In* R. G. Busnel (ed.), *Acoustic Behaviour of Animals*. New York: Elsevier.

WATANABE, T., YANAGISAWA, K., KANZAKI, J. and KATSUKI, Y. 1966. Cortical efferent flow influencing unit responses of medial geniculate body to sound stimulation. *Exper. Brain Res.* 2: 302–17.

WEVER, E. G. 1949. *Theory of Hearing*. New York: John Wiley and Sons, Inc.

WEVER, E. G. 1962. Development of traveling wave theories. *J. Acoust. Soc. Amer.* 34: 1319–24.

WEVER, E. G. 1966. Electrical potentials of the cochlea. *Physiol. Rev.* 46: 102–26.

WEVER, E. G. and BRAY, C. W. 1930. Action currents in the auditory nerve in response to acoustical stimulation. *Proc. Nat. Acad. Sci.* (U.S.) 16: 344–50.

WEVER, E. G. and LAWRENCE, M. 1954. *Physiological Acoustics*. Princeton: Princeton University Press.

WHITFIELD, I. C. 1968. Centrifugal control mechanisms of the auditory pathway pp. 246–58. *In* A. V. S. De Reuck and J. Knight. (eds.), *Hearing Mechanisms in Vertebrates*. Boston: Little, Brown and Company.

WHITFIELD, I. C. and EVANS, E. F. 1965. Responses of auditory cortical neurons to stimuli of changing frequency. *J. Neurophysiol.* 28: 655–72.

WIENER, F. M. and ROSS, D. A. 1946. The pressure distribution in the auditory canal in a progressive sound field. *J. Acoust. Soc. Amer.* 18: 401–408.

WOOLSEY, C. N. (1960). Organization of cortical auditory systems: A review and synthesis. *In Neural Mechanisms of the Auditory and Vestibular Systems*. Springfield: Charles C. Thomas.

WOOLSEY, C. N. and WALZL, E. M. 1942. Topical projection of nerve fibers from local regions of the cochlea to the cerebral cortex of the cat. *Bull. Johns Hopkins Hosp.* 71: 315–44.

WORTHINGTON, D. W. and DALLOS, P. 1971. Spatial patterns of cochlear difference tones. *J. Acoust. Soc. Amer.* 49: 1818–30.

ZEMLIN, W. R. 1968. *Speech and Hearing Science, Anatomy and Physiology*. Englewood Cliffs, N.J.: Prentice-Hall, Inc.

ZWISLOCKI, J. 1962. Analysis of the middle-ear function. Part I: Acoustic impedance. *J. Acoust. Soc. Amer.* 34: 1514–23.

ZWISLOCKI, J. 1963a. Acoustics of the middle ear. *In* J. Fletcher (ed.), *Middle Ear Function Seminar*. Fort Knox: U.S. Army Med. Res. Lab.

ZWISLOCKI, J. 1963b. An acoustic method for clinical examination of the ear. *J. Speech Hear. Research* 6: 303–14.

ZWISLOCKI, J. and FELDMAN, A. S. 1970. Acoustic impedance of pathological ears. *Amer. Speech Hearing Assoc. Monogr.* 15: 1–42.

9

PSYCHOACOUSTICS

Arnold M. Small

INTRODUCTION

Psychoacoustics is a part of psychophysics which is a study of the relation between the physical world and subjective awareness. In other words, psychophysics is the study of the relation between stimulus and response. Typically, the measurement and specification of the stimulus is encompassed by the science of physics and the measurement and specification of the response is within the realm of psychology; thus, the phrase psychophysics. Psychophysics is not unique in being a discipline where the interest is in the specification of the relation between stimulus and response. For example, all of experimental psychology is concerned with these relations.

One feature that distinguishes modern psychophysics from other disciplines with the same general stimulus-response aim is that it is possible to specify the exact nature of the stimulus to a much greater extent in this area than in others. We know a great deal about the physics of sound, light, and mechanics, therefore, the stimuli can be specified precisely and controlled easily. This is important since our ability to define a relation (for example, stimulus-response) depends upon our knowledge of the individual events that enter into the relation.

Psychoacoustics has traditionally dealt with the normal hearing process. However, there is nothing to prevent the use of traditional techniques and knowledge from being applied to experiments involving listeners with pathological auditory systems. Indeed, this is a very important contribution. Because of limitations of time and space this chapter will deal exclusively with the response of the normal-hearing listener to sound. In addition, since the history of psychophysics, and psychoacoustics in particular, is very long, we will limit our review to information that has been gathered since about 1930. The rationale of this lower chronological limit is that after 1930 the vacuum tube came into general use and the age of electronics began. Electronics allows a very precise control of the sound stimulus which was not possible previously (see chapter 2). Consequently, in research reported before 1930 we can never be quite sure what the stimulus was which produced a given listener reaction; thus, it is difficult to interpret the results. In other words, if we do not know what we are listening to, there is little point in trying to figure out what we hear.

PSYCHOPHYSICAL PROCEDURES

Rationale

We have mentioned that the careful specification of stimulus conditions is a distinguishing characteristic of psychophysics. We have also said that in order to establish a meaningful relation between two quantities we must know both quantities with acceptable precision. Thus it follows that if psychophysics in general, and psychoacoustics in particular, are to establish meaningful relations then both the response and the stimulus must be measured with rigor.

This is easy to say, but not easy to do. The stimulus for hearing, sound, is a physical event that can be measured with physical instruments. In contrast, the response to sound is subjective. It is not physical, it is psychological. Perception is a private, individual experience. That is, following the presentation of a sound to several listeners I may be aware of what I perceive, but there is no simple way in which I can tell what you perceive. How can I tell what you hear? One thing I can do is simply ask, "What do you hear?" If I were to ask this question the chances are excellent that I would get as many different answers as there were listeners to whom I addressed the question. In other words, it is entirely possible that even though all perceived the event, they might provide different responses because different words have different meanings to different people. You can imagine then that if in fact they heard slightly different things, the range of responses would probably be even greater.

How do we solve this problem? A step in the right direction would seem to be to structure the response situation; that is, rather than ask the person what he hears, allow him only certain choices of response. For example, ask him "Do you hear a soft tone, a loud tone, a high tone, a low tone?" or other appropriate categories. Such an approach, while possibly representing a move in the proper direction, still falls short of achieving the necessary precision of response measurement. The solution seems to lie in still further structuring the response situation and the development of particular procedures which go with these structured situations. These procedures are referred to as *psychophysical procedures* and several examples of these will be discussed in this section.

The experiment

Scientific observations are usually made in either of two situations. In one, which we refer to as *observational*, the scientist is completely passive and merely observes the world about him. The other method is the *experimental* method in which the scientist observes as he did previously but, in addition, takes an active role in that he changes certain aspects of the situation which he is observing. Since psychophysical methods are typically used in an experimental situation, let us describe the features of an experiment.

In most experiments there are three classes of variables. One variable, called an *independent variable*, represents that aspect of the experimental situation that the experimenter chooses to change. Another aspect of the situation is measured and this variable is called the *dependent variable*. Variables other than the independent and the dependent variables are held constant and are called *irrelevant variables*. Thus, an experiment may be defined as a situation in which the independent variable is changed, the dependent variable is measured, and the irrelevant variables are held constant.

What are the advantages of an experiment compared to simple observation? An experiment is usually more efficient than simple observation; that is, if a scientist had to wait for a certain event to occur before he could observe a particular reaction to that event he might wait a very long time. If, on the other hand, it was within his power to cause that event to occur, then he could observe the reaction to that event very much sooner and in this sense efficiency would result. Additionally, and probably more importantly, an experiment allows us to infer cause and effect relations. That is, if we change the independent variable but keep every other variable in the situation constant and, if under these conditions, we observe a change in the dependent variable, then we know that this change has been brought about by the variation of the independent variable since nothing else in the situation changed. As you might guess, one difficulty in carrying out a good experiment is to make sure that only one factor varies at a time. If more than one variable changes then it is very difficult to decide which of these changes is responsible for an observed difference in the dependent variable.

Graphs

The results of an experiment are often shown in graphical form. The primary reason for this is that graphs allow the visualization of relations more easily than many other forms of information presentation. However, in order to utilize graphs to their best advantage it is necessary to be familiar with their general form. One form of a graph is shown in Figure 9-1(*a*). There are two axes to this graph, the y-axis which extends in the vertical direction and is known as the *ordinate* and the x-axis which is in the horizontal direction and is called the *abscissa*. Typically, the values of the independent variable are plotted on the abscissa and the corresponding values for the dependent variable are located on the vertical axis. Thus, in Figure 9-1(*a*), if the independent variable was manipulated in such a way that it had a value of 4 we see that the dependent variable had a measured value of 2. The *function*, which is the line describing the relation between the independent and dependent variables, is composed of a connection of the points representing the values which define the function.

Next let us show how a graph can be used to illustrate the results of a very simple experiment. We are going to investigate the relation between the amount of light falling upon the eye and the size of the pupil. We may suspect that there is a relation between these two variables since casual observation shows that the brighter the light the smaller the pupil diameter. Thus, the independent variable which we will plot on the abscissa will be the amount of light falling upon the eye. On the ordinate we will plot the measured diameter of the pupil in response to specific amounts of light. Since this is an experiment

Figure 9-1   Graphical presentation of information. The fundamental aspects of an x-y plot are shown in (*a*) while the results of an experiment (see text) are represented in (*b*).

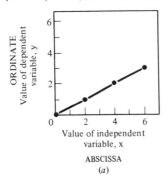

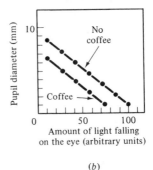

we have presumed that all variables, other than pupil size and amount of light, have been held constant. Now let us pick one additional variable for investigation. We might have a hunch that there may be other factors that influence pupil size in addition to the amount of light that falls upon the eye. For example, we might suspect that caffeine, which is found in coffee, could have an influence upon pupil size. How can we determine this? Let us assemble two groups of people; the first will consume no coffee and the second will consume five cups of coffee immediately prior to the experiment. A possible outcome of this experiment is shown in Figure 9-1(*b*). There are two functions shown, one corresponding to the no-coffee group and the other to the coffee group. These results show two things: first, that as the amount of light falling on the eye increases, the pupil size decreases regardless of the amount of coffee consumed; second, the group that consumed coffee showed a smaller pupil size than the no-coffee group regardless of the amount of light. The importance of this illustration for us is not whether caffeine has any influence on pupil size, but to show that different relations can be displayed on the same coordinate system. In this case there is an additional dimension to the graph which is referred to as a *parameter*. That is, in Figure 9-1(*b*) the amount of coffee consumed is the parameter. In this example, it represents a second independent variable. Notice that it was changed in such a way so as not to confuse the variation in pupil size caused by coffee and by light.

Problem areas of psychophysics

There are four different kinds of questions that may be asked in psychophysics. These questions define areas of investigation.

Detection. Detection represents that situation in which we ask what is the weakest stimulus to which a listener can respond. Upon presentation of a stimulus we make a judgment with respect to the apparent presence or absence of the stimulus.

Discrimination. In discrimination we ask what is the smallest stimulus difference between two stimuli that can be perceived. Typically the two stimuli being compared are identical in all respects except for the single dimension that is being varied. Examples of responses include same-different, louder-softer, or higher-lower. It is assumed that stimuli presented for discrimination tasks are in themselves detectable.

Identification. In an identification task the stimuli must be detectable and discriminable, and in addition we ask the listener to provide a specific and unique response to each different stimulus. For example in order for speech sounds to convey meaning not only must they be audible and discriminable one from another, but they must also be recognized (identified).

Scaling. Scaling represents that situation in which we ask the listener to make judgments regarding the perceived relation among a group of stimuli. For example, does one stimulus appear to be twice (or one-half, or four times) as loud as another?

Terms

Given a particular stimulus, we can choose to measure any of several responses to it. One of the most commonly used measures is that of threshold. *Absolute threshold* relates to the detection of the presence of a stimulus. Conceptually, a threshold refers to a stimulus value which, if exceeded, will result in positive response. However, if that value is not exceeded, a negative response occurs. Thus, threshold represents a unique point along the stimulus continuum. One of the aims of psychophysics (within the problem area of detection) is to estimate the stimulus value corresponding to threshold. Unfortunately, many factors operate in a situation in which we attempt to measure threshold. As a result, a certain variability exists in our threshold estimates. Thus, if the same stimulus value is presented a number of times, in some cases a listener may respond "Yes, I hear it" and in other cases will respond "No, I don't hear it." Often a threshold estimate is defined as that stimulus which the listener hears 50% of the time. Actually the definition of a threshold estimate depends upon the psychophysical method being used. The concept of *sensitivity* is related to threshold. When only a small stimulus value is required in order to obtain the threshold response, we say that the listener has high sensitivity. Conversely, if a large stimulus value is required for threshold estimate, then the listener is said to be displaying low sensitivity.

In addition to the absolute (detection) threshold there is a *differential threshold* which represents the size of the difference between two stimuli required in order for the listener to discriminate a difference. Again, with differential thresholds as with absolute thresholds, it is important to distinguish between the concept of the threshold and its measurement or estimation. The estimate of threshold is done on a probability basis, the exact definition depending upon the psychophysical method being used. The concept of *differential sensitivity* is analogous to that of absolute sensitivity (see previous paragraph).

Rather than asking the listener to perform a task which involves a judgment of the difference between two stimuli, we might ask him to judge the sameness of two stimuli. Again this is a discrimination problem, but the nature of the response differs from that previously discussed. The stimulus values at which two stimuli are judged to be perceptually equivalent is referred to as the *point of subjective equality* or *PSE*. It is not necessarily true that the PSE occurs when the two stimulus values are equal. The point at which the stimulus values correspond is referred to as the *point of objective equality* or *POE*.

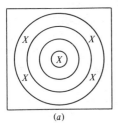 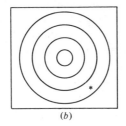 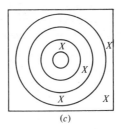

(a)   (b)   (c)

Figure 9-2 Target shooting. (a) Illustrations of variable "error." (b) Constant "error." (c) Combined constant and variable "error."

We will discuss the relation between the POE and PSE in a later section of this chapter.

Two types of variability have been mentioned in this section. We have said that in an attempt to estimate absolute threshold different responses to the same stimulus value are often obtained and we have indicated that the point of subjective equality does not necessarily correspond to the point of objective equality. This variability is referred to as *error* in the psychophysical literature. This term is unfortunate in that it incorrectly implies that there is something wrong with the measurement. The first mentioned "error" is *variable error* and the second "error" is *constant error*. In order to illustrate these two forms of psychophysical "error" let us assume we have a rifleman shooting at the target in an attempt to put each of his shots through the innermost circle. The black *X*s in Figure 9-2 show where his bullets actually entered the target. In Figure 9-2(a) we see that the marksman showed a certain degree of variability. He put one shot in the center and four others spread around rather evenly across the target face. There is no particular pattern to the marks and, on the average, we might say they tend toward the center. This is an example of variable error. Figure 9-2(b) shows a similar target with five shots again having been fired. In this case, however, all five shots went through the same hole, which was low and to the right of the center circle. All the shots were precisely in the same place; however, they did not go where they were intended. There is a bias or a systematic trend evident, namely, low and to the right; thus Figure 9-2(b) illustrates constant error. Of course, we usually find these two types of "errors" together such as shown in Figure 9-2(c) where we see a pattern similar to Figure 9-2(a) but displaced. The presence of constant and variable error simultaneously tends to be the rule not only for target shooting, but for psychophysics as well. In some psychophysical experiments it is possible to discover the source of the constant error. It may arise through some malfunction of the equipment, but more often constant error seems to be inherent in the listener and in nearly all cases variable error seems to be part of the listener's response.

One of the goals of psychophysical procedures, in addition to the measurement of thresholds and other performance indices, is to control, as best we can, the constant and variable errors. For example, if we have a large amount of variable error we will have a difficult time assigning a single number which meaningfully represents our estimate of threshold.

Traditional Methods

There are a number of psychophysical methods which have been in use over one hundred years and their usefulness continues undiminished. In this section we will discuss three of these traditional methods.

Adjustment

A factor which differentiates various psychophysical methods is the procedure by which the stimuli are presented. In the method of adjustment ascending and descending trials are used. That is, for an ascending trial the stimulus value would be small initially, but it would be gradually and constantly increased. A descending trial would be the converse; that is, with its initial value large, the stimulus would gradually be decreased. Value in this case refers to some dimension of the stimulus such as magnitude or frequency.

Another distinguishing characteristic of this method is that the listener actually controls the value of the dependent variable. That is, he controls the stimulus presentation on the ascending and descending series. Thus not only does he make judgments with respect to the stimuli, but he plays an active role in controlling the stimuli. With the method of adjustment the stimulus value is changed continuously as opposed to being changed in a discrete or step-wise fashion.

Each judgment that a listener makes is an estimate of whatever psychophysical index is being used in the particular experiment. If a threshold is being estimated, then each judgment represents such an estimate. If the point of subjective equality is being estimated, then each judgment represents an estimate of that quantity. To review, in a detection situation on an ascending trial, the stimulus begins at a small stimulus value, is increased continuously by the subject until he hears the stimulus, at which point the stimulus value is noted, and this constitutes an estimate of the threshold. On a descending trial the stimulus value is initially large and clearly audible. The listener then decreases the stimulus value until he can no longer hear the stimulus, at which point the stimulus value is noted and this corresponds to another estimate of threshold. A diagram of this method is shown in Figure 9-3.

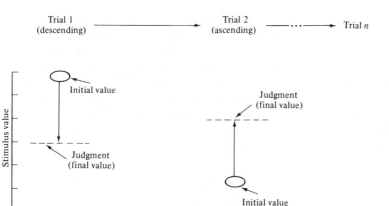

Figure 9-3 Summary of the method of adjustment.

Certain precautions should be taken in carrying out an experiment utilizing the method of adjustment. The reason that ascending and descending trials are used is that certain biases are often associated with both types of trials. For example, on a descending series it is not unusual for the listener to indicate he hears the stimulus at smaller stimulus values than for an ascending trial. Such a bias may be a form of a perseveration in that he may be thinking to himself, "I hear the stimulus, I hear the stimulus, I hear the stimulus" and accordingly he may continue beyond the stimulus value that might otherwise correspond to his threshold estimate. Similarly, on an ascending trial the listener does not initially hear the stimulus and very often the stimulus magnitude can be increased considerably with the same response being obtained until suddenly the listener says "Oh, I hear that stimulus" but didn't realize previously that he had been hearing it. In other words, there can be perseveration in the ascending trials as well. The hope is that any systematic trends associated with either of the types of trials will be averaged out if both types of series are utilized in the same experiment. Consequently, it is wise to use an equal number of ascending and descending series in order to optimize the probability that biases will be equal. It also is wise to start each ascending (or descending) trial at a different point. If we always start at the same stimulus value, listeners soon realize that threshold is a specific distance from the initial stimulus value and often begin to respond in terms of where they think the threshold should be rather than listening to the stimulus and making independent judgments.

What do we do with the threshold estimates (or other performance measures)? One of the most common procedures is to obtain an average of all the threshold estimates. This average represents our best estimate of threshold under the conditions of the experiment. We might also wish to see if there were systematic differences between ascending and descending trials. This could be done by averaging the two sets of trials separately and comparing the averages. If differences did exist this would be an example of a constant error. We are also interested in variable error and, although there are a number of ways in which we can specify the variability of the results, one of the simplest (and least satisfactory) is a measure of the *range* of stimulus values which corresponded to the threshold estimates. Another way is by calculating the *standard deviation*.[1] Whichever method we choose the aim is the same; that is, to provide a number which reflects the variability of the data.

Limits

In the method of limits ascending and descending series of trials are used; however, the stimulus value is changed in a step-wise fashion. The stimulus values which correspond to each of the steps is fixed and only certain equally spaced stimulus values are used during the course of an experiment.

Several kinds of judgments may be made. For example, if the task is one of detection the judgment may be "Yes, I hear it" or "No, I don't." If it is a discrimination task the listener's judgment might be "Yes, the second stimulus is louder than the first."

With the method of limits the measurement of the dependent variable is accomplished by the experimenter changing its value and the listener reporting appropriately. The listener is completely passive; he listens and responds; but plays no direct role in the manipulation of stimulus values.

A sequence of stimulus presentations for a detection task might be as follows. Let us assume that an ascending series of trials is to be used. The initial stimulus is presented and the listener is required to respond following its presentation. Since this is an ascending series his first response would probably be "No, I don't hear the stimulus." The second stimulus is then presented and the listener again must respond, perhaps also saying this time "No, I don't hear it." The stimulus-response process continues until the listener changes his judgment to "Yes, I hear it." At this point the series is terminated and the threshold is estimated as a value intermediate between the two stimulus values last presented. Sometimes different stopping rules are applied. A descending trial has the same features as the ascending trial just described except, of course, the ordering of the stimuli is in the opposite direction. Figure 9-4 summarizes the method of limits.

The same general cautions apply for the method of limits as in the case of the method of adjustment. Approximately equal numbers of ascending and descending series should be used. The initial stimulus values for either the ascending or descending trial should not be constant, but should be varied

---

[1] Standard deviation (SD) = $\sqrt{(\Sigma \bar{X} - X)^2/N}$, where there are N threshold estimates each of value X, the mean of which is $\bar{X}$.

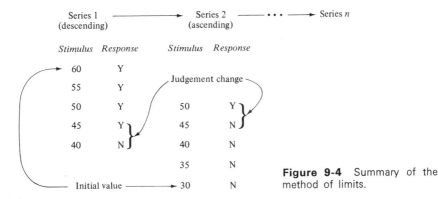

Figure 9-4 Summary of the method of limits.

from series to series. The treatment of the results of an experiment using the method of limits is similar to that of the method of adjustment. For example, to obtain a single value which best characterized the threshold, all the threshold estimates from both ascending and descending series are averaged. To estimate variability, the same kinds of procedures may be carried out as suggested for the method of adjustment.

Constant stimuli

In contrast to the two methods previously described, the method of constant stimuli does not use ascending and descending stimulus series. Rather a certain number of stimulus values are used, typically five or seven, and these constant stimulus values are presented in random order. Any of the previously mentioned psychophysical indices may be used, but let us illustrate the method in an experiment involving discrimination; that is, the determination of a differential threshold for intensity. The listener's task is a passive one in that he is only required to respond to each stimulus.

We present two stimuli which are identical except for intensity: the first we call the standard, the second we call the variable. The variable stimulus may take any of seven randomly chosen fixed values of any particular trial. For example, the standard stimulus might have a magnitude of 60 dB, the variable stimulus values of 57, 58, 59, 60, 61, 62, and 63 dB. The listener's task in this example would be to judge whether the variable stimulus is louder or softer than the standard stimulus. The stimulus-response process is continued until a substantial number of judgments are obtained (perhaps twenty for each value of the variable). The greater the number of judgments used, the more stable will be our estimate of differential threshold.

The process of estimating the differential threshold from the data is illustrated in Table 9-1. The results are expressed in percentage form; that is, for the variable stimulus of 57 dB, what percentage of the time did the listener judge this to be louder than the standard, for a stimulus of 58 dB what is the corresponding percentage, and so on? Thus, we have a per-

Table 9-1 Response tabulations

Stimulus	Responses	Percent times stimuli judged "louder"	Percent times stimuli judged "softer"
63	L L L L	100	0
62	L S L L	90	10
61	L S S L	70	30
60	S L S L	40	60
59	S L L S	10	90
58	S S S S	0	100
57	S S S S	0	100

Stimulus	Responses					Percent times stimuli judged "louder"	Percent times stimuli judged "softer"
63	L	L	L	L	....	100	0
62	L	S	L	L	....	90	10
61	L	S	S	L	....	70	30
60	S	L	S	L	....	40	60
59	S	L	L	S	....	10	90
58	S	S	S	S	....	0	100
57	S	S	S	S	....	0	100

(a)

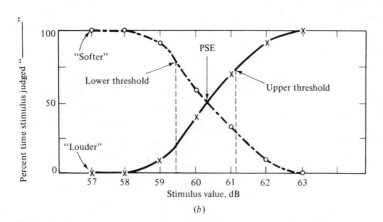

(b)

Figure 9-5 Procedures used with the method of constant stimuli; (a) Response tabulation. (b) Psychometric function.

centage associated with each of the stimulus values. Next, we ordinarily plot these percentage values as shown in Figure 9-5. A graph of this sort, in which we plot judgment percentage as a function of stimulus value, is called a *psychometric function*. How does the psychometric function help us estimate the differential threshold? It is at this point that the probabilistic nature of threshold estimation becomes clear. We might say to ourselves, "I do not believe that the listener really heard a difference until he can identify that difference with 100% certainty." However, we might think this criterion is too strict and perhaps a more reasonable rule would be to accept 50% discrimination. If the 100% rule was unreasonably stringent it is probably true that the 50% rule is unreasonably lax. The listener in this illustration has but two alternatives, he either says the second stimulus is louder, or softer than the first. If, without our knowledge, the listener removed his earphones and responded to the signal by flipping a coin and responding "louder" if the coin came up heads, he would be correct 50% of the time. Thus, in this response situation 50% discriminability is chance performance and could be achieved on the basis of flipping a coin and paying absolutely no attention to the signals. Although any point between 50% and 100% could be used, the most usual level is 75%, with the only rationale being that it lies half-way between the two extremes. Thus, threshold in this two-alternative forced-choice situation corresponds to that stimulus value for which the listener says "louder" (or "softer") 75% of the time. In Figure 9-5 a horizontal line has been placed coincident with the 75% point and at the position where it intersects the psychometric functions we have dropped perpendicular dotted line to the horizontal axis. These points on the horizontal axis then define the stimulus value corresponding to 75% judged "louder" and "softer." The use of a graph in this situation is advantageous in that it allows easy interpolation in case none of the data points happen to fall at the 75% point. The psychometric functions cross at the 50% point. That stimulus value for which one-half the time the listeners say "louder" and the other half of the time they respond "softer" may be taken as an estimate of the point of subjective equality. The distance between the PSE and either of the 75% points is a measure of differential threshold. For a judgment of "louder" the differential threshold is 61.1 dB − 60.2 dB or 0.9 dB. For a judgment of "softer" the differential threshold is 60.2 − 59.9 dB or 0.7 dB; the average being 0.8 dB.

Summary

The traditional psychophysical methods of adjustment, limits, and constant stimuli each provide unique advantages and disadvantages. Let us review some of these features. In the method of limits and constant stimuli the listener's role is completely passive; he merely listens to the stimuli and makes the required judgments. The method of adjustment provides an active role for the listener; not only does he make judgments, but he also controls the stimulus he is judging. An active role is advantageous in that it tends to keep the listener interested in his task. In contrast, the methods that require only passive participation tend to be dull, monotonous, and boring. However, the active role required by the method of adjustment provides a disadvantage in that the outcome of the procedure is dependent not only on the perceptual abilities of the listener, but also upon his ability to manipulate the stimulus. For example, if the manipulation of the stimulus value required the twisting of a knob, some listeners might be better knob twisters than others and as a result achieve a certain outcome, when in fact, we are interested in their ability to perform the judgment rather than in their motor skills.

The three traditional methods also vary in the degree to which fixed versus variable stimulus values are used. The method of constant stimuli requires a constant number of stimuli whose values are fixed. At the other extreme stands the method of adjustment in which the stimulus is continuously variable. The method of limits is intermediate in that the stimulus value is varied by fixed amounts but there is no necessity of using precisely the same initial value in successive series of trials. Those methods which involve continuous variability of the stimulus have greater flexibility but those methods utilizing fixed stimuli tend to yield higher reliability.

Psychophysical methods also vary with respect to the number of judgments required in order to estimate the psychophysical index being used (threshold, differential threshold, point of subjective equality). With the method of adjustment each judgment yields an estimate of the psychophysical index. With the method of limits each series of stimulus presentations yields an estimate of threshold. With the method of constant stimuli a very large number of judgments is required before the psychophysical index may be estimated. Thus, in general, the method of adjustment requires the least time for an estimate and the method of constant stimuli requires the greatest amount of time. However, we get what we pay for. Thresholds estimated with the method of adjustment tend to be more variable and less reliable than those estimates made on the basis of the method of constant stimuli. Thus, the method you choose to use depends upon the type of experiment you are doing. If you are interested in getting a threshold estimate in the quickest possible time and are not particularly interested in having extreme reliability, then clearly something like the method of adjustment is called for. On the other hand, if you are doing a laboratory study where precision is important and time and money are of secondary concern, then the method of constant stimuli is probably the best choice.

Psychophysical methods also vary with respect to the randomness of the stimulus sequence. With the method of constant stimuli the order of stimulus presentation is random by definition. On the other hand, with the method of limits the progression of stimulus values is extremely systematic (ascending and descending series). The stimulus order is probably quite systematic in the method of adjustment, but because it is under the listener's control, it is difficult to say precisely what he is doing. The advantage should lie with that method that utilizes the most random presentation of stimuli since with this method of presentation fewer biases should occur than with those methods which use a systematic stimulus presentation.

While we have described three specific traditional psychophysical procedures, it is perfectly acceptable to use what you consider to be the best features of each of these methods in devising your own optimum psychophysical method for a particular experiment. It is necessary, of course, that the features selected be compatible.

Adaptive Procedures

It is easy to see that if we picked stimulus values to which the listener always responded "Yes, I hear it" We would obtain no information about his threshold value. The precision of the method of constant stimuli rests on its ability to restrict the stimulus values used to those in the immediate vicinity of the expected threshold. This in turn requires some previous knowledge as to where the threshold might be. In other words, we really have to run two experiments, one in which we define the general region in which we expect to find the threshold and one using the method of constant stimuli in which we obtain a threshold estimate with the maximum possible precision. Thus the advantages of the method of constant stimuli are less than they might appear to be since preliminary experimentation is ordinarily required. Recently methods have been developed which attempt to arrive at the same precision of measurement as is possible with the method of constant stimuli, but that require no preliminary experimentation in order to fix the stimulus values. They attempt to achieve this goal by deciding, during the course of the experiment, which stimulus values are to be presented. Such methods are called *adaptive procedures*. This section reviews several of the adaptive procedures.

Up and down

The up and down method represents one of the earliest attempts at an adaptive procedure. It has never been widely used in psychophysics but by describing it we can illustrate some of the fundamental characteristics of adaptive procedures. The up and down method grew out of munitions manufacturing quality control. Samples of explosive material were taken from the production line into the laboratory and tested in order to determine whether they possessed the required characteristics. One of the specifications

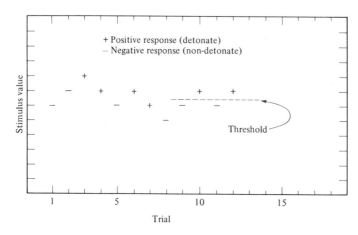

Figure 9-6 Example of results obtained with the up and down method.

was that the explosive material detonate when struck with given force. The tests not only had to specify as precisely as possible the force required for detonation, but they had to do this rapidly since the number of samples passing through the laboratory was large. The up and down method provided a reasonably good solution to this problem. The method consisted of dropping a metal ball onto the explosive material from a fixed height. If the material did not detonate under these conditions the ball was moved to the next higher step and dropped again. If the material still did not explode the ball was moved to a still higher position and dropped. If under these conditions the test sample detonated, the ball was lowered one position and dropped again on the next sample. If this sample also exploded the ball was moved down to a still lower test position and this continued until the sample failed to explode, then the process was repeated. In essence, the up and down method was one in which the stimulus (detonation device) could assume any of a number of stimulus values but the value presented on any given trial depended upon the response obtained to the previous trial. By its very nature the method presented stimulus values which were in the immediate vicinity of the threshold. This method is schematized in Figure 9-6.

Békésy tracking

Probably the most widely used adaptive procedure is Békésy tracking. This method, which is used on Békésy audiometers, is, in essence, an automatization of the up and down procedure. In the Békésy audiometer the intensity of the stimulus is constantly changing and the listener controls the direction of the stimulus change. The usual instructions to a listener go something like this. "You will hear a tone through the earphones. As long as you do not push the button, the tone will get louder. When you push the button the tone will get softer. Your job will be to keep the tone at the point where you can just barely hear it. That is, when you hear the tone push the button. The tone will get softer and softer and finally disappear. As soon as it disappears let up on the button until you again hear the stimulus, at which point again push the button." We see a typical result of this process in Figure 9-7. The Békésy method also concentrates the listener's judgments in the vicinity of the threshold. Notice that this tracking procedure also contains elements of the method of adjustment in that the stimulus is directly controlled by the listener.

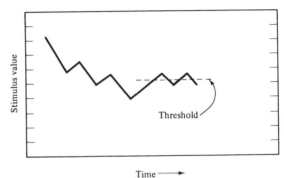

Figure 9-7 Example of results obtained with the Békésy tracking procedure.

PEST (Parameter Estimation by Sequential Testing)

The PEST procedure represents an extension of the up and down method with several interesting twists. Recall that the up and down method gets you to where you "need to go" by means of the rules applied for stimulus change. If one has the misfortune to pick an *initial stimulus value* which is far removed from the actual threshold value, the up and down method will still get you to that threshold value but it will take a long time to do so. One of the features of the PEST procedure is a process by which this time is minimized. For example, let us imagine that the initial stimulus is presented at a high intensity where the listener has no difficulty hearing it and thus responds positively. Because of his positive response the next stimulus is decreased in intensity by an amount equal to the *initial step size*. If the listener gives the same response on three consecutive trials a *doubling rule* is invoked and the next step size is twice that of the previous step size. If the subject still responds positively, the next stimulus will be again double the previous step size, four times the initial step size, and this process continues until the subject responds "No, I don't hear it." The doubling rule is designed to put the stimulus in the vicinity of the threshold in the shortest possible time.

By the time the stimulus reaches the region of the threshold, the step size may be extremely large. A large step size allows only a crude estimation of threshold and thus, ideally, there should be some means by which we could work with a smaller step size. The PEST procedure attempts to achieve these

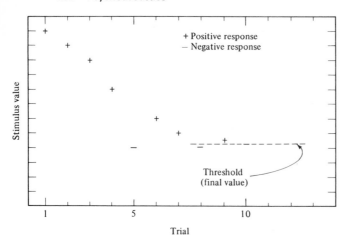

Figure 9-8 Example of results obtained with the PEST procedure.

conditions by invoking a step size *halving rule* each time there is a judgment reversal. In other words, every time the judgment changes from "Yes, I hear it" to "No, I don't hear it" the step size will be halved on the succeeding trial. This also occurs when the judgment changes from "No, I don't hear it" to "Yes, I do." Summarizing, if the initial stimulus is far away from the final threshold estimate, more appropriate stimulus values are rapidly obtained by the doubling procedure. Once the stimulus value reaches the region of the threshold, as defined by judgment reversals, the step size becomes small by virtue of the halving procedure and consequently the threshold estimate can be well defined. The PEST procedure is illustrated in Figure 9-8.

BUDTIF (Block Up Down Temporal Interval Forced Choice)

The BUDTIF method bears some similarity to several of the previous methods that we have mentioned. BUDTIF is a procedure in which the same stimulus value is presented for a number of trials. The results obtained on this block of trials is then analyzed, compared to a predetermined value, and the stimulus value for the next block of trials is selected as a result of the outcome of that comparison. For example, let us assume that we wish to find the stimulus value at which the listener correctly detects the presence of the signal 75% of the time. The smallest block size that we can use to estimate this 75% criterion is a block of four trials; that is, three correct out of a block of four is 75%. A trial in the BUDTIF procedure consists of two observation intervals, one of which contains the stimulus. The listener's task is to decide whether the stimulus is in interval *I* or interval *II*. Let us assume that on the first block of trials the listener achieved two correct responses out of the total of four. On the next block of trials then, the stimulus value would be increased by some fixed step and a second block of four trials presented. If, on the second block of four trials, the same number of correct responses was obtained, the stimulus value would be incremented still further. This process would continue until three out of four correct answers were obtained. If the results were four out of four, then on the next block of trials the stimulus value would be decremented.

This method is very similar to the up and down method previously described with two modifications; a forced choice method is employed and while the block size in the up and down method is one, the block size in the BUDTIF method is variable. That is, the block size depends upon the percentage correct point we are attempting to estimate. If we wanted to estimate the 66% point then we could get by with three trials (two out of three), or if we were attempting to estimate the 60% point we would need five trials (three out of five). BUDTIF is schematized in Figure 9-9.

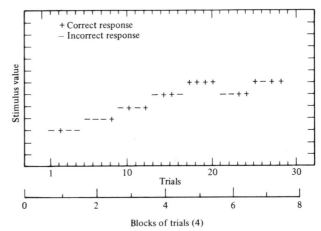

Figure 9-9 Example of results obtained with the BUDTIF procedure.

Summary

The general advantage then to adaptive procedures is that they allow considerable flexibility. The results obtained with the adaptive methods do not depend to any important degree upon the initial placement of the stimulus values. Thus, preliminary experimentation is unnecessary.

Scaling Procedures

Number systems

One of the very important things to keep in mind is that the meaning of any numbers that we obtain in an experiment is dependent upon the methods used to obtain those numbers. While that statement may sound reasonable, it does so only until we say that in some cases $2 + 2$ does not necessarily equal four. The material to be discussed in this section will attempt to show that $2 + 2 = 4$ only under certain conditions. There are four basic number systems with each system generated by a certain class of procedures.

Nominal. A number system in which $2 + 2$ does not equal 4 is the nominal system. One of the best examples of a nominal system is the numbers which we find on the jerseys of football players. The quarterback may have the number 14 on his back, the fullback may have the number 43 on his back, yet we know that we can not take the quarterback and somehow add him to the fullback and come up with the equivalent of football player number 57. The numbers are placed on the jerseys only for identifying or naming purposes. There is no implication that we can perform any arithmetic or logical operations with these numbers. Hence, the term nominal (naming) number system.

Ordinal. There exists still another number system in which arithmetic operations have no meaning. This is the ordinal system which may be described best by example. Let us assume that we have ten rocks. If we pick up a rock and attempt to scratch all the other rocks, we will find that perhaps some rocks are scratched and others are not. We then repeat this process for each of the ten rocks. When we finish this test we can arrange our rocks so that the rock on the far left is scratched by none of the other rocks, while the rock on the far right is scratched by all of the other rocks, and the rocks occupying intermediate positions do so on the basis that they scratch all rocks to the right, but none to the left. Thus, we have a system in which an ordering exists; the ordering being in terms of hardness. If the rocks are numbered 1 through 10 from left to right, the numbers form an ordinal number system. In this system we can not take a rock with a hardness of 1 and a rock with a hardness of 2 and combine them in some way so that they are equal to a rock of hardness number 3. The procedures that we have gone through to form our scale of numbers were simply not of a kind that allow us to perform arithmetic operations. With an ordinal scale we are restricted to making statements about the numbers which relate only to relative magnitude. We know that rock number 4 is harder than rock number 3, but we can say no more.

Interval. To obtain numbers forming an interval system, operations are performed such that numbers are separated by equal intervals. For example, let us assume that there are three tables in a lecture room, one large table and two smaller tables. The instructor, being a rather dramatic person, announces that he will measure the tables using his shoe. He takes off a shoe and places it end to end successively on the large table until he traverses the length of the table. He finds the table to be eight shoes long. In a similar fashion he measures the two smaller tables and finds each of them to be four shoes long. In this instance because of the operations which have been carried out, we are able to take these numbers, the units are immaterial, and say the 4 + 4 = 8. We can verify this by placing the two shorter tables end to end and seeing that, in fact, their total length is equal to that of the long table. Thus, with this procedure and the resulting numbers, we can perform the arithmetic operations of addition and subtraction.

Ratio. For a ratio number system the procedures by which the numbers are derived are such that equal ratios are formed between numbers, and also an absolute zero exists. Numbers from a ratio system can be used for the operations of division and multiplication as well as addition and subtraction. Thus, the ratio system represents the most powerful number system and the one which we generally assume in arithmetic operations. We saw, however, that there are several number systems in which the identical numbers are used but which have different meaning because of the methods used to obtain the numbers.

Methods

For those psychophysical tasks in which the judgments to be made involve the assessment of the perceived relations between stimuli, it is desirable to choose psychophysical methods which yield the most powerful possible number system. As an example of such methods, two illustrations will be discussed.

Equal interval. For some applications it is sufficient that the outcome of an experiment be expressed in numbers which form an interval number system. We can illustrate such a procedure by considering the following example. Let us assume that we are interested in assessing the perceived magnitude of an auditory stimulus. We might present one pair of stimuli, A and B, and indicate to the listener that a certain interval of perceived magnitude existed between stimuli A and B. We might then present a third stimulus C and ask that the subject adjust the value of C so the perceived interval between B and C was the same as between A and B. This same procedure could be repeated for as many sets of stimuli as we wished. We can see that this procedure will, of necessity, yield numbers which belong to an interval number system, since they were generated by a set of instructions which were designed to yield equal intervals between standard and variable stimuli. Although there are many variations on this procedural scheme, this example demonstrates one procedure which has been used successfully.

Direct magnitude estimation and direct magnitude production. Two methods that have been used to obtain numbers which form a ratio system are direct magnitude estimation and direct magnitude production. One is the inverse of the other and consequently we will limit our discussion to just one method. Again, let us proceed by example. Assume that we are attempting to assess the loudness of a stimulus. The methods that we are about to discuss allow us to express this loudness in numerical form. The method of direct magnitude estimation works as follows. A stimulus is presented to a listener and he is told that it has a loudness that corresponds to the number 100 (or any other arbitrary number). Any time during the course of the experiment that he hears a stimulus that sounds identical to the standard he is asked to assign the number 100 to the stimulus. He is further instructed that should he hear a stimulus whose loudness seems to be one-half that of the standard, he is to assign it the number 50. Correspondingly, should he hear a stimulus whose loudness was twice that of the standard, he should assign it the number 200. The instructions are designed so that the listener will make ratio judgments with respect to a standard stimulus and provide numbers consistent with his judgments. The data gathering consists of a series of stimulus presentations after which the listener responds in accordance with the instructions. After a sufficiently large number of judgments, the responses at each stimulus value are averaged and can be displayed as shown in Figure 9-10. We see that the result is a function which relates perceived magnitude (loudness) to stimulus magnitude. The numbers corresponding to the perceived magnitude are usually taken to represent a ratio number system because of the means by which they were collected. Consequently, the usual arithmetic operations may be performed with these numbers. Indeed, additional experiments have been carried out to verify that a stimulus with loudness value 2, for example,

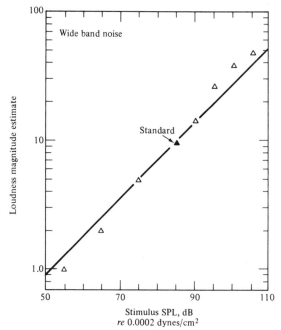

Figure 9-10 Results of a direct magnitude estimation experiment in which loudness is scaled. [*After J. C. Stevens and E. Tulving, "Estimations of loudness by a group of untrained observers,"* Amer. J. Psychol., *70 (1957),* 600-605.]

combined with another stimulus of loudness value 2, forms a stimulus with loudness value 4.

Although we have discussed only the scaling of loudness, any response dimension can be scaled, such as loudness, pitch, or quality. Indeed, psychophysical scaling procedures find usefulness in fields far beyond psychoacoustics or psychophysics. For example, they have been used in the scaling of the perceived severity of the handicap of persons with impaired speech.

AUDITORY SENSITIVITY

Absolute Threshold (Detection)

Detection of stimuli is one of the primary areas of psychoacoustics, and in this situation the threshold is the most generally used index of performance.

Factors influencing estimation of threshold

Stimulus variables: frequency. That frequency is an important determiner in the detection of stimuli has been known for some time. For example, whistles producing very high frequencies are readily responded to by dogs and cats, but are inaudible to humans. Less obvious, but still true, is the observation that frequency can be so low that the stimulus goes undetected. Detection or non-detection as a function of stimulus frequency is actually not an all-or-none phenomenon. That is, it is not simply a matter of failing to hear the stimulus if it is too high in frequency, but hearing it if the frequency is somewhat lower. Throughout a broad range of frequencies, the stimulus will be detectable provided it is presented at an appropriately intense sound pressure. Figure 9-11 shows a graph of such a relation. The solid curve shows the sound pressure level required for audibility in the middle range frequencies; frequencies which are ordinarily thought to be those to which the ear responds. It may be seen that as frequency is raised from 100 Hz the sound pressure required for threshold declines until the region of approximately 1,000 Hz is reached. In this region there is a broad minimum which extends to perhaps 3,000 Hz, but for higher frequencies the threshold again increases. The dotted extensions of this function represent thresholds for stimulus frequencies which are not ordinarily thought of as being within the range of hearing, but can elicit auditory sensations providing the sound pressure is sufficiently great. For example, we can hear sounds as low as 2 Hz, but for still lower frequencies the sound pressure required for detection is so great that the sound is felt rather than heard. The sound pressure level at this point is approximately 140 dB

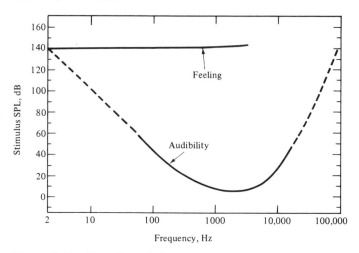

Figure 9-11 The effect of signal frequency on the threshold of audibility. [Audibility thresholds within the nominal limits are from *L. J. Sivian and S. D. White, "On minimum audible sound fields,"* J. Acoust. Soc. Amer., *4 (1933), 288-321; low frequency audibility thresholds and threshold of feeling are from G. von Békésy,* Experiments in Hearing (*New York: McGraw-Hill Book Company, 1960); and high frequency audibility thresholds are from J. F. Corso, "Bone-conducted thresholds for sonic and ultrasonic frequencies,"* J. Acoust. Soc. Amer., *35 (1963), Fig. 5.*] All measures are MAP (see p. 368).

relative to 0.0002 dyne/square centimeter. This is a sound pressure which is 10,000,000 times as great as the minimum sound pressure required for threshold (1,000 to 3,000 Hz). The dotted line at the other end of the frequency scale shows that above 15,000 Hz the function continues its upward climb until approximately 100,000 Hz. At this point the sound pressure is so great that any further increase would result in tissue damage to the auditory system. Although calibration at these higher frequencies is somewhat uncertain, the sound pressure required for threshold at 100,000 Hz is approximately the same as that required at 2 Hz.

It should be added that very special equipment and procedures are necessary to generate these very high or very low frequencies at the sound pressures required to elicit an auditory response. On the other hand, it is rather easy to measure threshold in that frequency range shown by the solid line in Figure 9-11. The dashed line shown across the top of the figure represents the *threshold of feeling*. Any stimulus whose frequency-intensity conditions are such that it falls between the threshold of audibility and feeling is perceived as an auditory sensation. Those stimulus conditions which lie below the threshold of audibility are not perceived in any form; those which lie above the threshold of feeling curve give rise to a tactual or pain response as well as an auditory response.

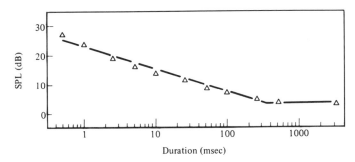

Figure 9-12 Effect of signal duration on the threshold of audibility using a wide band noise signal. [*From A. M. Small et al., "Loudness as a function of signal duration,"* J. Acoust. Soc. Amer., *34 (1962), 513-14.*]

Stimulus variables: duration. Another variable which is important in determining the audibility of a stimulus is the duration for which the stimulus is presented. Figure 9-12 illustrates the effect of stimulus duration upon audibility. It shows the sound pressure level required in order that the stimulus be audible for each of a number of stimulus durations. We see that if the stimulus duration is greater than about 0.3 second, the threshold sound pressure level is constant. On the other hand, as we shorten stimulus durations to less than about 0.3 second the sound pressure must be progressively increased in order to hear the stimulus. That is, our ability to hear the stimulus decreases as stimulus duration is shortened. In order to compensate for this decrease in sensitivity, we must increase the sound pressure level of the stimulus in order to detect its presence. If you are thinking that 0.3 second is too short to worry about remember that speech contains many sounds whose durations are 0.3 second or shorter. Stimulus duration can and does affect our ability to hear a sound.

Measurement variables: minimum audible field. The audibility function shown in Figure 9-11 is a general function, not representative of any particular set of procedures. Actually, the sound pressure required to hear a tone depends upon the way in which the sound pressure is measured. The minimum audible field technique is one in which the listener is placed in an acoustic free field, one in which there are no reflections from any surfaces and thus, all sound reaching the listener comes directly from the source. The transducer ordinarily used in this situation is a loudspeaker. The threshold estimates are made by any of the psychophysical procedures. For careful measurements, often only one ear of the listener is used, the other one being plugged. After the measurements are made, the listener is removed from the sound field. A microphone substitution is made, positioning it at the precise spot that the listener's active ear was located. With the calibrated microphone we are able

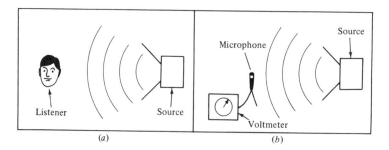

Figure 9-13   Estimation of threshold sound pressure by means of the minimum audible field procedure.

to measure the sound pressure at that position in space formerly occupied by the listener. Minimum audible field measurement involves certain assumptions, the most obvious being that the sound pressure as measured by the microphone is, in fact, the same sound pressure that is effective in eliciting a threshold response. Figure 9-13 illustrates this method.

Measurement variables: minimum audible pressure. Another way in which the sound pressure required for threshold can be estimated is by means of the minimum audible pressure technique. With this technique the sound is developed within a closed space rather than in a free field. The closed space is usually formed by an earphone and its cushion, tightly coupled to the listener's ear. A threshold estimate is obtained in accordance with any appropriate psychophysical procedure. The earphone is then removed from the listener's ear and is placed on a specially designed metal cylinder called an acoustic coupler. A calibrated microphone is located at one end of the coupler with the earphone at the other end. The microphone measures the sound pressure developed by the earphone within the coupler. Certain assumptions are made in inferring that the sound pressure measured with the

Figure 9-14   Estimates of threshold sound pressure by (a) the minimum audible pressure; (b) probe tube techniques.

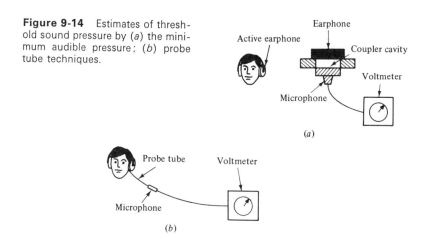

minimum audible pressure technique is the sound pressure that is effective in eliciting a threshold response. In this instance the volume of the coupler is designed to be equal to the equivalent volume enclosed under the earphone when it is being worn by the listener. Thus, it is assumed that the equivalent volume is of primary importance and other factors are relatively insignificant. Examples of other factors are the shape of the coupler and the extent to which the metal walls of the coupler simulate the acoustic properties of the soft tissue of the external ear and the external meatus. Figure 9-14(*a*) summarizes the procedures for the minimum audible pressure measurement. Typical results for minimum audible field and minimum audible pressure measures are seen in Figure 9-15. In general it is observed that the minimum audible field measurements are somewhat lower, particularly in the middle range of frequencies.

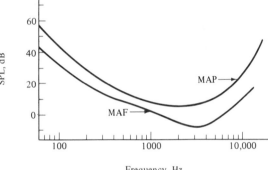

Figure 9-15 Threshold estimates obtained by minimum audible pressure (MAP) and minimum audible field (MAF). [*After L. J. Sivian and S. D. White, "On minimum audible sound fields,"* J. Acoust. Soc. Amer., *4 (1933), 288-321.*]

Measurement variables: probe tube. Where is the most appropriate point to measure the minimum sound pressure that is effective in eliciting a threshold response? The probable answer is: near the tympanic membrane since it is the sound pressure at this point which initiates mechanical motion in the ear. The measurement procedure is schematized in Figure 9-14(*b*) and is as follows. Earphones are worn by the listener and a threshold estimate is obtained by any appropriate psychophysical procedure. A very small plastic tube which leads to a calibrated microphone is slipped under the earphone cushion and inserted into the external auditory meatus. With appropriate care the tip of the probe tube may be moved to within a few millimeters of the eardrum and the sound pressure sampled at this point. There are a number of difficulties associated with technique; for example, the placement of the tip of the probe tube is critical. If it is inserted too far into the external meatus it may touch the eardrum which, in addition to blocking sound entrance into the tube, is very painful. If the tip is positioned at different distances from the eardrum, different values of sound pressure will be measured even though the stimulus level going into the earphone is constant. In other words, the sound pressure within the meatus is not uniform throughout its length.

There are assumptions involved in the use of the probe tube technique. For example, it is assumed that the insertion of the probe tube does not alter the sound field within the external meatus. It can be shown that this supposition is fulfilled as long as the diameter of the probe tube is small compared to the diameter of the external meatus.

The results of probe tube measurements correspond more closely to minimum audible pressure results than to minimum audible field results. The main reason for this is that the external auditory meatus acts as an acoustic resonator for the frequency range of approximately 2,000 to 5,000 Hz. An acoustic resonator, discussed in Chapter 2, is a device which, among its other characteristics, shows an increase in sound pressure within its cavity compared to outside, for a certain range of frequencies. The precise acoustic characteristics of a resonator depend principally upon its dimensions. The meatus' large opening to the outside results in a broad range of resonant frequencies. This resonance effect is seen only in the free field situation, and accounts in part for the difference between the minimum audible field and minimum audible pressure curves in Figure 9-15. Figure 9-16 shows the magnitude of the resonance effect as measured with a probe tube. It can be seen to amount to a maximum of about 12 dB.

It should be emphasized that we presume that the actual sound pressure required at the eardrum to elicit a threshold response is constant and thus the differences we see with the various techniques discussed in this section arise from the methods themselves. We should point out that sound pressure measurements are rarely made for those stimulus conditions that actually elicit a threshold response. The ear is considerably more sensitive than most microphones and, as a result, the usual procedure is to increase the sound pressure, perhaps 80 dB over what it is in the threshold situation. The sound pressure is then measured under these conditions and 80 dB is subtracted from this measured pressure, giving an estimate of what the original sound pressure would have been had we been able to measure it.

Figure 9-16 Resonance effect of the external auditory meatus. The ordinate is the increase in sound pressure at the ear drum compared to outside the meatus. [*After F. M. Weiner and D. A. Ross, "Pressure distribution in the auditory canal in a progressive sound field,"* J. Acoust. Soc. Amer., *18 (1946), 401.*]

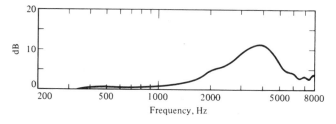

Frequency, Hz

In summary, although the probe tube procedure probably yields the most valid estimates of threshold sound pressure, such measurements are difficult to make. Since these results relate most closely to the minimum audible pressure measure and the minimum audible field technique is difficult to implement, requiring an echo free environment, the minimum audible pressure measure is most often used in a specification of threshold sound pressure. The use of the calibrated microphone and acoustic coupler is simple, reliable, and inexpensive. Consequently, it is the method of choice in most applications.

Instructional variables: criterion. Another factor which will influence the value of the estimated threshold is the criterion adopted by the listener. For example, if the listener says to himself, "I am not going to say that I hear a stimulus until I am absolutely sure that I hear it," he will show a higher threshold than if he adopts a lax criterion in which he says to himself, "I will not have to be sure, I will respond to practically anything." Still another criterion is whether listeners are instructed to respond when they hear a tone with a definite pitch or when they hear anything. Figure 9-17 shows results that were obtained with the "pitch" criterion versus "anything" criterion. We can see a small, but consistent, difference between the two curves.

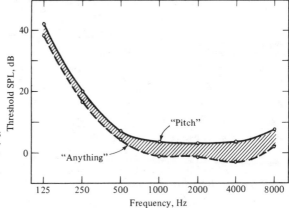

Figure 9-17 Effect of instructions upon the audibility function. [*After I. Pollack, "The atonal interval," J. Acoust. Soc. Amer., 20 (1948), 146.*]

Instructional variables: psychophysical method. The psychophysical method represents an instructional variable since it dictates the procedure and the listener's task. Large differences can often be obtained when estimating a particular function, depending upon the psychophysical method used. For example, forced choice response tasks typically yield lower threshold estimates than non-forced choice response tasks. Of those traditional psychophysical methods that we have described, the method of constant stimuli is most clearly a forced choice situation, while the method of adjustment is clearly the least forced choice-like situation.

Organismic variables: presbycusis. There are two subclasses of organismic variables, one pertaining to the psychological state of the organism and the other to its physiological state. Psychological variables include such things as motivation, importance of the task to the listener (in terms of monetary reward, for example) etc. Physiological variables include the anatomic and physiologic state of the ear itself. *Presbycusis* is an example of the influence of the latter class of variables. It refers to the deterioration of hearing with increased age and is seen as a reduction in sensitivity for the higher frequencies. For example, a young normal hearing person might require a sound pressure level of 20 dB in order to hear a tone of 10,000 Hz; a 40-year-old might require 30 dB, and 45 dB might be required for a 50-year-old. The exact cause of presbycusis is not known, but it occurs almost without exception as people grow older.

Audiogram

We have been discussing the ways in which hearing thresholds change as the stimulus frequency varies. A plot of sound pressure level required for threshold as a function of frequency is the most direct means of displaying this information. However, in some instances such a graph may not serve the needs of the user. For example, if we wish to see whether a group of people had normal hearing, then it would be advantageous to plot their threshold estimates so that they could be compared to those of normal hearing individuals. Such a graph is called an *audiogram.*

Audiometric zero. A necessary step in constructing an audiogram is to define normal hearing. We know that hearing sensitivity declines with age, therefore, in our definition of normal hearing we would probably wish to restrict our population to young people. We also know that various auditory pathologies can cause permanent damage to the hearing mechanism. Consequently, we would want to avoid those people who have known histories of auditory pathology. Further, individuals exposed to intense sounds suffer a deficit in their hearing sensitivity and thus we would want to avoid people with this type of exposure. Therefore, we might define normal hearing in terms of threshold estimates obtained under optimum listening conditions for a large group of people excluding those in the categories previously mentioned. Such a process has been carried out in a number of hearing surveys. Results from these works form a baseline against which we can compare the thresholds of people whom we suspect of having less than normal hearing.

Relation of sound pressure level graph to hearing loss graph. Figure 9-18(*a*) shows a typical audiogram. The solid line across the top represents the threshold of a person with normal hearing. The second line shows an audiogram of a person suffering from typical presbycusis. The third line shows an

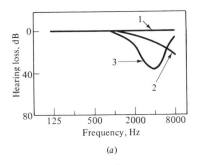 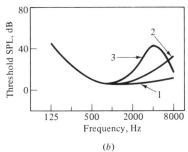

Figure 9-18 Examples of various hearing functions in terms of (a), an audiogram and (b), a sound pressure plot. Function 1 represents normal hearing ; function 2 shows thresholds typical of a person suffering from presbycusis ; function 3 is typical of thresholds obtained from people suffering from acoustic trauma.

audiogram of a person with a history of high level noise exposure. The coordinates of this graph are frequency and hearing loss. Hearing loss is defined as the difference between a person's threshold and audiometric zero. Thus, if audiometric zero for a particular frequency was 15 dB relative to 0.0002 dyne/cm² and the threshold of a particular person was 25 dB, his hearing loss at that frequency would be 10 dB.

It is important to remember that information with respect to thresholds can be presented either in a typical sound pressure level plot (Figures 9-11, 9-15, 9·17), or in a hearing loss plot. In either case the information is the same, it is simply represented in different forms. Figure 9-18(b) shows the information from Figure 9-18(a) replotted in terms of sound pressure level. Be sure you can follow how one graph is derived from the other.

Differential Thresholds (Discrimination)

Our ability to perceive small changes in a stimulus is extremely keen and very important. It is important because it is through discriminability that information is communicated. For example, if our only ability was to observe the presence or absence of a sound, then we would be limited to two pieces of information. However, because we are able to discriminate among various frequencies, intensities, and temporal patterns we recognize a large number of different stimuli, each of which has the potential to convey a bit of information. Were it not for this ability, speech would have no meaning since all speech would sound the same.

The differential threshold is a measure of our ability to discriminate small stimulus changes. Typically, two stimuli are made to differ along a single dimension, such as frequency, and the listener is required to respond to this difference. It is possible to obtain as many different kinds of differential thresholds as there are dimensions to a stimulus. Since there is an infinite variety of sounds which can be used as stimuli, we will restrict our discussion to three stimulus dimensions: frequency, intensity, and duration. The same factors that influence estimation of absolute thresholds also influence differential threshold; that is, organismic, instructional, measurement, and stimulus variables. However, the effect of the first three is similar for both differential and absolute threshold. Thus, we will confine our discussion to stimulus factors influencing differential sensitivity.

Figure 9-19 Differential threshold for frequency as influenced by (*a*) frequency, (*b*) sensation level. Sensation level is the number of dB a tone is above its own threshold. [*After A. M. Small and J. F. Brandt, "Differential thresholds for frequency," J. Acoust. Soc. Amer., 35 (1963), 785; and E. G. Shower and R. Biddulph, "Differential pitch sensitivity of the ear," J. Acoust. Soc. Amer., 3 (1931), 275.*]

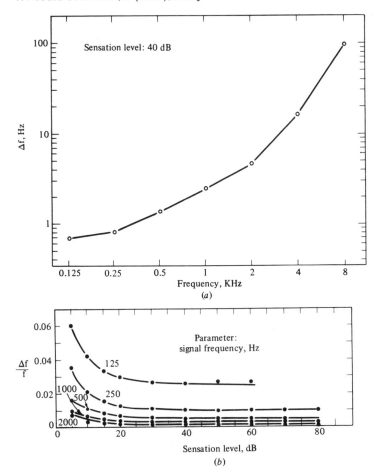

Frequency discrimination : stimulus factors

How far apart in frequency must two otherwise identical stimuli be before a listener can discriminate that there are in fact two different stimuli being presented? There are three major stimulus factors which determine this. Figure 9-19(*a*) shows the influence of one of these, frequency. As we increase the frequency of the stimuli, the difference between the stimuli must become larger in order for the listener to perceive the difference. The rate at which the differential threshold increases with increasing frequency is not constant, it is fairly slow until approximately 1,000 Hz and then increases more rapidly. A second factor in determining the differential threshold for frequency is the stimulus intensity. As we see in Figure 9-19(*b*), frequency discrimination tends to improve as sound pressure increases. This improvement continues only to a certain sound pressure, above which little further decrease in differential threshold occurs.

A third stimulus factor is the duration for which the stimulus is presented. The information in Figure 9-20 indicates that the differential threshold for frequency does not depend upon the stimulus duration until a fairly short duration is reached. Frequency discrimination deteriorates for durations less than this critical value.

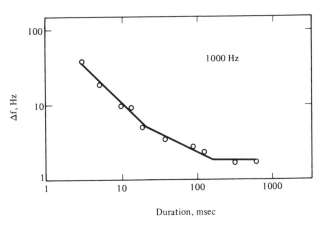

Figure 9-20 Differential threshold for frequency as influenced by stimulus duration. [*After L. Chih-an and L. A. Chistovitch, "Frequency difference limens as a function of tonal duration,"* Soviet Physics Acoust., *6 (1960), 75. Reprinted by permission of the American Institute of Physics.*]

Intensity discrimination : stimulus factors

When determining differential threshold for intensity, the stimuli are identical except for the factor measured. The intensity of one of the two stimuli is increased until they are sufficiently different so that the listener can perceive that difference. The same three factors that are influential in determining frequency discrimination are influential in determining intensity discrimination, but they act in a somewhat different fashion.

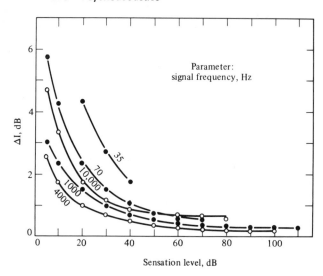

Figure 9-21 Differential threshold for intensity as influenced by intensity and frequency. [*After R. R. Reisz, "Differential intensity sensitivity for the ear for pure tones,"* Phys. Rev., *31 (1928), 867.*]

Figure 9-21 shows that as intensity is increased the differential threshold expressed in dB decreases. We also see that as stimulus frequency is increased the differential threshold decreases at least until 4,000 Hz, after which the threshold increases. This effect of frequency upon intensity discrimination resembles the effect of frequency upon absolute threshold. That is if we compare Figure 9-21 with Figure 9-11 we see that those frequencies for which absolute threshold is smallest are the same frequencies for which intensity discrimination is best.

Figure 9-22 shows the effect of stimulus duration upon intensity discrimination. For durations less than 0.25 sec the differential threshold increases as duration is shortened; that is discrimination becomes poorer. Duration has no effect on intensity discrimination for durations longer than 0.25 sec.

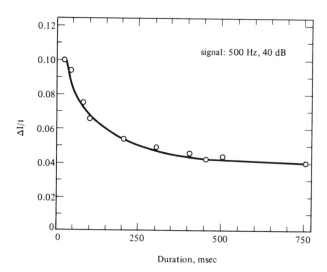

Figure 9-22 Differential threshold for intensity as influenced by stimulus duration. [*After G. A. Miller and W. R. Garner, "Effect of random presentation on the psychometric function . . .,"* Amer. J. Psychol., *57 (1944), 451.*]

Duration discrimination: stimulus factors

A third primary stimulus dimension which may be discriminated is the duration of the stimulus. How much longer must one stimulus be than another before a listener can discern that difference? Figure 9-23 illustrates the answer to that question. We see in Figure 9-23(*a*) that as duration is lengthened, the increment between the two stimulus values must be made greater in order for the listener to perceive the difference between the two stimuli. Except for very short durations, the frequency of the stimulus appears to be of little importance in differential thresholds for duration (Figure 9-23(*b*)). The differentiation between frequency conditions at the shortest duration is not related to frequency *per se*, but to the starting and stopping characteristics of the waveforms.

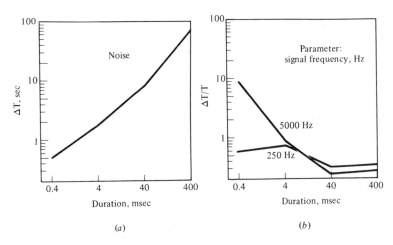

(*a*) (*b*)

Figure 9-23 Differential threshold for duration as influenced by (*a*) duration; (*b*) frequency. [*After A. M. Small and R. A. Campbell, "Temporal differential sensitivity for auditory stimuli,"* Amer. J. Psychol., *75 (1962), 401.*]

Comparison of discrimination ability

The material presented above indicates that for some situations the human auditory system is exceptionally well suited to the discrimination task. However, our ability varies markedly depending upon what aspect of the stimulus we are discriminating. We are capable of discriminating frequency changes as small as 1 or 2 parts in 1,000, intensity changes 1 or 2 parts in 100 and temporal changes 1 or 2 parts in 10. Thus, our ability to discriminate small differences in frequency compares favorably with sophisticated physical measuring devices, but our ability to detect temporal changes is very crude.

MASKING

Definition and Significance

Masking is the threshold shift in an auditory stimulus produced by the simultaneous presentation of a second auditory stimulus. Masking is measured by determining the detection threshold for a stimulus first in silence and then in the presence of a second auditory stimulus. The difference in those two thresholds is the *amount of masking*.

The significance of masking is that it is the manifestation of interaction between two stimuli. That is, if one stimulus can influence the threshold of another this means that somewhere in the auditory system their internal representations come together. Thus, there is considerable theoretical importance attached to the masking phenomenon. In addition, there are certain very practical implications for masking. For example, if it is necessary that we test hearing in other than a quiet environment, we must be aware that masking effects may take place. The thresholds that we measure may not be the same had we been able to estimate thresholds under conditions of quiet. Thus, we might judge a person to possess a hearing loss when really his hearing was perfectly normal but was influenced by simultaneously present auditory stimuli.

Examples of Masking Arising from Different Maskers

Typically the stimulus that we attempt to detect is called the *signal* and the stimulus that provides the interference is called the *masker*. In principle any stimulus can serve as a signal and any stimulus can be a masker. We will limit our discussion to several fundamental combinations in which the signal will always be a sinusoid and the masker either a sinusoid or noise.

Wide band noise

If the masker is a wide band of noise the results pictured in Figure 9-24 are obtained. The abscissa shows the frequency of the signal and the ordinate indicates the sound pressure level required to elicit a threshold response from the signal. The bottom curve corresponds to the threshold of audibility, that is, the threshold obtained under conditions of quiet. The next higher curve is obtained with a very small amount of noise; the next curve for somewhat greater amount of noise, and so forth. We see that for this masker, which contains an equal amount of energy at every frequency, the masking effect is not uniform at the low masker levels. That is, as we increase the masker noise level, we find that the threshold is first shifted in that frequency region to which the ear is most sensitive, the 1,000 to 3,000 Hz region. As we

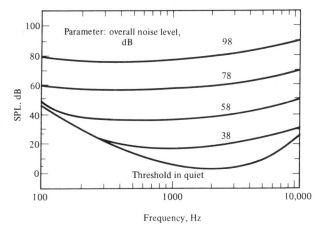

Figure 9-24 Masking of a sinusoid by another sinusoid. [*After J. E. Hawkins and S. S. Stevens, "The masking of pure tones and speech by white noise,"* J. Acoust. Soc. Amer., *22 (1950), 6.*]

further increase the masker, the threshold is shifted in the middle frequency region by an amount equal to the increase in masker level and the masking effect is extended to lower and higher frequencies. Eventually, as we move to high noise levels, the masking function is nearly flat indicating that the sound pressure level required for threshold is constant regardless of frequency. Thus at high masker levels the masking is perhaps what we might expect based on the spectrum of the signal, but at low masker levels the basic sensitivity curve of the ear in conjunction with the masker spectrum determines the threshold function.

Pure tone masking

Pure tone masking refers to that situation where both signal and masker are pure tones. When the masker was a wide band of noise it contained all audible frequencies in equal amount, but with a pure tone masker all the masker energy is concentrated at a single point in the spectrum. Figure 9-25 shows typical results obtained in a pure tone masking situation. Signal frequency is plotted on the horizontal axis, but in contrast to Figure 9-24, the amount of masking is plotted on the vertical axis. We see that the maximum amount of masking is obtained when the signal frequency is approximately equal to the masker frequency. We also observe that for the higher masker intensities the masking function declines more rapidly on the left or low frequency side, than on the right, or high frequency side. This pattern gives rise to the generalization that low tones mask high tones more effectively than vice versa. As the intensity of the masker is lowered the masking functions become more symmetrical. In all cases we see that there is a dip or irregularity when the signal frequency approximates the masker frequency. In some cases there are additional irregularities at higher signal frequencies. We will discuss the possible source of these irregularities in the next section.

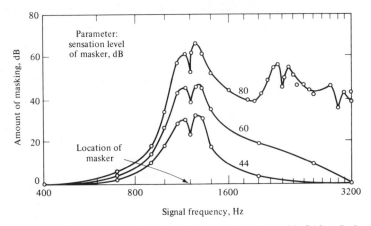

Figure 9-25 Masking of a sinusoid by another sinusoid. [*After R. L. Wegel and C. E. Lane, "The auditory masking of one pure tone by another and its probable relation to the dynamics of the inner ear,"* Phys. Rev., *23 (1924), 266.*]

Narrow band noise masking

Narrow band noise masking refers to the situation in which the masker is a narrow band of noise and the signal is a pure tone. It represents a situation intermediate between that of wide band noise masking and pure tone masking in that the noise energy is moderately dispersed in the frequency spectrum but not nearly to the same extent as the case for wide band noise. Figure 9-26 shows a typical result obtained with narrow band noise as a masker (the graph has the same coordinate system as was used in Figure 9-25). The narrow band noise masking function is similar to that for pure tone masking except for the absence of an irregularity when the signal is nearly equal to

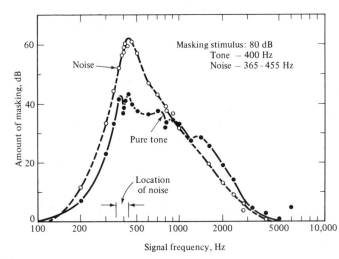

Figure 9-26 Masking of a sinusoid by a narrow band of noise. [*After J. P. Egan and H. W. Hake, "On the masking pattern of simple auditory stimuli,"* J. Acoust. Soc. Amer., *22 (1950), 827.*]

(or an integral multiple of) the masker frequency. We might suspect that there is something about the simultaneous presentation of two pure tones which leads to these irregularities. The most likely explanation lies in the production of beats, a phenomenon which will be discussed in the section on beats (p.386). At this time it is sufficient to say simply that when two frequencies are close together they interact in such a way that there is a periodic change in their loudness. We suspect that under these conditions the signal is more easily detectable than when beats do not take place. Since beats do not occur with a narrow band noise masker and we do not see the irregularity under these conditions, our idea appears reasonable.

The shape of the functions shown in Figures 9-25 and 9-26 would be similar even if different masker frequencies were used. In all cases the maximum amount of masking is obtained when the signal frequency approximates the masker frequency. The pattern of the response is the same although its absolute location in frequency will differ as masker frequency changes.

Critical Band Concept and Data

What would happen if we started out with a wide band of noise as a masker and a pure tone as a signal and in successive steps narrowed the band of noise? Some very interesting results occur which are of considerable importance in understanding the phenomenon of masking. As an illustration let us start out with a wide band of noise whose spectrum has been adjusted so as to provide equal masking at all frequencies. We locate our signal frequency at the center of this wide band of noise and determine its threshold under masking conditions. We then narrow the band of noise somewhat, chopping off a little at both the low and high frequency ends and redetermine the threshold of the signal. We would find it unchanged. Next we would narrow the masker noise band still further and reassess the threshold. This process is continued until eventually we come to a point at which narrowing the band further results in a change in the threshold of the signal. Continued narrowing beyond this point produces a greater decrease in the threshold.

What we have just described is shown in Figure 9-27. We see from the figure that the *critical bandwidth* at which this threshold change occurs depends upon the frequency of the tone. Of what significance is this result? It shows that only those noise frequencies within a narrow band centered about the signal frequency are effective in contributing to the masking of that signal. We know this because we can eliminate all frequencies outside of this band and see no effect upon the masked threshold. Yet, when we begin to eliminate frequencies within that band this causes a change in the masked threshold. Thus, only those frequencies contained within the critical band are effective in providing masking for a signal at the center of that band.

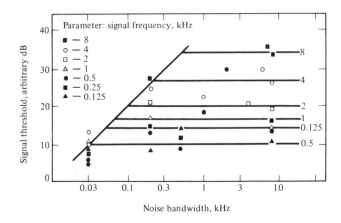

Figure 9-27 Determination of critical bandwidth. The point at which the horizontal line begins to slope downward to the left defines the critical bandwidth. For noise wider than the critical bandwidth masking is unaffected by bandwidth. [*After H. Fletcher, "Auditory patterns,"* Rev. Mod. Phys., *12* (*1940*), *47-65.*]

The practical implication of this finding is that masking is frequency specific. If we are testing hearing with a particular signal frequency, we know that only those frequencies in a simultaneously presented stimulus which are close in frequency to the signal will provide effective masking. Thus it may be possible to test hearing in a noisy environment if the frequencies contained in the noise are not close to the frequency of the signal. The theoretical importance of the critical band concept is that it appears as though there is something that acts like a bandpass filter within the ear. Although a wide band noise is presented to the input of this bandpass filter, it is the narrow band noise appearing at the filter output that is effective in providing the masking. This analogy has been found to be extremely useful in investigations of frequency selectivity in the auditory system.

LOUDNESS

Methods of Measurement

Direct

A direct method is any method in which judgments are made, or, stimulus values changed, relative to the perceived loudness of the stimulus. These methods are to be contrasted with those in which judgments are made with respect to loudness equality. The method of direct magnitude estimation, discussed on page 363, is one psychophysical procedure which yields a direct measurement of loudness. Typical results, shown in Figure 9-11 form a loudness scale. If a 1,000 Hz standard stimulus presented 40 dB above its threshold is assigned a loudness value of 1, then the loudness units of the resulting scale are called *sones*.

Indirect

Although there are a number of advantages to using a direct method of loudness measurement, there are also disadvantages. Direct methods show a considerable amount of variability. Both the same and different listeners assign varying loudness values to the same stimulus. Indirect methods yield less variable results, but are more difficult to relate to perceived loudness. Typically, indirect methods are those in which a psychophysical method is used such that a point of subjective equality can be estimated. For example, a listener is asked to adjust the intensity of a stimulus until its loudness is equal to that of another stimulus. Such a procedure is referred to as a *loudness balance*. In this situation the specification of the loudness of the unknown stimulus is in terms of the sound pressure of an equally loud comparison stimulus. In the subsequent discussion of loudness our information has been gathered primarily by the indirect method. Loudness as indicated by the indirect method is referred to as *loudness level* and has units that are called *phons*.

Stimulus Factors in Loudness Determination

Because there are a very large number of different kinds of stimuli whose loudness may be judged, we will confine our discussion to a consideration of the stimulus factors which influence the loudness of pure tones.

Intensity

While it is true that stimulus intensity is perhaps the primary stimulus factor in determining loudness, it is not the only factor. One function that shows the relation of loudness to intensity is the loudness scale of Figure 9-10. Another way of depicting the relation of intensity to loudness is shown in Figure 9-28. This figure shows both the effect of stimulus intensity and stimulus frequency on loudness level. The lowest curve on the graph represents the threshold of audibility. Next, a 1,000 Hz tone was increased in sound pressure so that it was 10 dB above its threshold, as shown by the open circle. The listeners then adjusted the intensity of a second stimulus until it was equally as loud as the 1,000 cycle tone 10 dB above the tone threshold. The sound pressure required to achieve a loudness equal to this standard at various frequencies is indicated by the filled circles. The line connecting all the circles represents an equal *loudness contour* since the stimulus value corresponding to any point on that line is equally as loud as a stimulus value represented by any other point. The next step was to raise the 1,000 Hz standard stimulus so that it was now 20 dB above its threshold. Its sound pressure under these conditions is shown by the open square. The listeners were asked to adjust stimuli of various frequencies until they again were

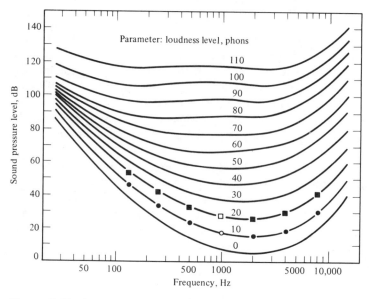

Figure 9-28   Loudness level as influenced by stimulus frequency and intensity. Each curve is an equal loudness contour. [*After H. Fletcher and W. A. Munson, "Loudness, definition, measurements and calculation," J. Acoust. Soc. Amer., 5 (1933), 82.*]

equally as loud as the new standard. The results of these matches are shown by the filled squares; the line connecting all of the squares represents another equal loudness contour. This process was repeated until all the contours shown in the figure were obtained. You will note that the method used in generating these curves was an indirect technique in which loudness balances were used. Thus, each equal loudness contour has a different loudness level which, when expressed in phons, is equal to the number of dB that the standard tone was raised above its own threshold. For example, the equal loudness contour formed by the circles has a loudness level of 10 phons while the equal loudness contour formed by the squares has a loudness level of 20 phons.

Frequency

In order to convince ourselves that loudness, or at least loudness level, is to some degree dependent upon frequency, all we need to do is to consider the 10 phon contour in Figure 9-28. We see that in order to maintain equal loudness as we change frequency it is necessary to change the sound pressure. In other words, if we kept the sound pressure constant and changed the frequency we would no longer have stimuli that fell on the same equal loudness contour, thus indicating that the stimuli have different loudnesses.

For very high loudness levels we see that the equal loudness contours are nearly a horizontal straight line. Under these conditions loudness is less dependent upon frequency than for moderate and low level stimuli.

Duration

Duration is another stimulus factor which influences loudness under some conditions. Figure 9-29 shows some of these conditions. The graphs are equal loudness contours in the same sense as in Figure 9-28. The listener's task was to adjust the intensity of a stimulus of a particular duration until it was equal in loudness to a stimulus of standard duration. Each curve represents stimulus values yielding equal loudness for various intensities of the standard stimulus. We see that as signal duration is shortened there is no change in the sound pressure required to achieve equal loudness until a certain critical duration is reached. For durations shorter than this critical duration it is necessary that the sound pressure of the comparison stimulus be increased in order to maintain equal loudness. Thus, for short durations, loudness declines as duration is shortened.

Figure 9-29   Loudness level as influenced by stimulus duration and intensity for wide band noise. Each curve is an equal loudness contour. [*After A. M. Small et al., "Loudness as a function of signal duration,"* J. Acoust. Soc. Amer., *34 (1962), 513-14.*]

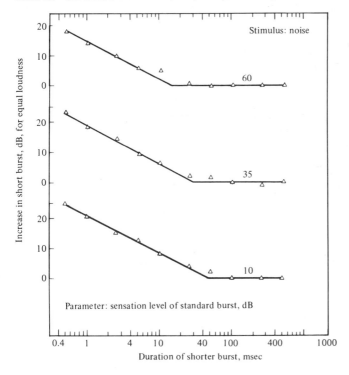

BEATS AND SUBJECTIVE TONES

Monaural Beats

It is important to distinguish between stimulus and response in the discussion of beats. In psychoacoustics the term beats refers to the perception of a certain type of stimulus. *Beats*, therefore, are defined in terms of response. They are generally thought of as a periodic variation in loudness related to corresponding variation in the physical stimulus.

Stimulus

A stimulus which gives rise to beating sensation is one composed of two sinusoids which are very close together in frequency. We remember from Chapter 2 that when two sine waves of identical frequency are combined, the resultant is dependent upon the relative phase of the two combining sinusoids. If the phase difference is 0°, reinforcement occurs; if the phase difference is 180°, cancellation occurs, and if the phase is intermediate the result is intermediate. Figure 9-30 shows the combination of two sinusoids of slightly different frequency. We see that the waveforms start in phase but as time progresses, because waveform A has a longer period than waveform B, an increasingly large phase shift occurs. If we compare the sum of these two waveforms at a point early in time, we see that the waveforms have reinforced each other. As we progress in time the phase differences are such the cancellation occurs. Thus, the resultant wave for two sinusoids close together in frequency shows periodic changes in its *envelope* resulting from the progressive phase shifts in the combining stimuli.

Figure 9-30 Waveforms of stimuli yielding beats of imperfect unisons. Sinusoids A and B have periods of T_1 and T_2 respectively and combine to form the resultant waveform R.

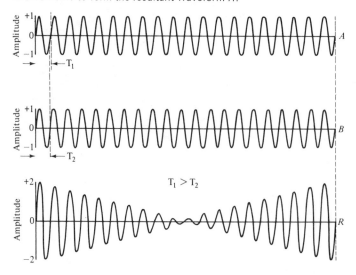

As the two stimuli are moved apart in frequency there is an increase in the rate of envelope changes. However when the frequencies are far apart, but form some simple ratio such as 2:1 or 3:2, the resultant waveform shows a slower pattern of envelope change similar to that seen when the frequencies were close together.

Imperfect unison

Beats of *imperfect unisons* occur when two sinusoids are close together in frequency. The rate at which these beats occur is equal to the frequency difference between the primaries. For example, if stimuli of 100 and 103 Hz were presented simultaneously we would find envelope changes occurring in the stimulus three times per second and perceptual loudness changes would also occur three times per second. The perception of beats depends very much upon the frequency difference between the two primaries. It is possible to have frequency differences so small that the change in loudness occurs so slowly that it is unrecognized. For example, if two frequencies differed by only 0.000001 Hz it would take more than 5 days for their resultant envelope to go from maximum to minimum amplitude. Beats are most pronounced for frequency differences of about 0.5 to 4 Hz. As the beat rate increases above about 5 Hz, the loudness variations occur so rapidly that they tend to blend together and are not heard as separate and distinct entities but rather as a roughness or trill. This general percept continues until the frequency difference between the primaries is perhaps 20 Hz. Beyond this point, even though the stimulus continues to show envelope variation, we simply hear two separate, distinct, and independent tones, just as though each were being presented separately.

Mistuned consonance

When two stimuli are quite far apart in frequency beats are perceived if the stimuli approximate the ratio of small integers, such as 2:1 or 3:2. Such beats are called beats of *mistuned consonance* and are generally less obvious than beats of imperfect unisons. In fact, they become increasingly difficult to perceive as the primaries form ratios of larger numbers, for example, 5:4 or 7:8.

Significance

Beats are a phenomenon which has long been recognized and which has been controversial in the sense that it plays a central role in the formulation of several theories of hearing. These theories of hearing will be discussed in more detail in the section on pitch, but the basic question is whether beats are a manifestation of imperfect frequency selectivity or simply represent the response to temporal changes in the stimulus.

Binaural Beats

What happens when a sinusoidal stimulus is put in one ear and a sinusoid of another frequency very close to the first is put in the opposite ear? Under these conditions periodic variations are perceived. However, measurements must be carefully made since sound energy delivered to one ear may find its way to the other ear. Thus, while sound is nominally delivered to opposite ears, in fact what may be perceived is nothing more than monaural beats. This crosshead leakage can occur by either air or bone conduction; in the first instance sound leaks out from under the cushion of one earphone, goes around the head and penetrates the cushion of the other earphone; in the second case sound may actually be transmitted through the bones of the head to the opposite ear. It is possible to minimize sound leakage and when this is done it is found that binaural effects still occur although they differ from the typical monaural beat. Instead of a periodic change in the loudness of the stimulus, binaural beats generally take the form of a change in the apparent location of the sound source. With earphone presentation sound appears to come from within the head, its apparent position moving across the head from one ear to the other and back again repetitively. The rate at which the sound's apparent position changes is equal to the frequency difference between the two primaries. It is important to emphasize, therefore, that binaural interaction does occur in a form which is referred to as beats but perceptually, binaural and monaural beats are not equivalent.

Aural Harmonics

Under some conditions a sinusoid may be put into the ear and, instead of hearing a pure tone, the original sinusoid plus a number of its harmonics are heard. The harmonics perceived under these conditions are referred to as *aural* harmonics because they are generated within the auditory system. The generation of harmonics is a well-known property of *nonlinear systems* and consequently, it is of interest for us to consider some elementary nonlinear systems.

Simple nonlinear systems

A system can be nonlinear (nonproportional) with respect to any of its dimensions such as amplitude, frequency, or time response. We will consider only amplitude nonlinearity in this section.

One of the simplest examples of nonlinearity can be developed from a children's teeter-totter, a diagram of which is shown in Figure 9-31(*a*). A teeter-totter, as you recall, is a board which is balanced on a fulcrum. A downward motion on one end results in an upward motion at the other end. Let us suppose the lengths on either side of the fulcrum are equal

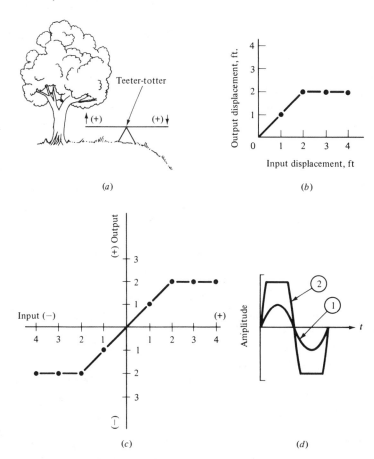

Figure 9-31 Example of a nonlinear system. A "teeter-totter" system is shown in (a) which has an input-output function as illustrated in (b) for positive displacement and as illustrated in (c) for positive and negative displacements. The output of this system is shown in (d) when the input is simple harmonic motion, if that motion is small, 1, or large, 2.

so that when the input is moved one foot the output also moves one foot. When the input is two feet, the output is also two feet. This relation is shown in Figure 9-31(b). Thus far the function displays a linear relation in that the output is proportional (in this particular instance identical) to the input. Now let us extend the input displacement to three feet. At this point the opposite end of the teeter-totter comes into contact with the branch of a tree. This restricts the movement of the output end of it with the result that, although the input is displaced one more foot, the output does not change. This implies, of course, that the board forming the teeter-totter is bending. We would probably find no change in output with further increase of input, except perhaps the board might break. Thus, Figure 9-31(*b*) indicates that a proportional relation for small amplitudes, and a nonproportional relation for higher amplitudes between input and output displacement. In general, a nonlinear system is any system in which the input-output function is not a simple straight line relation.

Thus far we have considered positive values of input. We have only moved the teeter-totter in one direction. We could, of course, move it in the opposite direction, which by convention we would assign a negative value. In this case the output end of the teeter-totter would hit the ground generating an inverse function to that seen in Figure 9-31(*b*). The complete function for positive and negative values of input is shown in Figure 9-31(*c*).

Rather than moving the teeter-totter with constant displacement, let us move the input end with simple harmonic motion. What kind of output would we expect? We can see intuitively that if the amplitude of the simple harmonic motion were small the output would also be simple harmonic motion. If, however, the input amplitude were large, then the motion of the teeter-totter would force it against the tree and the ground with the result that the motion of the output end would not be sinusoidal. The resulting outputs are shown in Figure 9-31(*d*) where waveform *1* corresponds to a small input value and waveform *2* to a larger input value. In the second case the amplitude is limited at the top and the bottom, as we would have guessed based on the presence of the tree and the ground.

Any waveform other than sinusoidal is a complex waveform and by definition contains more than one sine wave (see Chapter 2). Waveform *2* shown in Fig. 9-31(*d*), is a complex wave. Remember that the input was simple harmonic motion and its waveform was sinusoidal, but at the output of the system we see a waveform that is nonsinusoidal. The implication is, therefore, that the system has generated additional frequency components. A detailed examination of the output will show that added components are harmonics of the input signal.

Although we have talked about teeter-totters and trees, what we have said applies to most nonlinear systems. Because of the similarity of the output of the teeter-totter and the output of the ear, there is good reason to believe that the generation of aural harmonics is a result of nonlinear characteristics within the auditory system. Let us now examine the details of aural harmonics.

Methods of measurement

Although some people are able to pick out each of several aural harmonics that may be generated in a particular case, most of us can not do this. We do recognize that under some conditions the stimulus seems to have a different quality, but without training we do not have the ability to distinguish individual components of the complex sound. Thus, some additional means is required in order to establish the presence and measure the characteristics of aural harmonics. One method commonly used is called the *probe tone technique*. A second stimulus, the probe tone, is simultaneously presented and its frequency adjusted so that it very nearly corresponds to the expected frequency of one of the harmonics. The frequency and amplitude of the probe tone are then adjusted and an attempt is made to perceive beats. If beats occur it is presumed that the probe tone is beating with the aural harmonic, thus the frequency of the aural harmonic is established.

To determine the approximate amplitude of the aural harmonic, the probe tone is adjusted so as to obtain the maximum difference between the loud and the soft phase of the beat. If this adjustment is carried out with two pure tone inputs, the maximum difference between the loud and soft phase of the beats occurs when the amplitude of the two primaries are equal. Thus, in the probe tone situation it is presumed that when a maximum loudness difference between loud and soft phase occurs (called *best beats*) the amplitude of the probe and the aural harmonic are equal. The use of this technique for determining aural harmonic amplitude has been criticized, however, on the basis that the situation in which it is used with the probe tone represents a much more complex stimulus situation than with two externally presented sinusoids. There is little question, however, that the beat technique is a valid and valuable method for the establishment of the presence or absence of aural harmonics.

Figure 9-32   Sensation level at which aural harmonics of different fundamental frequencies can first be detected. [*From* Speech and Hearing *by Harvey Fletcher.* © *1929, 1953 by Litton Educational Publishing, Inc. Reprinted by permission of Van Nostrand Reinhold Company.*]

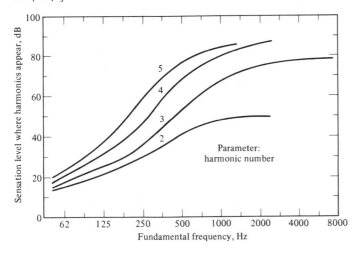

Stimulus factors

The primary stimulus factor in the generation of aural harmonics is the intensity of the stimulus. Figure 9-32 summarizes the situation. We see that for higher frequencies a sensation level of 50 dB is required before aural harmonics are detectable. At the lower frequencies aural harmonics are detectable at lower sensation levels. However, because of the shape of the audibility function aural harmonics become audible above 50 dB SPL regardless of frequencies. As the intensity continues to increase above 50 dB SPL, the aural harmonics increase in magnitude and number.

Difference and Summation Tones

In a nonlinear system such as was described above, when two frequencies are presented to the input simultaneously we find harmonics in the output and frequencies that are equal to the sum and the difference between the primary frequencies. Indeed, if the input-output function is sufficiently complex, we will find difference and summation frequencies occurring between the harmonics which have been generated. Consequently, we may have a very large number of "extra" frequencies.

The ear seems to operate in much the same fashion as we would expect with a simple nonlinear system, that is, under those same circumstances in which aural harmonics are generated, so also are difference tones generated. If the intensity is above 40 or 50 dB sound pressure level, we are easily able to detect the presence of a difference tone. The summation tone is more difficult to hear, perhaps because it may be partially masked due to the frequency position of the two primaries.

What part of the auditory system is responding in a nonlinear fashion and thus may be responsible for the generation of aural harmonics, difference tones and possibly summation tones? It appears as though most of the nonlinearity arises from within the cochlea. However, at sufficiently high intensities, perhaps over 90 dB sound pressure level, additional nonlinearity arises in the action of the middle ear. Thus, there are several sources, each of which contributes at different stimulus intensities.

BINAURAL EFFECTS

We would think that perhaps there was some good reason for having two ears rather than just one. We might guess that our auditory performance would be improved by the use of two ears. In this section we will explore that question and other phenomena associated with two-ear listening.

Summation

Threshold

If we compare the sound pressure required in order to detect the presence of a stimulus using two ears as opposed to doing the same thing using just one ear, we find that there is very little improvement in performance unless the two ears initially have equal sensitivity. That is, if the threshold in one ear is 10 dB higher than that in the other ear, the threshold obtained using both ears is simply that of the better ear. However, if by appropriate selection we obtain listeners with the same threshold in each ear we find that threshold improves by about 3 dB. As ears become less well matched in sensitivity the improvement declines rapidly. If somehow the sound power from one ear was being added to that from the other ear at some central location in the nervous system, then we would have twice as much sound power, or its representation, in the binaural as in the monaural case. You recall from Chapter 2 that a 2:1 increase in power is equivalent to a 3 dB increase. Since the improvement in threshold under optimum conditions also corresponds to 3 dB, this suggests that perhaps the equivalent of power summation is occurring someplace in the nervous system. It should be noted that this idea implies an interaction of the stimulus representation derived from each ear and thus regards the two ears really as part of a single auditory system.

The same experiment can be repeated, using one ear on each of two people. The listeners are instructed to respond whenever either of them thinks that they hear the stimulus while using the method of constant stimuli, for example. Again in this case if the sensitivity of the two ears is matched we find an improvement in threshold of 3 dB. Quite clearly, there can be no power summation in this case since there is no means by which the representation of the two stimuli can come together. However, it has been suggested that this result can be explained on a simple probability basis. If you add a second independent listener his chances of detecting the stimulus are just as good as that of the first observer. If you have two listeners observing simultaneously, their chances of detecting any given stimulus is twice as good as either one alone. A two-fold increase in this probability is equivalent to a 3 dB threshold decrease. It would follow from this analysis that if we added a third observer, performance should improve, and a fourth and so on. In fact, we find this to be so, although the increment in performance becomes increasingly small as we add observers.

This multiple observer result raises the question of whether the same effect might be occurring when a single listener is using both of his ears. Is his improvement in performance related simply to the use of two independent receivers? The power summation hypothesis implies a single auditory system with two receivers while the probability hypothesis suggests two independent auditory systems. Which of the two ideas is the correct interpretation is not clear; what is clear, however, is that given equal sensitivity two ears are clearly superior to one in the determination of an absolute threshold.

Loudness

Loudness also increases under binaural compared to monaural listening conditions. Figure 9-33 summarizes the situation. If listeners have ears of equal sensitivity, then once the stimulus is moderately intense, we need to adjust a monaural stimulus so that its value is 6 dB greater than that of a corresponding binaural stimulus in order to achieve equal loudness. This 6 dB monaural-binaural difference decreases as sensation level is decreased until we reach threshold at which point we are left with the 3 dB difference discussed in the previous section. Thus, the same stimulus presented to both ears is louder than that stimulus presented to one ear alone.

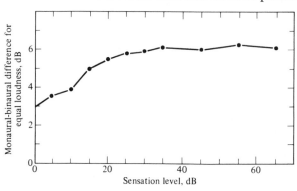

Figure 9-33 Binaural summation of loudness as influenced by stimulus sensation level. [*R. Caussé and P. Chavasse, Les Comptes-Rendus de la Société de Biologie, 136 (1942), 405. Reproduced by permission of Collège de France, Paris.*]

Discrimination

We find that both frequency and intensity discrimination improve if two ears are used rather than one. Differences in optimal performance in binaural and monaural listening are typically small, amounting perhaps to 0.2 dB for intensity discrimination, and perhaps a 30 % improvement in performance for frequency discrimination.

Masking

Since the masking situation requires two stimuli, the masker and the signal, and we have two ears, many combinations of ears and stimuli are available. The number of ear-stimulus combinations is increased still further when it is recognized that the relative phase of each stimulus at each ear may also be varied.

The relative phase of a given stimulus at the two ears is spoken of as *interaural phase*. We will illustrate just two phase conditions, although in fact there are an infinite number of such conditions. In Figure 9-34(*a*) there is a drawing of a listener's head. Assume that a sinusoidal stimulus is applied to the two ears in such a way that the earphone diagrams and consequently the tympanic membranes are moved inward at the same time. That is, the condensation phase of the sound wave occurs at the same instant in both ears.

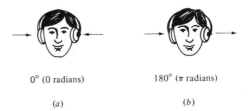

Figure 9-34 Examples of two different interaural phase relations: (*a*) the in-phase (0 radian) condition; (*b*) the 180 degree (π radian) out-of-phase condition.

0° (0 radians)   180° (π radians)

(*a*)   (*b*)

When the rarefaction phase of the sinewave occurs, both earphone diaphragms and both eardrums will move out together. Thus, the "inward together, outward together" pattern of activity repeats. Such a pattern of movement is spoken of as in-phase, 0 degrees, or homophasic. Figure 9-34(*b*) illustrates another possible phase condition in which the condensation phase of the sound wave arrives at one ear at the same moment that the rarefaction phase of the sound wave arrives at the other ear. As a consequence one earphone diaphragm and tympanic membrane moves inward while the other earphone diaphragm and eardrum moves outward. The movement is reversed as time progresses. This phase relation is spoken of as representing 180 degrees, π radians, out of phase, or antiphasic. Each of these interaural phase conditions (or any other) may be used for either signal or masker.

We have previously discussed monaural masking in which both signal and masker were in the same ear. If signal and masker are in opposite ears and we are careful to eliminate sound leakage from one ear to the other, only very small threshold shifts are obtained except under special circumstances. Other ear-stimulus combinations show quite different results. For example, we can determine a standard monaural threshold by putting a masking noise and a sinusoidal signal in the same ear. Now, with the signal still at monaural threshold intensity we add the same noise in the opposite ear as well. Under these new conditions the listener will hear the signal very clearly. At first glance this seems somewhat puzzling. We have added more noise and instead of making things worse, the signal becomes more clearly audible. If now we ask the listener to obtain a second threshold estimate, this time with the noise in both ears, we find that the threshold signal level is perhaps 10 dB lower than for the monaural noise condition. In this illustration 10 dB represents the *masking level difference* or MLD. It is the difference between the threshold obtained in the monaural and the binaural masking situation.

The largest MLDs are obtained with signal and noise in both ears, but with signal and noise having opposite interaural phase conditions. Under these circumstances, MLDs of about 15 dB are obtained. The MLD is highly dependent upon the frequency of the signal (Figure 9-35(*a*)). The maximum MLD occurs in the vicinity of 250 Hz, but decreases to a small and constant value for frequencies above about 1,500 Hz. The magnitude of the MLD also depends upon the intensity of the masking noise (Figure 9-35(*b*)). We see that the greater the intensity of the masker, the larger the MLD.

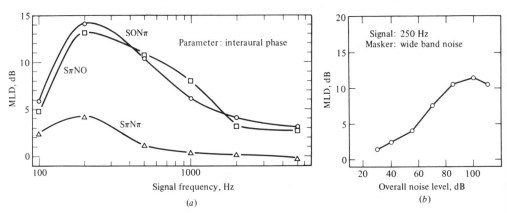

Figure 9-35 Effect of stimulus parameters on masking level differences (MDLs). MDLs for several phase conditions are shown (*a*) as a function of stimulus frequency; (*b*) as a function of stimulus intensity. [*After I. J. Hirsch, "The influence of interaural phase on interaural summation and inhibition,' J. Acoust. Soc. Amer., 20 (1948), 536; and J. A. Canahl and A. M. Small, "Masking-level differences as a function of masker level," J. Acoust. Soc. Amer., 38 (1965), 928.*]

The existence of a MLD demonstrates that information from the two ears is brought together at some central location. That is, if a sinusoidal signal applied to one ear can be made more audible by a noise applied to the opposite ear, this shows that the neural representation of these two stimuli interact at some point in the nervous system. This, of course, tends to support the concept of a single auditory system with two receivers rather than regarding the auditory system as consisting of two independent devices.

Localization and Lateralization

The localization of sound in space is an ability which is uniquely binaural. To the limited degree to which monaural localization occurs, it is accomplished mainly by moving the single ear to different points in space and, in a very inefficient fashion, simulating binaural listening conditions. The term *localization* refers to our ability to describe the location of a sound source based exclusively on auditory information. In attempting to pinpoint the acoustic cues that may contribute to our ability to localize sound, investigators have utilized the earphone presentation of sound in order that the input to each ear can be controlled independently. When earphone presentation is used, however, listeners indicate that the apparent source of the sound, rather than being outside the head such as is the case with loudspeaker sound presentation, is inside the head. This effect is referred to as *lateralization* in that the sound appears to come from one side of the head or the other.

Potential cues: geometric considerations

To help us determine what information might be used by the auditory system in order to localize sound sources, let us consider Figure 9-36 which is intended to illustrate possible acoustic cues arising from geometric considerations. If a sound source is located at point *S*, sound will reach the listener's ears directly by paths labelled *A* and *B*. Path *A* is longer than path *B*. This immediately suggests two things. If the sound source is emitting a transient sound such as a click, thump, or snap of the fingers, then, since sound travels with constant velocity, sound traveling path *A* to the left ear will take longer to arrive than sound traveling path *B* to the right ear. Thus, there will be a difference in time of arrival of the sound at the two ears. The difference in path length also produces a difference in sound pressure at the two ears if the source provides a spherical sound wave. The sound intensity at the left ear will be less than that at the right because of the greater distance it has to traverse. If the sound source provides a continuous output rather than a transient output, rather than speaking of a difference in time of arrival, it is more appropriate to speak of a difference in phase. For example with a 100 Hz sinusoid a time difference of 1 millisecond is equivalent to a 36° phase difference between the ears.

If the source is moved to a position *S'* the right ear has direct access to the sound, but the sound which reaches the left ear must curve around the head.

Figure 9-36 Geometry of a sound localization situation. Sound is received at the listener's ear from source, *S* (or *S'*) by paths *A* and *B*.

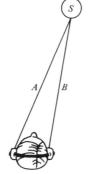

The extent to which waves will curve around an object is dependent upon their wavelength and the dimensions of the object. The higher the frequency the shorter the wavelength and the less effectively waves can curve around objects. Thus, in the present example, for high frequencies the sound pressure at the left ear will be considerably less than we would expect based simply upon the inverse square law. This effect is called a sound shadow by analogy to a light shadow which is formed in an identical manner.

At best, interaural phase differences can provide only limited information. That is, if the difference in path length is such that a phase delay of 380° exists between the two ears, the auditory system has no way of knowing whether the phase shift is 380° or 20°, or any other multiple of 360. Information is unambiguously provided only by interaural phase differences of 360° or less. Since the maximum difference in path length is determined by the size of the head, the upper limit of unambiguous phase difference is set by the frequency. This is so since, for a given fixed time delay, the corresponding phase shift increases as the stimulus frequency increases. Thus, based on geometric considerations, high frequencies have the potential of providing a very large interaural intensity difference, but can provide very little information via interaural phase differences.

Ability of the auditory system to utilize potential cues

In the previous section we discussed possible acoustic cues which might exist in a localization situation. Let us now decide whether the auditory system is capable of utilizing these cues. That is, assume that a sound source is positioned so that it generates an interaural intensity difference of 2 dB. If we can show that the auditory system must have an interaural intensity difference of 8 dB before it can discriminate a difference this would suggest that the 2 dB differential generated by the sound source could not be appreciated by the auditory system. Thus, we would have to look elsewhere for an acoustic cue for localization.

How different must two sounds be in intensity at the two ears before they may be distinguished? This is, of course, a question relative to interaural intensity discrimination. Results indicate that differences as small as 0.5 dB can be detected. Perceptually, how do we determine that a difference in interaural intensity exists? When two identical in-phase stimuli are presented, the sound image is at the center of the head but with a sufficiently large intensity differential the sound image is shifted from the center of the head toward the ear receiving the greater intensity.

Let us ask a similar question with respect to interaural time differences. Given two identical impulsive sounds (clicks) how much must one be delayed with respect to the other in time of arrival before a delay is observed? In the undelayed case the sound appears to reside in the middle of the head; but, if one click is delayed with respect to the other by as little as 0.000012 second the sound image moves toward the ear which received the click first. This represents exquisite responsiveness which indicates that the auditory system possesses more than enough sensitivity to allow it to utilize differences in time of arrival as a possible cue for auditory localization.

In the case of the interaural phase of sinusoids, a difference of 0.3 degree at 100 Hz is sufficient to cause the apparent sound source to move toward the ear which leads in phase. This, too, represents sufficient sensitivity to indicate the potential usefulness of phase information in auditory localization.

The data

Figure 9-37(*a*) shows the average size of the errors made in a localization task in which the listener pointed toward what he perceived to be the source of the sound. It may be seen that the size of the error is small at low frequencies, rises to a maximum in the vicinity of 3,000 Hz, and then declines again at higher frequencies. The shape of this error function is of interest because of the limitation in the information that can be provided by phase at the high frequencies and because of the sound shadow effect at high frequencies. Figure 9-37(*b*) indicates the magnitude of these intensity and phase effects. The peak in the error function occurs in that frequency region in which minimum information is available from either phase or intensity, thus suggesting the usefulness of these cues in localization.

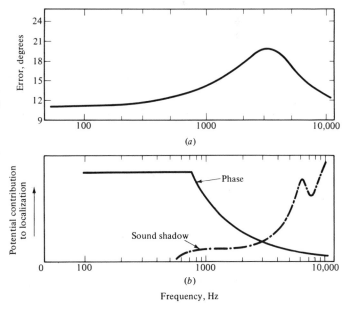

Figure 9-37 Sound localization as influenced by stimulus frequency: (*a*) actual performance; (*b*) potential contribution of several cues. [*From S. S. Stevens and H. Davis, Hearing, (New York: John Wiley & Sons, Inc., 1938), Figs. 74a and b. Copyright S. S. Stevens. Reprinted by permission.*]

ADAPTATION AND FATIGUE

The terms adaptation and fatigue have been used in many contexts and considerable confusion exists with respect to their meanings. Often the terms are differentiated on the basis of their potential usefulness to the organism. That is, adaptive effects are thought of as those which are beneficial and fatigue effects those which are detrimental to the organism. Others have classified effects as adaptive or fatiguing in terms of the duration of the effect, adaptation thought of as being a rapidly occurring effect and fatigue occurring more slowly. In hearing, the usage of these terms is also ambiguous. Consequently, we will make what we regard as operational definitions for our discussion. There have been a number of tasks devised which attempt to measure fatigue or adaptation, but we will confine our discussion to only two, namely, threshold and loudness determinations. In this context then, we will define *fatigue* as a reversible increase in threshold, brought about by the prior presentation of an acoustical stimulus. Similarly, we will define *adaptation* as a reversible decline in loudness of a stimulus brought about by prior exposure to an auditory stimulus. Thus, in terms of our definitions, adaptation and fatigue differ only in that we consider fatigue to be a threshold effect and adaptation a suprathreshold effect.

Threshold Fatigue

Long term effects

Threshold fatigue may occur as the result of the action of several different mechanisms. At least we seem to measure quite different effects depending upon whether the fatiguing stimulus is of long or short duration. Thus, it is convenient to discuss these effects separately.

Measurement. Measurement of long term threshold fatigue is schematized in Figure 9-38. A fatiguing stimulus is presented and terminated. Following an interval of silence a test stimulus is presented. The listener's task is to

Figure 9-38 Defining stimulus paradigm for long term threshold fatigue (TTS). The rectangles represent the occurrence of a stimulus at a particular moment in time (which progresses from left to right). The amount of fatigue is the difference in SPL required in order to hear the test stimulus in (a) the experimental conditions *versus* that required to hear the test stimulus in (b) the control condition.

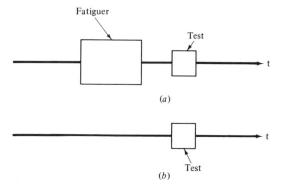

obtain a threshold estimate for this test stimulus. The amount of fatigue is the difference in sound pressure level required for the threshold in (*a*), the fatiguing situation, compared to that required in (*b*), the normal test stimulus situation. Since this threshold difference or shift is usually temporary, the effect is sometimes referred to as *temporary threshold shift* or simply TTS.

Four primary factors influence the amount of fatigue that we observe: the intensity and duration of the fatiguing stimulus, the interval of silence between the fatiguing and the test stimulus (recovery interval), and the frequencies of the fatiguing and the test stimulus.

The most usual way of gathering information about long term fatigue is not as shown in Figure 9-38, but rather with a Békésy audiometer p. 358. We present the fatiguer as in Figure 9-38(*a*), but upon its termination the listener immediately begins to obtain his threshold by varying the intensity of a continuously present test stimulus. Although his threshold may be changing as a result of exposure to the fatiguer, this procedure allows us to obtain continuous estimates of the listener's threshold. Indeed, that is its advantage: it effectively measures fatigue for many recovery intervals in a single trial. In order for us to obtain the same information with the method shown in Figure 9-38(*a*) we would need to use a large number of trials, each with a different recovery interval.

Recovery from fatigue. It may seem backwards to discuss the recovery from an effect that has not yet been described. However, the characteristics of the recovery process dictate the way in which we measure the onset of fatigue and therefore this ordering is desirable. Figure 9-39(*a*) shows a

Figure 9-39 Recovery from long term threshold fatigue. (*a*) Is the TTS for a 1,400 Hz test stimulus in the first few minutes of recovery following 2 min. of exposure to a 1,000 Hz, 100 dB SL fatiguer. (*b*) Is the TTS for a 4 KHz test stimulus following 27 min. of exposure to a wide band noise at 98 db SPL. [*After I. J. Hirsh and R. C. Bilger "Auditory-threshold recovery after exposure to pure tones,"* J. Acoust. Soc. Amer., *27 (1955), 1186; and W. D. Ward et al., "Relation between recovery from temporary threshold shift and duration of exposure,"* J. Acoust. Soc. Amer., *31 (1959), 600.*]

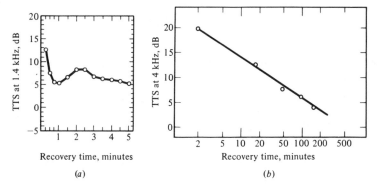

Recovery time, minutes

(*a*)   (*b*)

typical recovery curve as might be obtained from the midpoints of a Békésy tracking procedure. We see that recovery is initially rapid, but slows and even reverses its direction one or two minutes after the termination of the fatiguing stimulus. Thereafter as the recovery interval lengthens, the amount of fatigue declines in an approximately linear fashion. The bump at one or two minutes is not always present, but depends upon the stimulus conditions. When we specify the effect of stimulus variables upon fatigue it is convenient to do so for a particular point in the recovery function, since the amount of fatigue changes as recovery proceeds. Because the initial portion of the recovery function tends to be irregular in shape and shows considerable variability from person to person, the amount of fatigue at two minutes of recovery is the point usually specified. The recovery after two minutes is quite regular as is illustrated in Figure 9-39(b).

Onset of fatigue. For stimuli whose sound pressure level exceeds about 85 dB, threshold shift increases in a linear fashion as intensity is raised above this point. How fast it rises depends upon the duration of the exposure. The effect of these variables is shown in Figure 9-40.

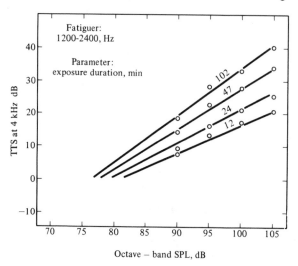

Figure 9-40 Growth of long term threshold fatigue. TTS of a 4 KHz sinusoid as influenced by the intensity and duration of a 1,200-2,400 Hz band of noise. [*After W. D. Ward et al., "Temporary threshold shift from octave band noise: Applications to damage-risk criteria,"* J. Acoust. Soc. Amer., *31 (1959), 522.*]

Threshold shift brought about by fatiguing conditions tends to depend, to a large extent, upon the frequencies involved. If the test stimulus is the same as the fatiguing stimulus, there is a small threshold shift at low frequencies, as frequency is increased there is an increasing magnitude of threshold shift. Analogously, if the fatiguer is a wide band of noise maximum fatigue is produced in the high frequency region.

To what extent does fatigue produced by a sinusoidal stimulus spread to adjacent frequencies? To answer this question we can present the fatiguer at one frequency and measure the amount of fatigue at various other test frequencies. Under these conditions the maximum amount of fatigue is often not found at the frequency corresponding to the fatiguer but rather at about one-half octave higher. This is in contrast to the frequency effects for simultaneous masking (p. 379), and is different from any phenomena we will be discussing in this chapter.

Short term fatigue

Measurement. The stimulus paradigm used in the measurement of short term fatigue is similar to that used for long term fatigue (Figure 9-38). The main difference is the duration of the stimuli. Typically the test stimulus is about 10 msec long and the fatiguing stimulus is 400 msec in duration. Because of its short duration, the listener does not have an opportunity to adjust the intensity of the test stimulus during its presentation when estimating his threshold. Figure 9-41 shows a common solution for this problem. The fatiguer and the test stimulus are presented, and about 500 msec later, the fatiguer is presented again by itself. The listener decides whether the two sets of stimuli sound different and, if they do, presumably it is due to the presence of the test stimulus in the first stimulus pair. The stimuli are then repeated, but with the test stimulus at a different intensity, another judgment is made, and the process is repeated until we obtain a satisfactory threshold estimate.

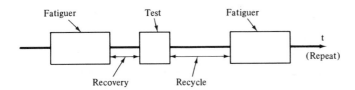

Figure 9-41 Stimulus paradigm for short term threshold fatigue. The rectangles represent the occurrence of stimuli at particular moments in time (which progress from left to right). The amount of fatigue is defined as the difference in the SPL of the test stimulus required for threshold with and without the fatiguer present.

In other words, the adjustment of the intensity of the test stimulus occurs between stimulus presentations. During a stimulus presentation the listener simply judges as to the presence or absence of the test stimulus. We measure the amount of fatigue in the same way as for the long term effects; that is, thresholds for the test stimulus are taken with and without the presence of the fatiguing stimulus. The difference between these two conditions represents the amount of fatigue.

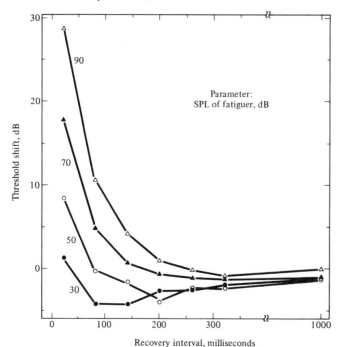

Figure 9-42 Recovery from short term threshold fatigue. Amount of fatigue for a 1,000 Hz, 10 msec test stimulus following exposure to a 400 msec, 1,000 Hz fatiguer. [*After A. M. Small and J. A. Canahl, "Loudness changes in a forward masking paradigm,"* J. Acoust. Soc. Amer., *38 (1965), 928.*]

Recovery. Recovery from short term fatigue is characterized by extreme rapidity. It is always completed within .25 sec even from threshold shifts as great as 50 dB, as Figure 9-42 shows. Recovery from smaller amounts of fatigue are even more rapid. As was the case for long term effects, it does not seem to make much difference how the fatigue was produced, the recovery time depends only upon the initial amount of fatigue.

Onset. Although exactly how much fatigue occurs depends upon the point in the recovery cycle we measure, the amount of fatigue increases linearly as the intensity of the fatiguer increases. The duration of the fatiguing stimulus is also important in determining the amount of fatigue, with the threshold shift increasing as fatiguer duration increases. However, if the fatiguer duration exceeds 400 msec, there is no further increase in threshold shift. In other words, fatiguer duration influences the amount of fatigue only for durations less than 400 msec. Thus, it becomes clear why this effect is called short term; the duration of test stimuli are extremely short, stimulus duration is effective only for durations below 400 msec and recovery from large amounts of fatigue is complete within 250 milliseconds. Short term fatigue develops quickly and recovery is rapid.

The frequency effects in short term fatigue are almost exactly the same as seen for simultaneous masking. The maximum threshold shift occurs when the test frequency approximates the fatiguer frequency and the spread of fatigue away from the fatiguer frequency tends to be asymmetrical, spreading further toward the high frequencies than to the low.

Loudness Adaptation

Long term effects

Measurement. The measurement of loudness adaptation is more difficult than the measurement of threshold fatigue. Although direct methods of loudness measurement probably could be utilized, almost without exception indirect methods have been used. That is, loudness changes in the adaptation situation have been assessed by means of loudness balances in which a comparison stimulus is adjusted so that its loudness is equal to that of the stimulus in question. Although there are several ways in which this could be done, the method outlined in Figure 9-43 is commonly used. An experimental run is divided into three sections: pre-stimulatory, per-stimulatory, and post-stimulatory. The first period represents normal auditory function; the second, auditory function during the presentation of the adapting stimulus;

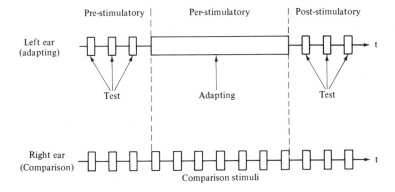

Figure 9-43 Stimulus paradigm for long term loudness adaptation. The figure construction is similar to Figures 9-38 and 9-41 with the rectangles representing stimuli and time progressing from left to right. The temporal segmentation of the run into pre-, per-, and post-stimulator divisions is also indicated.

and the third and final period represents the recovery process. During the pre-stimulatory period an attempt is made to obtain a loudness balance between the test stimuli presented in the adapting ear and comparison stimuli presented to the comparison ear when both stimuli are presented simultaneously. As many presentations are used as is necessary to obtain a stable estimate of loudness level. Typically, stimuli are on for 20 sec and off for

90 sec. During the per-stimulatory period the adapting stimulus is presented to the adapting ear and comparison stimuli are presented at about the same rate as during the pre-stimulatory period. The listener attempts to adjust the comparison stimulus each time it is presented so that an equal loudness balance is obtained between the two ears. Finally, in the post-stimulatory period a process similar to that of the pre-stimulatory period is carried out.

Onset. Figure 9-44 shows the time course of loudness adaptation as measured with the method just described. As soon as the adapting stimulus is turned on it begins to lose its loudness as indicated by the adjustment of the comparison stimulus to lower and lower intensities. After 3 to 6 minutes, depending upon the intensity of the adapting stimulus, the maximum amount of adaptation is obtained. Further continuation of the adapting stimulus beyond this point produces no additional effect.

The greater the intensity of the adapting stimulus, the greater the change in loudness we see under adapting conditions. There are two qualifications to this general statement; very little adaptation is seen for adapting stimuli whose sound pressure level is less than 50 dB. Also once the sound pressure level of the adapting stimulus exceeds 95 dB little further change is seen. Thus, the amount of adaptation is proportional to the sound pressure level of the adapting stimulus only through the middle range of stimulus intensities.

If the frequency of the test stimulus is the same as that of the adapting stimulus, as we increase frequency we obtain an increase in the amount of adaptation up to about 2,000 Hz. Above this frequency adaptation is constant and large. If the frequency of the test stimulus differs from that of the adapting stimulus, we find that the maximum amount of adaptation is obtained when the test frequency is equal to the adapting frequency and the spread of adaptation away from the adapting frequency is symmetrical. This, of course, is in contrast to what we saw for simultaneous masking, short term or long term threshold fatigue.

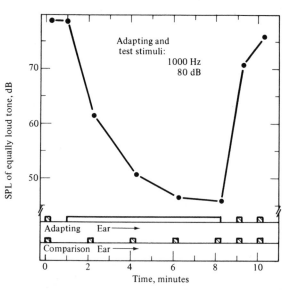

Figure 9-44 Time course of loudness adaptation. [*After E. J. Thwing," Spread of perstimulatory fatigue of a pure tone to neighboring frequencies,"* J. Acoust. Soc. Amer., 27 (1955), 741.]

Recovery. Recovery from auditory adaptation as illustrated in the post-stimulatory portion of Figure 9-44 seems to be more rapid than the onset of adaptation. That is, while the onset may take 3 to 6 minutes to reach its maximum, recovery is generally complete in substantially shorter time, perhaps 2 minutes or less. Again as was the case with threshold fatigue, the time required for recovery from adaptation seems not to depend upon the stimulus factors that brought about the adaptation, but only upon the amount of adaptation from which recovery must proceed.

Short term effects

Measurement. The measurement of short term loudness adaptation usually combines some of the features of the measurement techniques described for both fatigue and adaptation. Short duration stimuli similar to those used to measure short term fatigue are presented to one ear with a test stimulus of perhaps 20 msec and an adapting stimulus of 400 msec. In a manner similar to that used to measure long term adaptation, identical test and comparison stimuli are presented simultaneously in opposite ears. The listener's task is to adjust the intensity of the comparison stimulus until the coincident pair sound equally loud.

Results. The results obtained from these measurement procedures are about the same as those seen for short term fatigue except that the magnitude of the effects are much smaller. That is, for short term fatigue threshold shifts as large as 60 or 70 dB are not unusual. The maximum effects seen in the case of short term adaptation however, are the order of to 12 dB for the same stimulus conditions that give rise to the 70 dB effects for threshold.

PITCH

Methods of Measurement

Pitch as well as loudness is a primary response attribute of sound. The methods of measurement are also analogous.

Direct

The most direct way of measuring pitch is by means of a scaling procedure which assigns a numerical value to a given pitch. These methods are analogous to those used for loudness and are described on p. 363. An example of a pitch scale obtained by direct magnitude estimates is shown in Figure 9-45. If in the scaling procedure, the standard stimulus is a 1,000 Hz tone, 40 dB

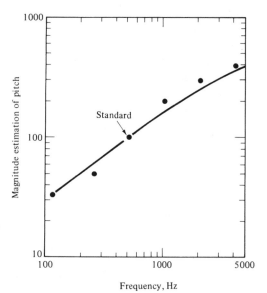

Figure 9-45   Pitch scale. [*After J. Beck and W. A. Shaw,* "*Single estimates of pitch magnitude*," J. Acoust. Soc. Amer., *35 (1963), 1722.*]

above its threshold, and is assigned a pitch value of 1,000 then the units of the pitch scale are called *mels*. The advantages and disadvantages of direct methods of pitch measurement are similar to those for loudness. An advantage of the direct approach is the generation of numbers which may be manipulated according to the standard arithmetic operations. Indirect methods provide small variability and high precision.

Indirect

The indirect measurement of pitch involves the use of two stimuli: one is the stimulus whose pitch is to be determined and the other is a comparison stimulus. The listener's task is to adjust the comparison stimulus, usually by changing its frequency, until the pitch of the two stimuli are equal. The indirect method is preferred in most situations.

Stimulus Factors (Sinusoids)

Frequency

Pitch is often thought of as being related, in a 1:1 fashion, to stimulus frequency; this, however, is not the case. The precise manner in which pitch is related to frequency is shown in the pitch scale (Figure 9-45). While it is true that stimulus frequency is a prime determiner of the pitch of simple stimuli, other stimulus parameters are also important.

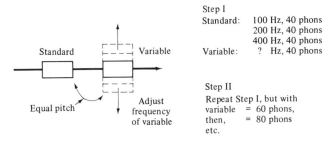

Step I
Standard: 100 Hz, 40 phons
           200 Hz, 40 phons
           400 Hz, 40 phons
Variable: ? Hz, 40 phons

Step II
Repeat Step I, but with
variable = 60 phons,
then,   = 80 phons
etc.

Figure 9-46 Stimulus paradigm for monaural pitch matching. Steps I and II describe the procedure used for measuring pitch changes occurring as stimulus intensity is changed. (See Figure 9-47.)

Intensity

Intensity is one of those stimulus factors, in addition to frequency, that influences pitch. The procedure outlined in Figure 9-46 is one commonly used to assess pitch changes caused by variation in intensity. A commonly used procedure employs a standard stimulus presented at a loudness level of 40 phons while variable stimuli are presented at different loudness levels. Any pitch change induced in the variable stimulus by changing its loudness level (from 40 phons) is compensated for by readjusting its frequency so as to maintain equal pitch for variable and standard. The results of this procedure are shown in Figure 9-47. They indicate that as the loudness level of the variable stimulus is increased from 40 phons, the pitch of the variable stimulus decreases. The numbers shown on the ordinate indicate the percentage change in the frequency of the variable necessary to bring the pitch of the variable stimulus back to that of the standard. We see that the change in pitch induced by a change in loudness level is confined to the low frequencies.

Figure 9-47 Pitch as influenced by stimulus intensity at various frequencies. Each curve is an equal pitch contour. [*After W. B. Snow "Changes of pitch with loudness at low frequencies,"* J. Acoust. Soc. Amer., *8 (1936), 14.*]

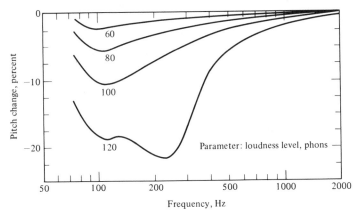

More recent information suggests that the magnitudes of the pitch shifts are smaller than shown in Figure 9-47 but there is little doubt that the effect itself is real. In addition, there is some data to suggest that for frequencies above 2,000 Hz an increase in loudness level brings about an increase in pitch. This latter effect is less well documented than the lowering of pitch of low frequencies as their loudness level is increased.

Duration

There seems to be no evidence that the stimulus duration influences the pitch; that is, pitch does not seem to become higher or lower as stimulus duration is changed. However, there is good evidence to suggest that the precision of the pitch judgments depends upon the stimulus duration, since as stimulus duration is shortened it is necessary that frequency differences between two stimuli must be increased for them to remain perceptually distinct.

Masking and fatigue

If the pitch of a sinusoid is compared under conditions of quiet and under conditions of masking, we often find that the pitch is systematically changed depending upon the masking conditions. This represents another situation in which the stimulus frequency remains constant but its pitch is changed.

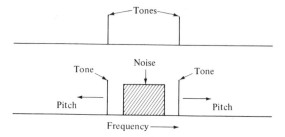

Figure 9-48 Pitch as influenced by the simultaneous presentation of other stimuli. The pitch of sinusoids near a band of noise shifted away from the band compared to the pitch without the noise present.

In Figure 9-48 we see that if a tone is presented so that its frequency is immediately below that of a band of noise, at a position where it is partially masked, its pitch will be shifted downward. On the other hand, if the tone is located immediately above the band of noise and again positioned so that it is partially masked, the pitch of the tone is shifted upward. The same general pattern is seen in a short term fatigue situation. That is, the band of noise need not be present simultaneously with the tone in order for the pitch shift to occur. In addition, if a permanent hearing loss exists in a restricted frequency region it is not unusual to find (by comparison to a contralateral normal ear) pitch shifts occurring in spectral regions adjacent to the loss.

Taken as a whole, these results suggest that the important factor in the generation of a pitch shift is that the sensitivity of the auditory system be reduced in a localized frequency region. How this desensitization is brought about seems unimportant, whether it be by simultaneous masking, short term fatigue, or auditory pathology. If, under these conditions, a tone is presented in a frequency region adjacent to the region of desensitization its pitch is different from that which would occur were the region not desensitized.

Place Theory

Why do these effects, described in the previous section, occur? Indeed, more generally, what is it about the auditory system that allows us to perceive a particular pitch upon the presentation of a certain stimulus? There have been many explanations advanced throughout the years however, place theory has been one of the most prominent theories of pitch perception.

Although the elements for a place theory have existed for some time, it remained for Helmholtz in 1863 to draw together its various features and state them explicitly and authoritatively. Helmholtz' theory of hearing has been an important concept which has stimulated a considerable amount of research. Let us describe his theory. Helmholtz conceived of the basilar membrane as being comprised of a large number of stretched transverse fibers whose length, tension and mass varied from the base to the apex of the cochlea. This concept is roughly analogous to the strings on a piano or a harp. When a sinusoid of a particular frequency was presented to the ear, one of these stretched fibers would be set into vibration in accord with the principle of sympathetic resonance. The vibration of this fiber would cause the response of the sensory cell associated with that fiber which, in turn, would excite the neuron connected to it. At some central point in the nervous system the excitation of that particular neuron would be recognized as signaling a particular pitch. Thus, in this theory the important factor in the determination of pitch is which neuron is stimulated. The neuron, in turn, occupies a particular spatial location and consequently a particular place—thus the idea of a place theory. We should note that in Helmholtz' theory, as in other place theories, it is presumed that a peripheral analysis is carried out at the level of the basilar membrane and it is by virtue of this analysis that particular neurons are stimulated. However, a theory would still be a place theory so long as specific neurons denoted particular pitches, even if there were not an analysis carried out at the level of the cochlea.

We know now that Helmholtz' theory is almost certainly wrong in detail since there are no well-developed transverse fibers on the basilar membrane and since the membrane is not under tension. Further, we know that usually single neurons do not go to single hair cells, rather a single neuron receives

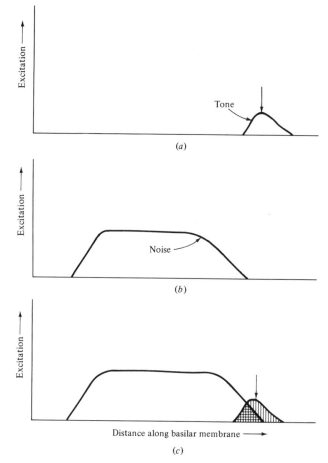

Figure 9-49 Hypothetical excitation patterns: (*a*) response to a sinusoid alone; (*b*) to a noise alone; (*c*) to a combination of sinusoid and noise. The arrow shows the position of maximum effective excitation. [*After J. P. Egan and D. R. Myer, "Changes in pitch of tones of low frequency as a function of the pattern of excitation produced by a band of noise,"* J. Acoust. Soc. Amer., 22 (*1950*), 827.]

stimulation from many hair cells representing a fairly large area of the basilar membrane. However, we do have broadly tuned resonance effects occurring in the cochlea in which low frequency sinusoids cause a maximum movement of the basilar membrane in the apical region, while high frequency sinusoids cause maximum amplitude movement in the basal region. Thus, while the specificity of analysis proposed by the Helmholtz theory appears not to occur, there does exist the potential of peripheral analysis of a more general sort.

Let us examine the pitch shifts which occur under certain conditions of masking and see to what extent we can explain these effects by means of a place principle of pitch perception. Let us assume that when a single sinusoid is presented to the ear it forms an *excitation* pattern which may be represented as in Figure 9-49(*a*). We presume that although this excitation covers a substantial distance along the basilar membrane there is more excitation at one particular point than at any other. The pitch which is perceived corresponds to this position of maximum excitation since we assume it is translated into the excitation of a specific group of neurons. This maximum is denoted with an arrow. In Figure 9-49(b), we show the excitation that might be associated with a fairly narrow band of noise. Because it has no single point of maximum excitation, we presume that it possesses little or no pitch quality, as is in fact the case with such bands of noise. In Figure 9-49(c) we have combined (a) and (b). The frequency of the signal has been located slightly above the band of noise so that we have overlapping excitation patterns. Let us assume that the effective part of the signal excitation is only that part which lies above the noise excitation function. The part of the signal excitation that lies below the noise excitation function and is crosshatched is assumed to be no longer effective in eliciting a response. Since the pitch is presumably dependent upon the position of the maximum, the question is where is the maximum excitation for the *effective* signal excitation? To determine this we can draw a series of vertical lines through the effective excitation function of the signal; the longest vertical line will indicate the position of maximum excitation. The arrow shows the position of the maximum under noise conditions. We see that it has shifted upward relative to its position in quiet; thus indicating a pitch shift.

What we have shown is that by utilizing the assumptions derived from a place theory of pitch perception we can predict pitch shifts of the sort which occur under conditions of narrow band noise masking. This increases our confidence that there may be merit to this particular theoretical point of view.

Stimulus Factors (Complex Stimuli)

We have previously discussed some of the factors which influence the pitch of simple sinusoidal stimuli. However, in real life, we rarely hear simple sinusoidal stimuli, rather we hear complex stimuli such as speech and music. Consequently, it is important that we consider the pitch perception of complex stimuli.

Periodicity pitch

An adult male voice is usually characterized as having a low pitch. An adult female voice or a child's voice is usually thought of as having a higher pitch. If we examine the spectrum of speech we find that in general an adult male voice has a lower fundamental frequency and, consequently, more closely spaced harmonics than does a woman's or child's voice. Indeed, the pitch assigned by listeners to these voices corresponds approximately to the fundamental frequency. Let us consider what happens to speech when we talk through a telephone. Telephone circuits are commonly designed so that frequencies below about 300 Hz are not transmitted or reproduced. What do men's and women's voices sound like over the telephone? Well, the pitch of the male voice is still perceived as low and that of a female voice is relatively high. The significance of this observation is that for the male voice in particular, the fundamental frequency, and indeed a number of the lower harmonics, are not present at the other end of the telephone wire. Thus, a pitch is assigned to a stimulus which contains no energy at the frequency ordinarily corresponding to that pitch. This is particularly significant in terms of a place theory of pitch perception. This theory suggests that the pitch assigned to a complex signal is that which corresponds to the place of maximum excitation. Thus, if a complex signal has most of its energy in a particular frequency region we would presume the pitch would be assigned to that region of maximum stimulus energy and excitation. In the example of the telephonic speech material we see that according to the place theory it would be impossible for the pitch to be assigned to the fundamental frequency since, in fact, the fundamental frequency does not exist. This example is not unique. For example, pocket-sized radios contain loudspeakers about the size of a quarter which do not reproduce low frequencies. Yet, when we listen to these radios we perceive low pitches; tubas, trombones, and bass drums produce their appropriate sounds. Still another example is the pitch of natural vowels, unmodified by telephone circuits. In spite of the fact that there may be a number of harmonics that are of greater magnitude than the fundamental, almost without exception the pitch assigned to these vowel sounds corresponds to the fundamental frequency. Thus there appears to be a basic difficulty in explaining the pitch of complex signals utilizing the place theory of pitch perception.

It is possible to provide other complex stimuli under more controlled conditions which display the same type of pitch perception we have been discussing. For example, if we interrupt a sinusoid (turn it off and on) perhaps 100 times per second and ask a listener to adjust an uninterrupted sinusoid until its pitch is equal to that of the interrupted stimulus, we find

Figure 9-50   Periodicity pitch. (*a*) A high frequency sinusoid interrupted at a low rate yields a pitch sensation corresponding to the interruption rate even though its spectrum (*b*) contains no energy at that frequency. [*After W. R. Thurlow and A. M. Small, "Pitch perception of certain periodic auditory stimuli," J. Acoust. Soc. Amer., 27 (1955), 132.*]

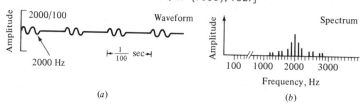

that under most conditions the listener will adjust the comparison stimulus so that its frequency corresponds to the rate of interruption. This indicates that the pitch of the interrupted stimulus corresponds to the interruption rate rather than to the frequency of the basic sinusoid. If we examine the spectrum of the interrupted signal as shown in Figure 9-50 we find that energy is located in the vicinity of the steady sinusoidal signal with little or no energy at the rate of interruption. Thus, this situation is similar to that discussed previously where the pitch assigned to a stimulus corresponds to a frequency that is not present in the stimulus. Because the pitch corresponds to the rate of interruption, which in turn corresponds to the periodicity of the waveform envelope, the pitch perceived under these conditions is often referred to as *periodicity pitch.*

Time separation pitch

If two trains of an interrupted sinewave, such as shown in Figure 9-50, are combined as shown in Figure 9-51 we hear at least two pitch effects. One, the basic periodicity pitch, represents the periodicity of the individual pulse trains shown in Figure 9-50. This corresponds to the reciprocal of the time period labelled T. In addition, we hear a pitch which corresponds to the reciprocal of the time period denoted by τ, which is the delay between pulse trains A and B. If we move pulse train B with respect to pulse train A we change the value of τ; the smaller τ, the higher the pitch. This effect has been called *time separation pitch* but perhaps might be better called *time delay pitch* since it corresponds to the time delay of corresponding points in waveform B and A. Again there is no energy in the frequency spectrum at $1/\tau$, the frequency corresponding to the pitch assigned.

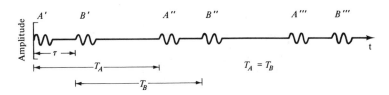

Figure 9-51   Time separation pitch. A double pulse train is formed by delaying identical pulse trains A and B by a time, τ. A pitch is heard corresponding to $1/\tau$. [*After A. M. Small and M. E. McClellan, "Pitch associated with time delay between two pulse trains,"* J. Acoust. Soc. Amer., *35 (1963), 124-55.*]

One of the striking aspects of pitch perception for complex stimuli is that the pitch appears to correspond to temporal rather than spectral features of the stimulus. This suggests that for a complex stimulus at least, perhaps a mode of analysis other than spectral (place principle) is occurring.

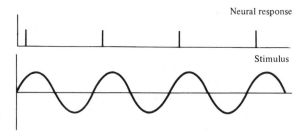

Neural response

Stimulus

Figure 9-52   Synchronous neural discharge to a sinusoid.

"Rate of Neural Discharge" Theory

A theory that succeeds to some degree in accounting for the pitch of complex stimuli is the *rate of neural discharge theory* which is sometimes called the volley or telephone theory. Let us consider first how this theory might apply to simple stimuli and then discuss its application to complex stimuli. We assume that neurons will fire at a certain point in a sinusoidal stimulus waveform when some threshold value is exceeded and that they will fire regularly when this event occurs. Such a possibility is shown in Figure 9-52 and has, in fact, been observed to be the case. Notice that the temporal separation between adjacent bursts of neural response is the same as the separation between corresponding points on the input sinusoid. The rate of neural discharge theory says that it is this information that determines the pitch of the stimulus. If the signal is a sinusoid then the distance between neural bursts is equal to the period of the sinusoid and the pitch is assigned on this basis.

Figure 9-53   Volley principle of neural discharge.

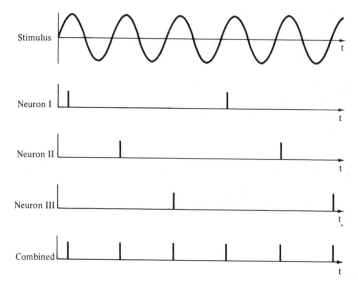

Stimulus

Neuron I

Neuron II

Neuron III

Combined

Because of the nature of the neural response, it is necessary that a neuron recover following each discharge; thus the rate at which it can respond is limited. We find that single neurons can not respond more rapidly than about 1,000 times per second; however, we perceive pitches which correspond to frequencies above 1,000 Hz. To account for this discrepancy it has been proposed that something like the process shown in Figure 9-53 occurs. Let us assume that the input frequency is 3,000 Hz, but neuron *I* is limited to a maximum response of 1,000 Hz, therefore it is unable to respond to every cycle of the input sinusoid. It responds as rapidly as it is able which, in this case, is every third cycle. Neuron *II*, because of a similar response limitation, responds to every third cycle at a maximum rate of 1,000 times per second, but by chance does not respond to the same cycle as did neuron *I*. Neuron *III*, with similar limitations, also responds to every third cycle, but if we look at the combined response of all three of these neurons we observe a rate of 3,000 responses per second. Thus, aggregates of neurons are able to represent, in their combined response, higher stimulus rates than is possible by a single neuron alone. Such a process is referred to as *volleying*, and has been observed to occur in the nervous system although on a probabilistic rather than a fixed basis. By probabilistic we mean that a single neuron may not respond to every third cycle, but sometimes might respond to a third, sometimes a fourth, or a fifth cycle. However the action of large numbers of neurons results in the pattern shown in Figure 9-53.

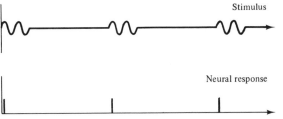

Stimulus

Neural response

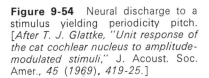

Figure 9-54 Neural discharge to a stimulus yielding periodicity pitch. [*After T. J. Glattke, "Unit response of the cat cochlear nucleus to amplitude-modulated stimuli,"* J. Acoust. Soc. Amer., *45 (1969), 419-25.*]

For periodicity pitch it is reasoned that the neural response is similar to that shown in Figure 9-54 where there is neural activity corresponding to the onset of each burst of the stimulus. The separation between neural responses is the same as the separation between stimulus bursts. If pitch is determined by the time difference between adjacent responses it should correspond to the interruption rate of the stimulus, which of course it does. Time separation pitch is explained in much the same way in that neural activity occurs coincident with the onset of each burst in the stimulus, thus the time intervals are interpreted as signaling pitch. It should be added that this theory is not specific about the mechanism that actually extracts the pitch. It only says that pitch information is contained within the timing pattern of the neural response and is not related to the activity of any specific neuron or a group of neurons.

Summary

How do we relate the data and the presumed mechanisms of pitch perception? On the one hand we have a group of results obtained primarily with simple stimuli that are explained most straightforwardly with a place theory of pitch perception. On the other hand, the pitch associated with complex stimuli is difficult to explain on this basis and seems most easily defined by the rate of neural discharge coding of pitch information. We should mention that effects seen with simple stimuli such as pitch shifts with masking are not easily explained by a rate of neural discharge theory. Thus, it seems as though we have two theoretical positions, neither of which can explain all the effects.

It is entirely possible that we have at least two mechanisms of pitch perception operating and that the auditory system chooses information derived from one or the other depending on the circumstances. In general, periodicity pitch and time separation pitch are effects that are limited to fairly low pitches. Thus it may be that a temporal analysis utilizing the rate of neural discharge principle is operative for low pitches. On the other hand, for higher pitches it may be that a place representation is utilized. Thus, a dual mechanism of pitch perception may exist. Of course, it may be that other mechanisms are operational, either in conjunction with, or instead of, the ones we have discussed.

REFERENCES

BECK, J. and SHAW, W. A. 1963. Single estimates of pitch magnitude. *J. Acoust. Soc. Amer.* 35: 1722–24.

BÉKÉSY, G. VON 1960. *Experiments in Hearing.* New York: McGraw-Hill Book Company.

CANAHL, J. A. and SMALL, A. M. 1965. Masking-level differences as a function of masker level. *J. Acoust. Soc. Amer.* 38: 928.

CAUSSÉ, R. and CHAVASSE, P. 1942. Différence entre l'écoute binauriculaire et monauriculaire pour la perception des intensités supraliminaires. *C. R. Soc. Biol.* (Paris) 136: 405.

CHIH-AN, L. and CHISTOVITCH, L. A. 1960. Frequency difference limens as a function of tonal duration. *Soviet Physics-Acoust.* 6: 75–79.

CORSO, J. F. 1963. Bone conducted thresholds for sonic and ultrasonic frequencies. *J. Acoust. Soc. Amer.* 35: 1738–43.

EGAN, J. P. and HAKE, H. W. 1950. On the masking pattern of simple auditory stimuli. *J. Acoust. Soc. Amer.* 22: 622–30.

EGAN, J. P. and MYER, D. R. 1950. Changes in pitch of tones of low frequency as a function of the pattern of excitation produced by a band of noise. *J. Acoust. Soc. Amer.* 22: 827–33.

FLETCHER, H. 1929. Speech and Hearing. Princeton, N.J.: D. Van Nostrand Co., Inc.

FLETCHER, H. 1940. Auditory patterns. *Rev. Mod. Phys.* 12: 47–65.

FLETCHER, H. and MUNSON, W. A. 1933. Loudness, its definition, measurement, and calculation. *J. Acoust. Soc. Amer.* 5: 82–108.

GLATTKE, T. J. 1969. Unit response of the cat cochlear nucleus to amplitude-modulated stimuli. *J. Acoust. Soc. Amer.* 45: 419–25.

HAWKINS, J. E. and STEVENS, S. S. 1950. The masking of pure tones and speech by white noise. *J. Acoust. Soc. Amer.* 22: 6–13.

HIRSH, I. J. 1948. The influence of interaural phase on interaural summation and inhibition. *J. Acoust. Soc. Amer.* 20: 536–44.

HIRSH, I. J. and BILGER, R. C. 1955. Auditory-threshold recovery after exposure to pure tones. *J. Acoust. Soc. Amer.*, 27: 1186–94.

MILLER, G. A. and GARNER, W. R. 1944. Effect of random presentation on the psychometric function: Implications for a quantal theory of discrimination. *Amer. J. Psychol.* 57: 451–67.

POLLACK, I. 1948. The atonal interval. *J. Acoust. Soc. Amer.* 20: 146–49.

RIESZ, R. R. 1928. Differential intensity sensitivity for the ear for pure tones. *Phys. Rev.* 31: 867–75.

SHOWER, E. G. and BIDDULPH, R. 1931. Differential pitch sensitivity of the ear. *J. Acoust. Soc. Amer.* 3: 275–87.

SIVIAN, L. J. and WHITE, S. D. 1933. On minimum audible sound fields. *J. Acoust. Soc. Amer.* 4: 288–321.

SMALL, A. M. and BRANDT, J. F. 1963. Differential thresholds for frequency. *J. Acoust. Soc. Amer.* 35: 787.

SMALL, A. M., BRANDT, J. F. and COX, P. G. 1962. Loudness as a function of signal duration. *J. Acoust. Soc. Amer.* 34: 513–14.

SMALL, A. M. and CAMPBELL, R. A. 1962. Temporal differential sensitivity for auditory stimuli. *Amer. J. Psychol.* 75: 401–10.

SMALL, A. M. and CANAHL, J. A. 1965. Loudness changes in a forward masking paradigm. *J. Acoust. Soc. Amer.* 38: 928.

SMALL, A. M. and McCLELLAN, M. E. 1963. Pitch associated with time delay between two pulse trains. *J. Acoust. Soc. Amer.* 35: 1246–55.

SNOW, W. B. 1936. Changes of pitch with loudness at low frequencies. *J. Acoust. Soc. Amer.* 8: 14–19.

STEVENS, J. C. and TULVING, E. 1957. Estimations of loudness by a group of un-trained observers. *Amer. J. Psychol.* 70: 600–605.

STEVENS, S. S. and DAVIS, H. 1938. *Hearing*. New York: John Wiley & Sons, Inc.

THURLOW, W. R. and SMALL, A. M. 1955. Pitch perception of certain periodic auditory stimuli. *J. Acoust. Soc. Amer.* 27: 132–37.

THWING, E. J. 1955. Spread of per-stimulatory fatigue of a pure tone to neighboring frequencies. *J. Acoust. Soc. Amer.* 27: 741–48.

WARD, W. D., GLORIG, A. and SKLAR, D. L. 1959a. Temporary threshold shift from octave band noise: Applications to damage risk criteria. *J. Acoust. Soc. Amer.* 31: 522–28.

WARD, W. D., GLORIG, A. and SKLAR, D. L. 1959b. Relation between recovery from temporary threshold shift and duration of exposure. *J. Acoust. Soc. Amer.* 31: 600–602.

WEGEL, R. L. and LANE, C. E. 1924. The auditory masking of one pure tone by another and its probable relation to the dynamics of the inner ear. *Phys. Rev.* 23: 266–85.

WEINER F. M. and ROSS D. A. 1946. Pressure distribution in the auditory canal in a progressive sound field. *J. Acoust. Soc. Amer.* 18: 401–8.

10

LANGUAGE

Charles E. Cairns/Frederick Williams

SPEECH COMPARED WITH LANGUAGE

Thus far in this volume the chapters have dealt primarily with the acoustical and physiological aspects of speech. In this chapter we consider language as the speaker's knowledge of the relationship of sounds and meanings. As compared with the description of speech, the description of language necessitates our dealing with generalizations of a more abstract nature. We have organized this chapter in a way that the introduction of linguistic concepts takes advantage of a reader's existing knowledge of the articulatory and phonetic aspects of speech behavior. Accordingly, we begin with a discussion of how the sounds of speech can be considered from the viewpoint of linguistic structure. Given examples of linguistic generalizations about speech sounds, the concept of linguistic knowledge, or *competence*, is introduced. Examples of the description of competence in the forms of syntactic and phonological rules are next provided. Finally, the chapter concludes with an overall view of the organization and aims of a *grammar*—the description of linguistic knowledge.

The Sounds of Language

For any given language, it is possible to select a set of phonetic features which can be used to describe the sounds of that language and which have the function of keeping meaningful utterances distinct from each other. The concept of *minimal pairs* is a convenient illustration of what we mean by "distinct."

Consider the two English words "pill" and "bill." They differ from each other only in terms of their initial sounds. Moreover, even these initial sounds are very similar to each other; both are bilabial stops. The only difference lies in the fact that in articulating "b" the vocal folds are in vibration; whereas, in "p" they are not. It can therefore be said that the feature of "voicing" plays a distinctive role in our distinguishing "p" from "b," or "pill" from "bill." For that matter we can think of other such voicing distinctions, as in "dip-tip," "vat-fat," "Jill-chill," and so on. This kind of distinction illustrates the linguistic concept of a *minimal pair*. A minimal pair can be defined as any two words or utterances which contain the same number of phonetic segments and which differ from each other *only* in one segment. Not every minimal pair will illustrate the distinctive power of a single phonetic feature for the distinguishing segment. For example, the English words "rake" and "race" constitute a minimal pair because the only phonetic difference between them lies in the final segment. However, more than one phonetic feature characterizes the distinction between the segments.

It is important to note that not every phonetic feature plays a distinctive role. Consider, for example, all the phonetic differences between the two words "spill" and "pill." The initial "p" in the word "pill" is aspirated; whereas, there is no aspiration in the "p" in the word "spill." The presence or absence of the aspiration in these examples is, of course, completely conditioned by the neighboring sounds. Any voiceless stop in initial position immediately before a stressed vowel is aspirated. Stops which occur in clusters, however, are never aspirated. It is impossible to find a minimal pair of English words or utterances which are similar in every respect except that in one of them there occurs an aspirated sound and in the other there occurs an otherwise similar sound which is not aspirated. Accordingly, there are no two utterances (or minimal pairs) in English which can be distinguished from each other solely on the basis of the feature of aspiration. Hence, aspiration is not a distinctive feature of English, but is a predictable feature which occurs under specific conditions.

The Phonological Level

The preceding description of the concept of minimal pairs illustrates the concept of *distinctive* features as well as of *nondistinctive*, or *redundant* features. Taken together, these two types of features may be referred to as *phonetic* features. A complete analysis of the sound pattern of English would contain a description of all the features which play a distinctive role in English, as well as of the nondistinctive features. In addition, a set of rules stating the conditions under which the redundant features occur would have to be provided. Other rules, which will be described shortly, are also necessary for an adequate description of the sound structure of most languages.

Consider now a representation of an utterance where only the distinctive features are indicated. Such a representation would consist of a sequence of segments, where each segment is defined as a bundle of distinctive features. This is called a *phonological* (or *phonemic*) *representation*, and each segment is referred to as a *phoneme*.[1] It is also possible to represent an utterance as a sequence of segments in which all the phonetic features—the distinctive as well as the redundant—are indicated. Such a representation is referred to as a *systematic phonetic representation*. We will return below to a more detailed examination of systematic phonetics, including an explanation of the term "systematic." Observe now, however, that the relationship between the systematic phonetic and the phonological representations can be described by a set of rules. These rules will include those which supply the redundant features, as well as others which will be described later. It is important to note that the systematic phonetic representations contain all the phonetic information which is governed by linguistic regularities. That is, an utterance represented at this level contains all the linguistically significant phonetic information pertinent to that utterance. A phonemic or phonological representation is said to underlie a phonetic representation in the sense that a set of rules—known as *phonological* rules—maps or transforms the phonological into the phonetic representation. A phonological representation of an utterance contains only those features which, coupled with the phonological rules of the language, are minimally necessary for specifying the phonetic representation of the utterance. In addition to describing the set of phonetic features, a central concern of phonology, which is a branch of linguistics, is the specification of the nature of the rules which relate the phonological and phonetic levels. As we shall see below, the relationship between these two levels is quite complex.

To recapitulate briefly, observe that at both the phonological and the phonetic levels the individual segments (i. e., phonemes at the phonological

---

[1] There is considerable dispute among linguists about the theoretical status of the concept "phoneme." For the interested reader, the term "phoneme" is used here in roughly the sense of "systematic phoneme" in Chomsky, 1964, *Current Issues in Linguistic Theory*.

Table 10-1 Phonetic features

Feature	Description
Consonantal	A speech sound is consonantal if it is produced with a constriction along the center line of the oral cavity. Only the vowels and the glides (/w/, /h/, and /y/) are nonconsonantal.
Vocalic	Vocalic sounds are those which have a largely unobstructed vocal tract. The liquids /l/ and /r/, which are consonantal, are also vocalic. This is true because while there is a central obstruction for the liquids, there is a large unobstructed area to either side of the tongue. Although there is no central obstruction for glides, the most narrow area in the vocal tract during the production is not large enough to qualify them as vocalic. The glides, therefore, are nonvocalic.
Anterior	A sound is anterior if the point of articulation is as far front in the oral cavity as the alveolar ridge. Thus, all the labial and dental sounds are anterior, while sounds produced farther back are nonanterior.
Coronal	A sound is coronal if its articulation involves the front (or corona) of the tongue. A sound is noncoronal if another part of the tongue is used (such as in /k/) or if the tongue is not involved in the production of the sound at all (such as in /p/).
Continuant	A sound is noncontinuant if it is produced with a complete obstruction in the oral cavity. Only the nasals, stops and affricates are noncontinuant. (The nasals are considered to be noncontinuant because while there is an opening in the nasal cavity, the oral cavity is completely obstructed.)
Strident	A strident sound is produced by an obstruction in the oral cavity which forces the air through a relatively long, narrow constriction. As the air rushes out of the opening of this constriction, its turbulence serves as a primary noise source. This turbulent air is then directed against a second obstruction which causes a secondary noise source.
Voice	Voiced sounds are those in which phonation (vibration of the vocal folds in the larynx) takes place as the sound is articulated.
Lateral	A lateral sound is one which involves a contact between the corona of the tongue and some point on the roof of the mouth, along with a simultaneous lowering of the sides of the tongue. In English, /l/ is the only lateral sound, and this feature differentiates it from /r/, the only other liquid, which is nonlateral.
Nasal	Nasals are characterized by a lowering of the velum, which opens the nasal cavity for sound resonation.
High	High vowels are those which involve the highest tongue position, and thus the narrowest constriction in the oral cavity. /u/ and /i/ are the only high vowels; all others are nonhigh.
Low	Low vowels are those which involve the lowest tongue position, /æ/, /a/, and /ɔ/. All other vowels are nonlow. Note how the so-called middle vowels are classed in this system; /e/ and /o/ are nonlow and nonhigh.
Back	The traditional back-front distinction is accounted for by the back/nonback distinction. Thus, /u/, /o/, and /ɔ/ are classed as back, while /i/, /æ/, and /e/ are nonback.
Round	As in traditional classifications, the rounding of the lips is a feature for vowel differentiation. Thus, /u/, /o/, and /ɔ/ are round. Others are nonround.

level and phonetic segments at the phonetic level) are represented as bundles of features. At the phonological level, only those features which are necessary for distinguishing among the relatively small set of phonemes are indicated. At the phonetic level, every relevant feature for specifying the actual pronunciation of the segment is indicated. Consider, as an example, the pronunciation of the word "cat." The aspiration of the initial sound is not indicated in a phonemic transcription, since it is predictable by a general rule of English which states that all voiceless stops of English are aspirated when they appear before a stressed vowel and not in a consonant cluster. A transcription of the utterance at the phonetic level, however, must indicate the aspiration of the initial stop, because the aspiration is a phonetically relevant feature of the sound. At the phonological level, only those features are indicated which are necessary to distinguish the form "cat" from other meaningful forms in English. At the phonetic level the phonological rules have applied and specified all the feature values, as well as the feature of aspiration. The alphabetic symbols at the phonological and the phonetic levels are to be interpreted as shorthand notations for bundles of features.[2]

Although the study of the features at each of the levels of analysis is important, there is not agreement among linguists about what features of speech sounds should be selected as most pertinent for linguistic study. For that reason, we will forego a detailed description of any one system of features, and present, in tabular form, one of the systems which is in current use in the linguistic literature. The reader should bear in mind that it is quite likely that the technical literature in linguistics will probably show change in the set of phonetic features considered most appropriate. Table 10-1 illustrates the features necessary for a specification of the phonemes of English, which are given in feature notation in Table 10-2. The features necessary for a complete specification of the phonetic transcription of English would be essentially similar, although more complicated in a number of details which are not relevant here. For one thing, it should be noted that the limited choice between a "+" and a "−" value for a feature is an oversimplification. A more accurate phonetic transcription would indicate a number of possible values—representing varying degrees—for some features.

The Phonetic Level

What is the status of the phonetic transcription of an utterance? There are two ways of looking at phonetics, and the difference between them is very important. So far in this book, the reader has seen detailed descriptions of various physical and physiological aspects of speech sounds. For example, the dependence of formant frequencies on the volumes of various vocal tract

---

[2] Note that phonological transcriptions are enclosed within slanted lines, whereas phonetic transcriptions are enclosed within square brackets.

Table 10-2 Distinctive features of English phonemes

	l	r	n	m	ŋ	z	s	ð	θ	d	t	v	f	b	p	ž	š	ĵ	č	g	k	u	ə	a	o	i	æ	e	w	y	h
consonantal	+	+	+	+	+	+	+	+	+	+	+	+	+	+	+	+	+	+	+	+	+	−	−	−	−	−	−	−	−	−	−
vocalic	+	+	−	−	−	−	−	−	−	−	−	−	−	−	−	−	−	−	−	−	−	+	+	+	+	+	+	+	−	−	−
nasal	−	−	+	+	+	−	−	−	−	−	−	−	−	−	−	−	−	−	−	−	−										
lateral	+	−	−	−																											
anterior	+	+	+	+	−	+	+	+	+	+	+	+	+	+	+	−	−	−	−	−	−										
coronal	+	+	+	−	−	+	+	+	+	+	+	−	−	−	−	+	+	+	+	−	−										
continuant	+	+	−	−	−	+	+	+	+	−	−	+	+	−	−	+	+	−	−	−	−										
strident						+	+	−	−	−	−	+	+	−	−	+	+	+	+	−	−										
voice	+	+	+	+	+	+	−	+	−	+	−	+	−	+	−	+	−	+	−	+	−	+	+	+	+	+	+	+	+	+	−
back					+															+	+	+	+	+	+	−	−	−	+	−	+
high					+															+	+	+	−	−	−	+	−	−	+	+	−
low																						−	+	+	−	−	+	−	−	−	+
round																						+	+	−	+	−	−	−	+	−	−

Consonants

/l/	l:	/θ/	thigh	/š/, /ʃ/	shall
/r/	ril	/d/	drill	/ĵ/, /dʒ/	Jill
/n/	nil	/t/	till	/č/, /tʃ/	chill
/m/	mill	/v/	ville	/g/	gill
/ŋ/	tang	/f/	fill	/k/	kill
/z/	zeal	/b/	bill		
/s/	sill	/p/	pill		
/ð/	thy	/z,ʒ/¹	rouge		

Vowels and glides²

/u/	boot	/w/	will
/ə/	saw	/y/	yet
/a/	cot	/h/	hoe
/o/	boat		
/i/	beet		
/æ/	bat		
/e/	bait		

¹ Alternative symbols are given.

² The simplified system portrayed here is meant to illustrate the application of the feature concept to vowels in general rather than a complete description of the vowel system of English. English also contains a distinction between tense and lax vowels as in "bait" [bet] and "bet" [bɛt]. Moreover, there are several different phonetically occurring vowels, such as the vowels in the words "cut" [kʌt], "bird" [bɔrd], "sofa" [sofə]. Students who wish to see the feature system applied in detail should consult Chomsky and Halle, *The Sound Pattern of English*, 1968.

cavities has been described. Similarly, the dependence of fundamental frequency on the mass and tension of the vocal folds in the larynx was also described. All of these factors, and many more, are necessary for a full specification of the physical characteristics of an utterance. However, the phonetic transcription which interests the linguist does not include any direct reference to such factors which may be dependent on individual characteristics such as sex, age, and vocal tract size. The linguist's phonetic transcription is really an idealized representation of an utterance in that it contains only (and all) that information which is linguistically significant. The level at which such transcriptions are found is called the *systematic phonetic* as contrasted with the *physical phonetic*, which is far more concrete. The systematic phonetic level is a level defined by linguistic theory, whereas the physical phonetic level of description is much more a product of the experimental phonetician's laboratory. Systems of phonetic transcription, such as the International Phonetic Alphabet (IPA), are alphabets for transcribing utterances at the level of systematic phonetics, as contrasted with physical phonetics. The IPA, for example, does not include any symbols for indicating physical characteristics due to age, sex, or vocal tract size. The IPA is followed in this chapter, with only one exception: the symbols [č] and [ǰ], for the affricates, are used instead of the IPA [tʃ] and [dʒ], in order to be consistent with our analysis of these sounds as unitary segments.

So far we have seen three levels of interest to the phonologist and phonetician. The most abstract of these is the phonemic. Utterances represented at the phonemic level are mapped into systematic phonetic representations by means of a set of general phonological rules. The systematic phonetic representation is, in a sense, the "lowest" linguistically significant level. As was explained previously, this level provides a description of *all* the rule-bound phonetic properties of an utterance. Properties of speech sounds due to nonlinguistic factors such as sex, age, etc., are described at a third level, that of physical phonetics.

From the preceding discussion it is possible to discern two distinct roles played by phonetic features. On one hand, they serve as vehicles for the description of speech sounds at the systematic phonetic level. On the other, they play the more abstract role of keeping meaningful utterances perceptually distinct from each other at the phonological level.

The Morpheme

Roughly, a *morpheme* is an indivisible or minimal meaningful item. Sometimes a morpheme is coextensive with the word; more frequently it is not. For example, the word "cats" contains two morphemes. One of these is the stem "cat." The other is the plural morpheme, which could be represented by the phonetic symbol [s]. The word "cat" consists of just one morpheme.

Linguists distinguish between several types of morphemes on the basis of the linguistic roles they play. For example, it is necessary to distinguish between *lexical* morphemes (such as "cat" and "dog") and *grammatical* morphemes (such as "plural," "past tense," etc.).

Phonological Processes

Frequently a morpheme will have a variety of phonetic forms. Consider, for example, the lexical morpheme "wife." In the singular, where there is no suffix, we find that this morpheme has roughly the phonetic shape [waɪf]. However, in the plural (spelled "wives") we find that the morpheme in question has the phonetic form [wāɪv], which is followed by the plural morpheme having the phonetic shape [z]. (The bar written above the [ā] indicates that the vowel is long.)

As a further example, notice that the grammatical morpheme used to indicate plurality in nouns also has a variety of phonetic shapes. Thus, the plural morpheme is represented by the phonetic [s] when it follows a grammatical morpheme which ends in [p, t, k, θ, or f]. When the plural morpheme follows a noun morpheme which ends in [s, z, š, ž, č, or ǰ], it takes the phonetic form [ɨz]. In other environments, the plural is represented simply by [z].

It is possible to establish a single underlying representation of a morpheme such that the various phonetic representations can be predicted by phonological rules. (We will see an example of phonological rules later in this chapter.) A morpheme is given in its underlying representation, such as we have referred to "plural" here, at the *phonological* level. Although the phonological level is an abstraction, linguists claim that it corresponds to a perceptual reality. We may go our whole lives never being conscious of the details of the phonetic diversity of plurals. The perceptual significance is plurality itself, with all the redundant or predictable information of the different phonetic variations unconsciously filtered out. Phonological theory is concerned with the relations between the phonological and systematic phonetic levels. Again, these relations can be described by rules which transform the phonological representation of an utterance into its phonetic representation.

To sum up, we have seen that a phonological description of a language contains two linguistically significant levels, the phonological and the (systematic) phonetic. In addition, the description must contain a set of rules which convert the phonological into the phonetic level. These rules describe two main kinds of regularities which occur in the sound patterns of languages: (1) the regular occurrence of redundant phonetic features and (2) the variety of phonetic representations which a single morpheme may assume, depending on its environment in the utterance.

This chapter started from the readers' knowledge of physical properties of speech sounds, based on previous chapters. It was shown that as speech sounds were viewed from the standpoint of linguistic structure, it became necessary to posit the existence of a variety of levels of analysis and rules for relating these levels. It is fair to say that the main goal of linguistic theory is the specification of all the rules and levels which a descriptively adequate linguistic analysis of a language must contain. In order to gain an appreciation of the full scope of linguistic concerns, it is necessary to stand back from the material presented so far in this volume and examine some very broad questions about the nature of language.

LINGUISTIC THEORY

Competence, Performance, and Grammar

The distinction between linguistic competence and performance is an important one in contemporary theory. This distinction is essentially that between the knowledge of a language (*competence*) and the use of that knowledge (*performance*). The reader should be aware that the use of these terms in linguistics is specialized and in many respects different from their usage in everyday speech and in other disciplines. For example, in ordinary usage, competence is taken to mean something like adequacy, skill, or proficiency. Performance usually refers to specific actions or specimens of behavior. These terms have different referents in linguistics. As we will see in the following paragraphs, *linguistic competence* refers only to an abstract mental component—namely, knowledge of linguistic rules. By contrast, *linguistic performance* refers to the set of skills and strategies employed by the language user as he applies his linguistic competence to the actual production and comprehension of sentences. Linguists are typically concerned with the study of linguistic competence, whereas psychologists who study language are usually concerned with the study of linguistic performance.

One of the major advances in contemporary linguistic theory has been the view that it is possible to describe linguistic competence by means of a list of rules. In the terminology of linguistics, these rules comprise a *grammar*— that is, a set of rules which is a model of linguistic competence. If a linguist presents a grammar of a language, he is thereby making the claim (either rightly or wrongly) that his grammar is a model of the linguistic knowledge possessed by the native speaker of that language. It should be clear, of course, that the linguist is concerned with a *descriptive* grammar rather than a prescriptive grammar (rules of "correctness").

The distinction between competence and performance can be made more clear with the use of an analogy between language and the game of chess.

One important aspect of the game can be described by the rules which regulate the possible moves of the chess pieces. These rules are analogous to the rules of grammar (which are considerably more complicated, of course). Given only these rules of chess, it is possible to generate all and only the legal configurations of pieces on the board. To put this another way, it is always possible to determine whether any given arrangement of pieces on a chess board is attainable by a sequence of legal moves, starting from the initial position. If a given configuration of pieces is illegal, then it is so because it would not be possible to attain that position without violating a rule of the game. The rules for moving the chess pieces are analogous to the rules of grammar. The set of legally attainable configurations of chess pieces is analogous to the sentences of a language. The rules of chess generate the set of all and only the possible arrangements of pieces in the same way as the rules of grammar generate all and only the sentences of a language. The rules for moving the pieces might be called chess competence, using the term competence in this specialized sense.

What, then, is performance in the analogy with chess? If all you knew about chess were the rules for moving the pieces, you would be a very poor player! You might never make an illegal move, but your opponent, if he or she had any experience in the game, would very quickly have you checkmated. The point is that in addition to knowledge of the rules of the game, the chess player must also possess skills and strategies for harnessing this knowledge and applying it to given situations in order to achieve specific ends. Obviously, possession of such strategies is necessary for adequate chess play. These strategies are analogous to linguistic performance. Thus, just as knowledge of the rules of chess is not sufficient for successful play, so knowledge of the rules of grammar is insufficient for actual language use.

The analogy between chess and language, like every other analogy, has its limitations. One important difference is that the rules of chess are made explicit and conscious to the person learning to play the game. That is, every chess player has been explicitly told the rules of the game and could, on demand, state the rules. This is not at all the case with the rules of grammar. Young children somehow infer the rules of their native language without explicit linguistic instruction. Speakers of natural languages, unlike chess players, are not able to state the rules of their grammar; in fact, even professional linguists do not agree on what is the most accurate statement of many of the rules of grammar. In the case of chess we are dealing with an aspect of knowledge which is explicit and can easily be brought to consciousness, whereas linguistic knowledge is tacit and remote from conscious inspection. It is a task of linguistic science to seek evidence which can yield insight into the nature of the rules of grammar and, on the basis of such evidence, provide a theoretical description of linguistic competence.

The reader may well wonder how it is possible to gain any insight into the form of linguistic competence. After all, competence is obviously a highly abstract structure, embodied somehow in remote aspects of human mental life. Linguists have discovered, however, that detailed study of some of our linguistic abilities which are due solely to our possession of linguistic competence can yield significant insights into the nature of grammar.

The task faced by the linguist is not very dissimilar to that faced by a hypothetical engineer confronted with an unfamiliar and alien computer. Suppose the engineer had no knowledge of the physical constitution of the computer, but wished to describe its information-processing capacities. He would study the properties of its logical operations and, on the basis of this study, he could make inferences concerning the organization of the machine's information-processing structures. The linguist proceeds in roughly the same way: He studies the results of the information-processing structures which we call grammar, or linguistic competence, and makes inferences about its organization on the basis of such studies.[3]

The first question one might ask in attempting to study the general nature of linguistic competence, then, is: What operations can the native speaker of a language perform which are due only to his knowledge of his language? Or, in other words: What can the native speaker of a language do which someone who does not know his language cannot do? The first and most obvious answer to this question is that someone who knows a language can comprehend and produce meaningful sentences of that language. The native speaker can regularly pair sequences of sounds of certain kinds with semantic interpretations in both production and comprehension. This ability is due to possession of linguistic competence. Let us now turn to some further human abilities which reflect linguistic competence in their explanation.

Competence: Five Characteristics

We can gain some insight both into the structure of particular languages and into the nature of language in general if we look at some of the capacities and abilities possessed by native speakers of English. We will discuss five such abilities, all of which are common to speakers of any natural language.

Infinite sentence capacity with finite linguistic knowledge

One of the most remarkable characteristics of our knowledge of English is that we deal every day with sentences not identical to any we have ever seen, heard, or uttered before.

---

[3] The analogy between the linguist and the computer engineer is something of an oversimplification. Later in this chapter we discuss linguistic methodology in more detail.

Reflect a moment on the fact that you have probably never before encountered an exact replica of any of the vast majority of the sentences in this book. It is probably also true that most of the sentences you have uttered today are equally novel to you. Yet the novelty of these everyday sentences is no occasion for surprise; the sentences may seem very ordinary indeed. This might appear paradoxical. On the one hand we are dealing with structures (sentences) which we have never seen before, yet on the other hand they seem perfectly familiar to us. What makes the sentences familiar, of course, is not their specific content, but rather that they are all generated by a set of familiar rules.

The rules which comprise the grammar are considered finite in number; it is quite unlikely that a human would possess a component of knowledge which consists of an infinitely long list of rules. Yet the number of sentences which the grammar can generate is so vast that we consider this number infinite. In short, the set of possible sentences is infinitely large, whereas a finite set of rules comprises the linguistic competence for the generation or interpretation of these sentences.

Since it is the object of linguistic theory to describe the nature of linguistic competence, a theory of the structure of a knowledge of English (or of any other language) must incorporate the capability of infinite sentence creation. It should be mentioned that the property of infinite sentence capacity with finite rules is unique to human communication; no other animal communication system reflects it.

The considerations which we have already discussed lead to the more precise definition of the term grammar as *a set of rules, which is finite in number, which produces all and only the well-formed sentences of a language, and which must provide for each sentence generated the appropriate structural description*(s).[4]

This definition includes two concepts which have not yet been sufficiently discussed. One of these is *structural description*, a concept to be discussed in the context of the third characteristic of competence. The other is *well-formed*, which is discussed next.

The ability to distinguish sentences from non-sentences

We can gain insight into some of the details of the structure of English if we look at the speaker's ability to distinguish well-formed English sentences from ill-formed ones. By *well-formed*, we mean a sequence of linguistic symbols which is generated by the grammar of the language in question. Of course, the practicing linguist, in trying to describe the linguistic competence of a native speaker, does not start off knowing what the rules are. The judgments

[4] Some sentences may have alternative descriptions as discussed on pp. 434 *ff.*

of the native speaker concerning the grammaticality of strings of linguistic symbols serve as data to the linguist in his attempt to evaluate a set of rules which he has proposed as a model of the linguistic competence of the native speaker. Since we assume that linguistic competence is describable by means of a grammar as defined here, then those strings which the native speaker would judge to be sentences of his language must be in the set of sentences generated by the grammar. That is, the grammar must specify that they are well-formed. Strings which the native speaker would judge as non-sentences must not be in the set generated by the grammar.

It is important to recognize that grammatical well-formedness is distinct from that of meaningfulness. Consider the following sentences:

(1)   The children are sleeping comfortably.
(2)   *Comfortably the children sleeping are.[5]

Any native speaker of English would recognize (1) as a perfectly ordinary sentence of English. Example (2), however, is obviously deviant, although it is possible to impose an interpretation on it. What is it about (1) which tells us that it is a sentence of English? It cannot simply be that sentence (1) makes sense, because example (2), which is ill-formed, also makes some sense. Thus it is possible to utter a string of words which makes sense but is not a well-formed sentence of English. It also is possible to utter a string of words which is a well-formed sentence of English but which does not make sense. Sentences (3) and (4) illustrate this.

(3)   The man standing near the doorway is holding a child on his lap.
(4)   John shattered the ice cube right after Mary melted it.[6]

These strings are grammatically acceptable, but the semantic conflicts cause us to question their sense. The point of these examples is that semantic sense, or meaningfulness, is neither necessary nor sufficient for the grammatical well-formedness of a string. It is often possible to make some sense out of grammatically ill-formed sentences; similarly, it is often possible to find grammatically well-formed sentences which are semantically anomalous.

The ill-formedness of example (2) is due simply to the occurrence of the words in an ungrammatical order. Some further properties of linguistic competence can be revealed by examples of ill-formed sentences which require a deeper explanation of illegality than that for sentence (2). Consider, for example, the strings in examples (5) through (8).

[5] An asterisk is typically used to denote an illegal or ill-formed construction.

[6] Assume, of course, that "it" refers to the ice cube John shattered.

(5a) I expected the doctor to examine John.

(5b) I persuaded the doctor to examine John.

(6a) I expected John to be examined by the doctor.

(6b) I persuaded John to be examined by the doctor.

(7a) John expected to be examined by the doctor.

(7b) *John persuaded to be examined by the doctor.

(8a) I expected that the doctor would examine John.

(8b) *I persuaded that the doctor would examine John.

Examination of pairs of sentences such as in (5a) and (5b) or (6a) and (6b) might lead one to suspect that the sentences in these pairs have similar syntactic structures. The ill-formedness of (7b) and (8b) would then seem surprising. It is impossible to explain the ill-formedness of these examples by claiming that words are in the wrong order. Their illegality can only be explained by reference to subtle aspects of the syntactic structure. Since the ill-formedness of (7b) and (8b) is immediately apparent to any native speaker of English (although, again, any English speaker would know what was meant), then the rules proposed by the linguist as a model of the English speaker's linguistic competence must specify that they are not well-formed— i. e., that they are not in the set of sentences generated by the grammar.

It is not very difficult to think of a set of rules which would account for the illegality of (2), or of any other string which deviates because of obvious violations of word order. The ill-formedness of (7b) and (8b), however, presents more of a challenge, since it involves deeper aspects of grammatical structure. An adequate account of these deeper aspects requires the concepts of *structural description* and of *deep* structure, which are next discussed in connection with examples of syntactically ambiguous sentences.

Recognition of syntactic ambiguity

Another ability native speakers of English possess solely by virtue of their knowledge of the language is the capacity to perceive that some sentences can be interpreted in more than one way. Consider sentence (9):

(9) Old men and women stay in the east wing.

It is easy to account for the syntactic ambiguity of sentence (9) in terms of how the words are grouped together. Any native speaker of English would readily agree that the sentence is ambiguous in that the adjective "old" can modify either the phrase "men and women" or it can modify only the noun "men." The alternative groupings of the elements of the ambiguous phrase in (9) can be formally represented by means of parentheses, as follows:

(9a) (old (men and women)) . . .

(9b) ((old men) and women) . . .

This use of parentheses can be taken as an introduction to structural description. The logically equivalent notation exemplified in (9c) and (9d) is more frequently shown as:

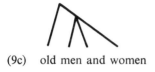

(9c) old men and women

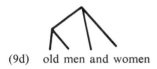

(9d) old men and women

Structural descriptions depicted in (9c) and (9d) are called *phrase markers*. Further notational refinements will be made throughout this section.

Since native English speakers would judge (9) as ambiguous in the way described above, then the rules which constitute the linguist's model of the English speaker's competence must provide two ways of generating the string of words in (9). More precisely, there must be two ways that the rules for the construction of noun phrases in English can be applied. One of these ways must generate structures as illustrated in (9a) or (9c), the other must yield structures like (9b) or (9d). It is now possible to give a formal definition of the term *syntactically ambiguous:* A sentence of a language is ambiguous if (and only if) the grammar of that language provides for more than one way of generating it. For each way of generating a sentence, there is a unique structural description. Therefore, a syntactically ambiguous sentence is one which has more than one structural description associated with it.

Sentence (9) illustrates how the judgments made by a native speaker can serve as data to the linguist. Those sentences which are judged as ambiguous by English speakers must be ambiguous with respect to the grammar the linguist proposes for English. Furthermore, the grammar must explain the way in which a sentence is ambiguous. This is accomplished by providing more than one structural description for ambiguous sentences.[7]

[7] We are now in a position to explain why the last word in the definition of "grammar" on page (432) is written "description(s)." There must be two (or more) structural descriptions for ambiguous sentences.

Recall that in the discussion of the native speaker's ability to distinguish well-formed from ill-formed sentences we saw examples of ill-formed sentences which seemed to reveal that English (and, presumably, all other languages as well) possesses aspects of grammatical structure which are more subtle and abstract than can be accounted for by means of rules of word order. The following examples are a few of the many examples that could be presented which can shed some light on the nature of these deeper features of grammar.

(10)   The boy looked up the street.

Superficially, it appears that it might be possible to account for the ambiguity in terms of the two ways of grouping the words indicated in (10a) and (10b):

(10a)   The boy (looked (up the street)).
(10b)   The boy ((looked up) the street).

In (10a) the grammatical relationships are different from the grammatical relationships which occur in (10b). In (10a), "up the street" is a prepositional phrase where "up" is a preposition and "the street" is a noun phrase. The main verb of the sentence is "looked." In (10b), however, there is no prepositional phrase, and "up" is not a preposition but a verbal particle. The main verb of the sentence is "looked up," and "the street" is the direct object of the sentence.

Recall that we stipulated that a descriptively adequate grammar must account for the ways in which a sentence is ambiguous. It follows from this example that we must augment our structural descriptions in order to account for the information given in the preceding paragraph. This can be done simply by adding labels to the branching points (called *nodes*) of the phrase markers which were illustrated in (9c) and (9d). The *labelled phrase markers* which constitute the two structural descriptions of (10) are given below:

(10c)

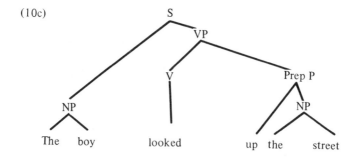

(10d)

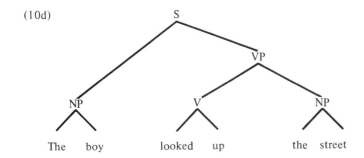

These symbols are to be interpreted as follows: S means sentence; VP means verb phrase; Prep P means prepositional phrase; and NP means noun phrase. The diagrams can be read as stating that in both cases the sentence consists of a noun phrase followed by a verb phrase. In (10c) the verb phrase consists of a verb followed by a prepositional phrase, whereas the verb phrase of (10d) consists of a verb followed by a noun phrase. The relational notions of direct object and main verb mentioned above will be defined later in this chapter.

In all, example (10) differs from example (9) in an important way. The ambiguity of example (9) can be accounted for solely in terms of a specification of the manner in which the constituents of the sentence group together. In order to account for the ambiguity in sentence (10), however, it is also necessary to specify the syntactic labels associated with the constituents which occur.

There are also many examples of syntactically ambiguous sentences for which it is not possible to discover alternative constituent structures. Consider, for example, sentence (11). The only way to account for the ambiguity of sentence (11) is in terms of the grammatical relationships between the word

    (11)   Visiting relatives can be a nuisance.

"relatives" and the word "visiting." Thus, in the reading of sentence (11) which can be paraphrased "It can be a nuisance to visit relatives," the word "relatives" is the object of the verb "visiting." In the other reading of sentence (11), however, which can be paraphrased "relatives who visit can be a nuisance," the word "relatives" is the subject noun phrase of the verb form "visiting." The only way to account for the ambiguity of sentence (11) is in terms of these different grammatical relations. There is not a concomitant alternative grouping of the words within constituents as in sentences (9) and (10). The phrase marker in (11a) is an approximate description of the gram-

(11a)

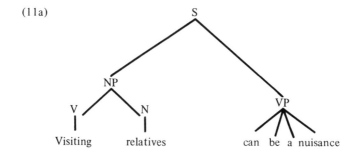

matical structure of (11). It is important to note that there is only one such phrase marker. Although one might quibble about the precise assignment of some of the labels to the nodes in (11a), there is only one reasonable way to group the morphemes. In any case, there is no way of devising two phrase markers for the string of morphemes which appears in (11), each of which would be one of the two ways in which the sentence is ambiguous.

In order to account for the ambiguity it is necessary to examine the grammatical relationships which seem to underlie each of the interpretations of (11). Consider the relationships depicted in abstract structures in (11b) and (11c):

(11b)

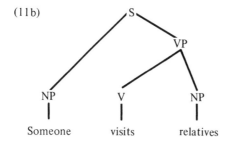

(11c)

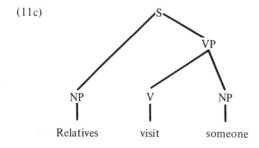

Although (11b) and (11c) do not represent any actually occurring constituents of (11), their presence does seem to be implied. In (11b), "relatives" is the object of "visit," whereas "relatives" is the subject in (11c).[8]

Examples (11b) and (11c) represent what linguists call the *deep structure* phrase markers of (11). Deep structure is to be contrasted with *surface structure*. These two terms refer to different levels of analysis; we have been dealing only with surface structures in examples (1)–(10). Surface structure is the apparent syntactic structure revealed, for example, in sentence (9). It specifies the hierarchical relationship among constituents as they appear in the sequence of actually occurring sentences. Example (11) reveals, however, that not all of the relevant syntactic information can be captured within clusterings of the word sequence. The relevant syntactic facts in example (11) can only be revealed by appeal to what linguists refer to as deep structure. It is at the level of deep structure that grammatical relationships such as object of a verb phrase or subject of a verb phrase are defined. We will see the distinction between deep structure and surface structure revealed in considerable detail in subsequent sections of this chapter. For the time being, it will suffice to say that the grammar of English contains what we refer to as *transformational rules*. Such rules automatically convert deep structures into surface structures. The necessity for distinguishing between the deep structure and surface structure in a descriptively adequate grammar of English is revealed in part by the distinction between the kinds of syntactic ambiguity illustrated above.

Recognition of syntactic relationships and synonymous sentences

As indicated in the previous section, an ability possessed by native speakers of English is the capacity to perceive syntactic relationships. Consider, for example, sentences (12) and (13).

(12) John is eager to please.

(13) John is easy to please.

In sentence (12) the subject of the verb "please" is quite clearly the word "John." In sentence (13), on the other hand, it is John who is to be pleased. Whereas "John" is, at a superficial level, the subject of the sentence, the word "John" is also the object of the word "please" at the level of deep structure. These sentences further illustrate the distinction between surface structure and deep structure. Although most native speakers of English would not be able to describe the difference in the syntactic structure of (12)

---

[8] Subject and object will be given more precise definitions later. For the time being, the traditional usage of these terms will suffice.

and (13) in these terms, any normal mature speaker of English is aware that in sentence (12) it is John who is to do the pleasing, and in sentence (13) it is John who is to be pleased. A descriptively adequate grammar of English must accommodate these representations.

Native speakers of English also possess the capacity to recognize certain pairs of sentences as paraphrases of each other. Consider, for example, sentences (14a) and (14b). Sentence (14a) is a simple active declarative sentence, whereas (14b) is the passive form analogous to (14a). Although one

(14a) The doctor examined John.

(14b) John was examined by the doctor.

might argue that there is a difference in emphasis or focus between the two sentences, the two sentences do mean essentially the same thing. In (14a) the phrase "the doctor" is the subject of the sentence, whereas in (14b) at the level of surface structure it is the word "John" which is the subject of the sentence. At the level of deep structure, however, it is clear that "the doctor" is the subject of the sentence in both (14a) and (14b). The similarity in meaning between (14a) and (14b) is accounted for in contemporary linguistic theory by the claim that they both have the same deep structure. The difference between (14a) and (14b) is that (14b) has been subject to a transformation called the *passive* which transforms the deep structure which underlies both (14a) and (14b) into the surface form represented in (14b).

The ability to perceive deleted elements

A further ability of the native speakers of English which illustrates the necessity to postulate a level of deep structure is the ability to perceive linguistic elements which have been deleted by the rules which relate deep structures and surface structures. Consider, for example, sentence (15). Any native speaker of English who hears sentence (15) knows that the subject of the verb "examine" is "the doctor." At the level of deep structure, sentence

(15) The doctor promised to examine John.

(15) consists of two component sentences. One of these sentences states that the doctor promised something and the other one states that the doctor is to examine John. In the process of relating the deep structure representation of (15) to the surface structure representation, however, the subject of the second sentence has been deleted by transformational rule.

Consider sentence (16): any native speaker of English would recognize

(16) The doctor invited John to stay.

that the subject of the verb "stay" is "John." At the level of deep structure sentence (16) also consists of two complement sentences, one of which states that the doctor invited John to do something and the other one, that John is to stay. In this case, also, the subject of the verb "stay" is deleted. If we look at the superficially similar sentence (17), which differs from (15) only

(17)   The doctor promised Bill to examine John.

in the specification of to whom the doctor made the promise, we recognize that the subject of the verb "examine" remains "the doctor." A descriptively adequate grammar of English must account for the speaker "knowing" at some level what the subject of the embedded sentence is. At the level of deep structure the subject of the embedded clauses is explicitly present. The level of deep structure may be related to the level of surface structure by an explicit formal set of rules. These rules are such that there is only one possible deep structure for each of the sentences (15), (16), and (17). Therefore the ability of the native speaker of English to assign the appropriate interpretation to each of these sentences is accounted for by his possession of the set of rules which relates their deep structure and surface structure. When confronted with the surface structure representation of these sentences, the native speaker can reconstruct the deep structure representations which contain explicitly the subjects of the embedded sentences.

Syntactic Rules

So far we have noted that linguistic theory concerns the competence of the ideal speaker, that the characteristics of competence are described by a grammar, and that the description is in the form of rules. In this section we turn to representative examples of how the syntactic aspects of competence are described by rules.

Simple structural descriptions

We can begin by considering a relatively simple view of syntactic structure as involving combinations of morphemes as constituents in phrase structures, and a hierarchy of phrase structures serving in turn as constituents in sentence structures. Let us temporarily restrict attention to those sentences which can be seen as having two primary phrase constituents, a noun phrase (NP) followed by a verb phrase (VP). For example:

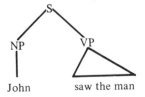

These are the highest level or largest constituents of any such sentence, and are often analyzable into smaller constituents. Thus, the verb phrase can consist either of a verb (V) followed by a noun phrase or of a copula followed by an adjective. For example:

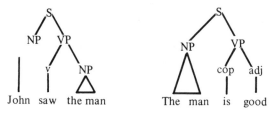

In the former case the verb would be analyzed by a traditional grammarian as the main verb of the sentence, and the noun phrase as the direct object of the verb phrase. In the second case, the copula would be some form of "be" and the adjective would be what a traditional grammarian would label a "predicate adjective." The noun phrase can also be analyzed into smaller constituents; it may consist either of an article followed by a noun or of the complementizer "that" followed by an embedded sentence or clause. For example:

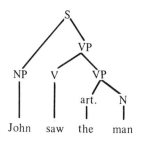

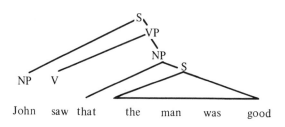

Simple rule examples

Every structural combination that has been discussed in the preceding paragraph could be described in terms of the following simple rules:

(i)   S $\longrightarrow$ NP + VP

(ii) VP $\longrightarrow$ $\begin{cases} \text{V} + \text{NP} \\ \text{cop.} + \text{adj.} \end{cases}$

(iii) NP $\longrightarrow$ $\begin{cases} \text{art.} + \text{N} \\ \text{that} + \text{S} \end{cases}$

Here *S* is the abbreviation for the sentence construction. The arrow means either *consists of* or *rewrite as*. (*Rewrite as* may be preferable since it implies the dynamic qualities of the grammar.) The brackets which appear in rules (ii) and (iii) indicate that there is an optional choice among the sequences of constituents which appear as rewrites. Thus, in rule (ii) VP can be rewritten either as a verb followed by a noun phrase or as a copula followed by an adjective.

These rules simply state the constituent structures of a subset of the sentences of English. The sentence diagram (or *phrase markers*) in Figure 10-1 illustrate rule applications. Any of these phrase markers can be derived from the rules listed above.

Relative to the phrase markers in Figure 10-1, a constituent may be defined as any word or string of words which can be traced back to a single labelled intersection of branches (*node*) in the structure. Thus, in sentence (1) the phrase "the boy" is a constituent since it can be traced back to the node labelled NP. Similarly, the phrase "examined the boy" is a constituent since this string of words can be traced back to the node labelled VP. The phrase "the doctor" is a constituent since it can be traced back to a node labelled NP. The phrase marker reveals that the highest level constituent cut exists between the phrase "the doctor" and the phrase "examined the boy." The highest level constituent is, of course, the entire sentence which is traced back to the node labelled S.

Notice that it is possible to generate any of an infinite number of sentences with this model of linguistic description. This is true because within the constituent labelled NP it is possible to generate a symbol S which in turn contains another NP which might contain another S, and so on. Thus in the sentence labelled (2) in Figure 10-1, there is the constituent "the doctor examined the boy" which is embedded within the noun phrase, which in turn is contained within the main sentence. This embedding is also illustrated in sentence (3) in Figure 10-1. Sentence (4) illustrates that this process could be

Figure 10-1 Phrase markers derived from the sample rules.

(1)

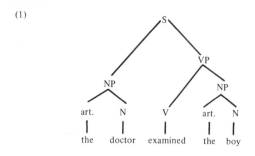

(2)

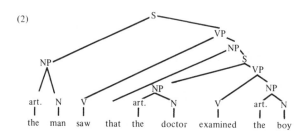

(3)

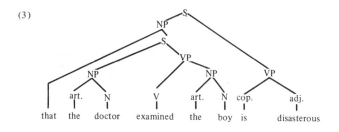

(4)

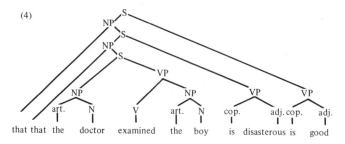

repeated essentially indefinitely, although cumbersome and awkward sentences would result. The main point is that this approach can be construed so as to capture the essential properties of what is called *recursiveness*, which is one of the basic properties of all human language.

Transformational rules

At the level of surface structure, the elements of some constituents are not adjacent with each other. In order to analyze such *discontinuous constituents*, it is necessary to introduce transformational rules, which are quite different from the phrase structure rules discussed above. Note the difference between sentences (5a) and (5b) in Figure 10-2 relative to their verb phrase constructions. Sentence (5a) might lead the linguist to revise the noun phrase rule (iii) to the form (iv) below:

$$\text{(iv)} \quad NP \longrightarrow \begin{cases} \text{art.} + N \\ \text{that} + S \\ \text{to} + VP \end{cases}$$

Figure 10-2 Additional phrase markers derived from sample rules.

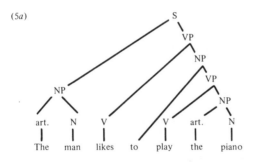

(5a)

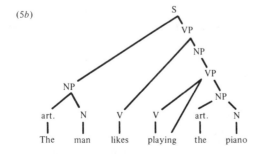

(5b)

Rule (iv) indicates that the noun phrase constituent contained within the verb phrase can optionally consist of a particle "to" followed by the verb phrase "play the piano." Sentence (5b) poses a more major problem, however. This lies in analyzing the noun phrase constituent contained within its main verb phrase. It appears that this noun phrase is similar to that in (5a) in that it contains the verb phrase "play the piano" plus an extra morpheme "-ing." However, there is no natural way of determining where the major constituent break within this noun phrase takes place. In sentence (5a) the major constituent break within this noun phrase was between the particle "to" and the verb phrase "play the piano." However, since the morpheme "-ing" actually occurs within the verb phrase, it is not possible to analyze it in this manner. Although it is evident that this noun phrase should be analyzed into two constituents, namely "-ing" plus the verb phrase "play the piano," there is no natural, non-arbitrary way of doing this. This is an example of the problem of discontinuant constituents. The verb phrase "play the piano" is interrupted by the particle or morpheme "-ing."

The answer to the problem lies in adopting a different view of the rules illustrated in (i) through (iv). If we were to look at them not as simply a shorthand notation for describing the constituent structure of actually occurring sentences, but rather as abstract elements in a general theory which describes the principles of construction of English sentences, it is possible to find a solution to the problem. Suppose you were to view the rules in (i) through (iv) as statements of a dynamic process whereby phrase markers such as illustrated in sentences (1) through (4) in Figure 10-1 or sentence (5a) in Figure 10-2 may be regenerated. Suppose further that we would replace rule (iv) with rule (v):

$$
\text{(v)} \quad \text{NP} \dashrightarrow \left\{ \begin{array}{l} \text{art.} + \text{N} \\ \text{that} + \text{S} \\ \left\{ \begin{array}{l} \text{to} \\ \text{-ing} + \text{VP} \end{array} \right\} \end{array} \right\}
$$

This revised set of rules would then generate all of the sentences (1) through (5a) plus the phrase marker illustrated for sentence (6) in Figure 10-3. However, observation of sentence (6) reveals the necessity to posit further rules in order to relate the structure indicated in (6) to actually occurring sentences. We need a rule which will move the "-ing" to the right of the verb "play." Such a rule is illustrated in (vi):

(vi)   Transpose: ing + V to V + ing

The application of rule (vi) to the phrase marker in (6) yields the phrase marker shown for sentence (7) in Figure 10-3. This rule is only one example

(6)

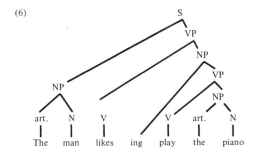

(7)

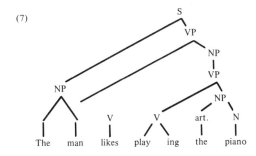

Figure 10-3 Phrase markers involving discontinuous constituents.

of the general concept of transformational rules. Transformational rules are also needed to handle a far wider range of syntactic phenomena from those illustrated here.

It is now possible to define the noun phrase constituent which is the object of the verb phrase in the sentence "The man likes playing the piano." As shown in Figure 10-3, it consists of the constituent labelled verb phrase ("play the piano") plus the morpheme "-ing," where "-ing" and the verb phrase are themselves a noun phrase constituent. This can only be done, however, by reference to the phrase marker shown in (6) prior to the application of rule (vi). That is, in order to give a reasonable specification of the constituent structure of this sentence, it is necessary to refer to an abstract phrase marker which is related to the structure of actually occurring sentences only by the application of rule (vi).

The main point here is that a descriptively adequate grammar of English must go beyond a mere listing of the classificatory principles of actually occurring sentences. It is necessary to look upon the rules illustrated in (i) through (vi) not as merely a shorthand notation for the list of constituents out of which sentences may be constructed, but rather as statements of dynamic processes for the generation of sentences.

The examples also generally illustrate the distinction between *surface* structure and *deep* structure. Structures such as appear in (6) are analogous to what linguists refer to as deep structure, whereas sentences such as (7) are analogous to surface structure representations of sentences. Deep structure phrase markers are converted into surface structure phrase markers by the application of rules such as illustrated by (vi).

There is an important difference between rule (vi) and those previously illustrated. Rules such as in (i) through (v), called *phrase-structure* rules, generate phrase markers starting with the symbol S. Rules such as in (vi) are *transformation* rules, and do not generate phrase markers but rather transform phrase markers. They receive as input a phrase marker which has been previously generated by phrase structure rules and convert it into another phrase marker. Also, there are some transformational rules that receive as input phrase markers which have been operated on by prior transformational rules. Again, phrase structure rules generate phrase markers, whereas transformational rules transform phrase markers from one form into another.

Phonological Rules

We noted earlier that the variety of phonetic forms assumed by individual morphemes can be accounted for largely by regular rules. That is, the phonetic shape of a morpheme is partly a function of the environment in which that morpheme occurs. Phonological rules account for those aspects of the phonetic shape of a morpheme which are due to its environment. Again, these are the rules which transform the phonological representation of an utterance into the phonetic representation.

In an earlier example, we mentioned that the phonetic form for the plural morpheme for regular English nouns was conditioned by the stem environment. We can represent this conditioning by some simple rules where Plu represents the phonological level of the plural morpheme; the arrow can be read as *realized as* (as a dynamic process such as in syntactic rules); brackets enclose the stem environment; and the plus indicates a morpheme boundary. Consider the following rules:

(1) Plu → /ɨz/ in environment {s, z, š, ž, č, ǰ} + ____

(2) Plu → /s/ in environment {p, t, k, θ, f} + ____

(3) Plu → /z/ in environment
$$\left\{\begin{array}{l} \text{l, r, n, m, d,} \\ \text{ð, v, b, g, u,} \\ \text{ɔ, a, o, i, æ} \\ \text{ŋ, e, w, y} \end{array}\right\} + \underline{\quad}$$

We can improve upon the above rules by using phonetic features to designate relevant stem environments and by taking advantage of the order of the rules. Rule (1), for example, applies to environments where the final stem segment is both strident and coronal. Rule (2) refers to environments which are unvoiced. But if rule (2) referred to *all* unvoiced segments, then it would also refer to s, š, and č found in rule (1). However, if we assume that rule (1) is always applied prior to rule (2), then this excludes s, š, and č from rule (2), thus "unvoiced" is all that is needed to designate the stem environment. Finally if we consider that rules (1) and (2) are always applied prior to rule (3), then the environmental designation for this rule could be simplified to "any." In this new form, using phonetic features and rule order, the rules are stated as follows:

(1) Plu → /ɨz/ in environment $\begin{bmatrix} + \text{ strident} \\ + \text{ coronal} \end{bmatrix}$. + ____

(2) Plu → /s/ in environment [− voiced] + ____

(3) Plu → /z/ in any environment

As a further example of the operation of phonological rules, consider the behavior of the stems in the following examples:

constituent	constituency
democrat	democracy
pirate	piracy
advocate	advocacy
aristocrat	aristocracy
clairvoyant	clairvoyancy
complacent	complacency

Notice that whenever the noun-forming suffix-y is added to a noun, verb, or adjective stem which ends in a /t/, the /t/ changes into an /s/. Below is a regular phonological rule which applies to the stems just given:

t ⟶ s/ ____ + y#

Or, in feature notation:

$$\begin{bmatrix} + \text{ coronal} \\ + \text{ anterior} \\ - \text{ voiced} \\ - \text{ sonorant} \end{bmatrix} \longrightarrow [+ \text{ continuant}]/ \underline{\quad} + \begin{bmatrix} - \text{ consonantal} \\ - \text{ vocalic} \\ - \text{ back} \end{bmatrix} \#$$

Of course, there are a few exceptions to this rule, such as honest-honesty. Also, it is important to stipulate that the suffix in question is a noun-forming suffix, rather than the homophonous suffix which forms adjectives. Thus, chocolate, chocolatty and brat, bratty do not show the /t/–/s/ alternation.

An alternative analysis of the above situation is to establish an underlying form for the stem morphemes which end in /s/ and establish a rule which converted /s/ to /t/ in word final position. The problem with this, however, is that there are many words which do end in /s/ which do not convert to /t/. All these words would have to be exceptions to such a rule. The analysis given above, with the single underlying form with a final /t/ which converts to /s/ in the environment before noun-forming /y/, has many fewer exceptions.

The Organization of a Generative Grammar

Up to this point we have seen a number of illustrations of the linguist's concerns with syntax and phonology. Theories of syntax and phonology are in turn components of the more general theory of language. In this section we will describe the overall organization of this general theory as well as discuss the theoretical goals adopted by linguists.

Based on the generative idea, extensive research into the structure of language has revealed that it is expedient to envisage three coordinated components which relate sound and meaning. These are the phonological, syntactic, and semantic components of a grammar; all are shown in Figure 10-4.

Chomsky (especially, 1964, 1965) has proposed that a revealing theory of language contains, as a central component, a set of syntactic rules. This

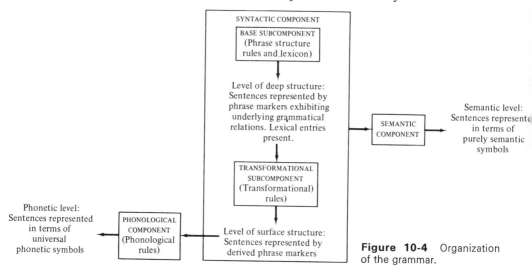

Figure 10-4 Organization of the grammar.

component generates a set of abstract structures which represents all and only the sentences of a language as well as their structural descriptions. The phonological and semantic components are viewed as interpretive, rather than generative in their own right. They receive structures generated by the syntactic component and encode them into (1) a set of instructions for their phonetic realization, and (2) a set of conceptual elements (of a yet undetermined kind) which correspond to semantic readings of sentences.

The syntactic component

The *base* and the *transformational* subcomponents constitute the syntactic component of the grammar. In previous sections of this chapter we have seen that it is necessary to distinguish between two levels of syntax—namely, the levels of deep and surface structures. The base subcomponent generates deep structure representations of sentences. The transformational subcomponent maps the deep structures generated by the base into derived phrase markers (as in Figures 10-1, 10-3) at the level of surface structure. The base subcomponent consists of phrase structure rules (examples on pp. 443 ff.) as well as a lexicon.

The transformational subcomponent consists of rules which operate on the phrase markers created by the base subcomponent. For each sentence generated by the base, the first applicable transformational rule (example p. 446) applies, carrying out the appropriate transformations on the phrase marker. The next applicable transformational rule then applies to the result of the first transformational operation, and so on, until the list of transformational rules has been exhausted.[9]

The semantic component

Note how Figure 10-4 illustrates that the output of the base subcomponent —i. e., sentences represented at the level of deep structure—serves simultaneously as inputs to two sets of rules. Not only do deep structures feed into the transformational subcomponent, as discussed above, they are also input to the semantic component of the grammar. Although little is known about the structure of the semantic component or about the nature of the semantic representations they produce, it is believed that the semantic component consists of a set of *projection rules*. These rules assign to every deep structure a semantic interpretation. Speculations on the nature of the semantic component can be found in Katz and Fodor (1963).

---

[9] It is important to note that the description given of syntax, as well as of the rest of the grammar, is greatly simplified for purposes of exposition. Although the basic ideas expressed are accurate, important qualifications are necessary on many of the descriptions of the operation of the rules. The interested reader is referred to the references listed at the end of the chapter.

The phonological component

As described above, syntactic surface structure is the input to the phonological component. The phonological component consists, essentially, of a set of rules which assigns to every syntactic surface structure a phonetic representation. In order to properly assign the phonetic features of stress and sentence intonation (and, perhaps, other phonetic phenomena as well), the phonological rules must refer to the constituent structure provided by the surface structure representation of sentences. This is why it is believed that the output of the transformational subcomponent is the input to the phonological component. There is no evidence that phonological rules must, in order to correctly assign phonetic features, refer to syntactic information at the level of deep structure.

As we have seen, the phonological component consists of rules which are given partly in terms of phonological or phonetic features. These rules apply to syntactic surface structures represented in terms of morphemes (both grammatical and lexical) and the syntactic organization imposed by the syntactic rules. The morphemes are realized in terms of sequences of distinctive feature bundles. Each bundle describes a separate phoneme. Thus, syntactic surface structure is equivalent to the phonemic level defined previously. The total set of phonological rules makes all the changes of feature representation necessary to render the correct phonetic output. As we have seen, many of these changes can be predicted on the basis of the phonological constituency of the neighboring morphemes.

There is much more that could be said concerning the character and internal organization of phonological rules. Phonologists have not reached universal agreement concerning many basic aspects of the organization of the phonological component. For further information concerning the theoretical problems involved, see Postal (1968) and Chomsky and Halle (1968).

On the Goals of Linguistic Theory

Linguistic as against psycholinguistic study

The overall goal of the scientific study of language—including both linguistics and psycholinguistics—is to explain the processes and capacities which underlie man's ability to associate sound and meaning. Again, linguistic theory only attempts to provide that aspect of these processes and capacities which can be accounted for by one's knowledge of one's language—that is, by *competence*. Psycholinguistics, on the other hand, attempts to explain the nature of the strategies and heuristics which play a role in the use of this knowledge. Again, this is the study of *performance*.

In the contrast of competence and performance study, it is important to know that the set of rules put forth by the linguist as a theory of linguistic knowledge does not necessarily represent, in any concrete way, rules which are actually used in everyday production and generation of sentences. Grammatical rules are put forth as formal and precise descriptions of the interrelationships among the various levels of language. It has been shown experimentally that the levels described by linguistic theory play an important role in the psychological processing which takes place in language use. However, the same can not be said for the individual rules of grammar. It is not presently known how language users actually relate these levels during speech acts. The next chapter, however, will present some speculations on this topic.

Linguistic universals

The grammar of English is a theory of the linguistic knowledge possessed by those who have mastery of English. Similarly, grammars of French, Navajo, Chinese, and so on, are theories of the linguistic knowledge possessed by speakers of those languages. It is a very important observation that all human languages show basic similarities. All languages seem to be cut from the same mold, as it were. For example, every human language which has been investigated in any depth has a grammar which is organized in the manner described in Figure 10-4. This is a particularly significant point, since it reveals that the general theory of grammar reflects a universal linguistic property common to all human beings.

It is important to distinguish between the theory of grammar and the grammar of a particular language. The latter is also a theory (i. e., a theory of the linguistic competence of a speaker of that language), whereas the former is really a meta-theory which determines the general form of grammars. Linguistic meta-theory embodies all that is known to be universal among languages of the world. Moreover, it is assumed that if any feature of language is universal, its universality stems from innate characteristics of human beings. Since there are so many unrelated languages of the world, it would not be plausible to maintain that such features as the organization of grammar depicted above could be explained by cultural transmission.

There are two basic kinds of linguistic universals, *formal* and *substantive*. Formal universals are those which specify the general form and organization of grammars and the rules which comprise them. For example, the organization depicted in Figure 10-4 is a formal universal, as is the statement that the grammars of all languages have transformational and phrase structure rules. Such statements as the latter specify the type of rules which languages must have. Substantive universals, on the other hand, refer more to the content rather than to the form of grammars, although the distinction is not always easy to draw. A substantive universal would be the claim, believed to be true by contemporary linguists, that all languages have nouns, verbs, and adjectives. A comparable universal from the field of phonology is the statement that all languages have consonants and vowels, or that no language fails to have the consonant /t/ and the vowel /a/. The list of known linguistic universals is considerably longer than space allows here.

The general theory, or meta-theory, specifies the form and, to some extent, the content of the grammar of any particular language. The meta-theory represents all that is assumed to be common to all languages and, hence, innate. If the meta-theory reflects innate features of human beings, then it can be assumed that all human beings are born "preprogrammed" in such a way that the communication system they develop will conform to the universal constraints on human languages. When one considers the monumental task of the child in learning his native language, as well as that normal children develop the knowledge of their own language in an amazingly short period of time, then it is reasonable to assume that the child already has a predisposition to learn the general pattern of a grammar. The study of linguistic universals—i. e., the study of the linguistic meta-theory, is considered the most important and interesting aspect of linguistics.

The epistomology of linguistics

To what extent can the linguist claim that the statements he makes about linguistic universals or even about the grammar of a particular language are consonant with a speaker's actual linguistic knowledge? In order to approach this problem, it behooves us to consider the general relationship between facts and theory. A theory—by which we mean not only a linguistic theory or meta-theory, but any theory—is a model of processes or relationships believed to underlie observable events. The tasks of the scientist are to develop the theory or model which best describes as broad a range of observables as possible and to seek evidence which can aid him in deciding between alternative theories which predict the same range of phenomena. Although linguistics does not proceed with carefully constructed laboratory experiments as in the physical sciences, linguistic theory does proceed in a scientific manner. In constructing a grammar of English—i. e., a theory of the English speaker's linguistic competence—the linguist attempts to devise sets of rules which can generate all and only the sentences of English and their structural description(s). Any such set of rules will generate strings of symbols, and it is an empirical question whether English speakers will accept any such string as a well-formed sentence. The set of proposed rules constitutes the hypothesis. The validity of the hypothesis can be tested by determining whether a native speaker of English (frequently the linguist himself) accepts the strings of symbols generated by the rules as English sentences. Moreover, the rules should also predict other properties of sentences, such as that some will be ambiguous, some will exhibit deep grammatical relationships which differ from the surface relationships, and so on. It is empirically determinable whether speakers of English will indeed make the same judgments concerning these properties of sentences as predicted by the rules established by the linguist. Support for the theory is in the form of a congruence of speakers' judgments and the predictions made by the rules. If speakers were to fail to make predicted judgments, this would be evidence against a proposed set of rules.

Proceeding by the method of hypothesis formation and testing, linguists have formulated partial grammars of a number of languages. The universal linguistic theory has been based largely on these theories. Obviously, there is no way in which the meta-theory can be tested directly. The only empirical test for the meta-theory is a test of its compatability with descriptively adequate grammars of actual languages. It should be pointed out that, although the study of linguistics dates back several centuries, it has not developed a formal and explicit theory with as much explanatory power as in many of the physical sciences. The reasons for this are diverse and to some extent obscure. It is generally true, however, that the scientific study of human beings has lagged considerably behind the physical sciences.

In linguistics the problem of subjectivism can be overcome to the extent that the linguistic judgments which serve as evidence are unequivocal. One major problem is that there is no completely reliable way to test the judgments which native speakers may make concerning various properties of sentences. Linguists frequently notice that, when working with a set of rules, continual exposure to a set of sentences or sentence types distorts their own set of judgments. Although this problem can sometimes be resolved by informal questioning of native English speakers concerning the status of strings of sentences, no highly reliable testing procedure has been worked out for this. The relatively clear sentence examples, such as those used in this chapter (pp. 433–40), pose no problem. However, for some of the fine points about alternative sets of rules, it may well become necessary to develop an established set of experimental procedures for determining speakers' judgments.

REFERENCES

CHOMSKY, N. 1964. *Current Issues in Linguistic Theory*. The Hague: Mouton.

CHOMSKY, N. 1965. *Aspects of the Theory of Syntax*. Cambridge, Mass.: M.I.T. Press.

CHOMSKY, N. and HALLE, M. 1968. *The Sound Pattern of English*. New York: Harper & Row, Publishers.

JAKOBSON, R. 1941. *Kindersprache, Aphasie, und Allgemeine Lautgesetze*. Uppsala, Universitets Aarsskrift.

KATZ, J. J. and FODOR, J. A. 1963. The structure of a semantic theory. *Language* 39: 170–210.

POSTAL, P. M. 1968. *Aspects of Phonological Theory*. New York: Harper & Row, Publishers.

11

LINGUISTIC PERFORMANCE

Frederick Williams/Helen S. Cairns

INTRODUCTION

It is difficult to discuss all aspects of language behavior within the confines of a single chapter. Accordingly, one aim in preparing this chapter was to be selective rather than exhaustive in the choice of topics. The main emphasis is upon the current approach to linguistic performance which attempts to relate language behavior to generative linguistic theory. This approach is known as *cognitive psycholinguistics* in contemporary nomenclature. Two other topics are discussed for purposes of providing the reader with an orientation toward other approaches to linguistic performance. One of these is an overview of several of the learning-theory-based perspectives on verbal behavior. The other is the recent approach to urban language study which illustrates a contemporary trend in sociolinguistic research.

THE COGNITIVE APPROACH[1]

As discussed in the preceding chapter, there is a complementary relationship between the linguist and the psychologist of language (or *psycholinguist*) in that both are concerned with the account of how humans are able to relate sounds with meaning. Whereas the linguist is primarily concerned with determining the nature of linguistic knowledge that accounts for this relation, the psycholinguist is concerned with the psychological processes by which this knowledge is used to effect linguistic performance—that is, the understanding and creation of sentences. Because linguistic knowledge, or grammar, plays such a central role in this approach to the study of linguistic performance, it is not unusual that a major question has been the type or degree of relationship between the details of generative grammar and the details of performance theories.

When generative grammar was developed in the late 1950s, it was of great interest to a number of psychologists concerned with language study because the linguist seemed to be making very strong psychological claims about the nature of the language user. Psychologists, particularly Miller (1962, 1965), argued that a productive approach to the study of language behavior would be to attempt to discover psychological correlates of the various constructs of linguistic theory. Much of the psycholinguistic research of the early 1960s found psychologists interested in ascertaining which elements of linguistic theory might be said to have psychological reality, as contrasted with which elements could not. In question form, the research issue was: What is the psychological relation between competence and performance? After a decade of research into the matter, this relationship has been clarified considerably, but certainly not conclusively. The sections which follow present some of the highlights of this research and the implications for the competence-performance relationship.

The Psychological Reality of Linguistic Rules

Early studies: the complexity thesis

The prevailing hypothesis in psycholinguistic research of the early 1960s was that there was great similarity between linguistic and psychological processes. In particular, the role of the transformational rule as a psychological entity was investigated in detail. The research focus upon transformational rules was prompted, in particular, by an earlier version of generative

[1] This section draws heavily upon concepts introduced in the preceding chapter; hence if the reader is not familiar with generative grammatical theory, he should read Chapter 10 prior to reading this section.

theory which held that such surface forms of sentences as "The boy did not hit the ball," "The ball was hit by the boy," and "The ball was not hit by the boy," were differentiated by single transformations. In particular, the theory held that these were optional transformations and represented variations of the same basic underlying structure. If no optional transformations were applied to the underlying structure, a simple, active, declarative sentence, referred to as a *kernel* sentence, would result. "The boy hit the ball" is the kernel sentence derived from the same underlying structure as the transformed sentences above. Since sentences of the above types were linguistically related in terms of transformational rules, it seemed reasonable to hypothesize that the language user was actually using these rules when creating or understanding these sentences. In a variety of studies investigating this hypothesis, it was reasoned that the more transformations an individual had to use in the creation or understanding of a sentence, the more demands would be made upon psychological-processing mechanisms. Researchers speculated that such an increased processing load might be revealed by a person's taking more time to create or understand a sentence, having more problems in remembering the sentence, or making more mistakes in other behaviors involving the sentence.

A study illustrative of the foregoing approach was one undertaken by Mehler (1963) in which subjects attempted to memorize lists of variously transformed sentences. The errors which they made in this task were used as an index of the increased processing load associated with individual transformations. Mehler found that when subjects made memory errors, they tended to err in the direction of substituting a less transformed sentence for a more complex one, as in erroneously recalling "The ball was not hit by the boy" as "The boy hit the ball." Based on these findings, Mehler advanced the *coding hypothesis*, which said that when a person stores a sentence in memory he decodes it and stores a kernel (or untransformed) version of the underlying structure, plus notations about which transformations have to be applied to regain the original surface structure. Thus, for example, when a person attempted to store in memory the sentence "Was the ball hit by the boy?" the hypothesis said that he stored it in the form of "The boy hit the ball," with the notations that its surface structure was to incorporate a passive and a question transformation. It was also held that when the sentence was recalled, the kernel was retrieved, the appropriate transformational variations applied, and the sentence was reconstituted as "Was the ball hit by the boy?" Mehler speculated that when forgetting occurred, it was the notations about the individual transformations which were most susceptible to loss. Thus one would expect the less transformed versions of a sentence to be produced when recall of transformationally complex sentences was less than perfect.

Another early and illustrative experiment in this area was one (Miller,

1962) which required subjects to match variously transformed versions of the same sentence. Subjects were presented lists of sentences such that the sentences on the lists were derived from common underlying structures. For each basic structure, the lists would include kernel sentences as well as various transformed versions. For example, "The boy did not hit the ball" might appear on one list and "The ball was hit by the boy" appear on another. The subject's task was to match the two transformed versions of the "same" sentence on two lists. It was assumed that a subject would have to decode the transformed versions of the sentences to their basic structures then make a comparison of the kernel level in order to find the matches. Accordingly, if decoding involved actively making transformations, then the more transformations that separated the two sentences of a pair, the longer it should take to make that match. The results of this study (Miller, 1962) lent support to the hypothesis that transformational rules have psychological reality. Generally, the more transformations which separated a pair of sentences, the longer it took people to match them.

A subsequent study (Miller and McKean, 1964) consisted of essentially the same experimental design (carried out by a more sophisticated technique) and replicated the findings of the earlier study. The explanation of the results of that subsequent study was a great deal more cautious, however. These authors warned against the oversimplified interpretation of their results as "proof" of the psychological reality of transformational rules. The only two transformations incorporated in both these studies were the negative and the passive. Miller and McKean pointed out that negation as a syntactic operation is closely related to the semantic variables of truth and falsity. The conclusion of the authors was that researchers would be ill-advised to attribute a great deal of theoretical importance to results obtained with only one transformation—the passive.

Another study (Savin and Perchonock, 1965) in this early series incorporated an imaginative strategy for testing implications of the recoding hypothesis. Subjects were again required to remember various transformed sentences. In addition, however, they were required to recall a list of eight monosyllabic words presented to them after each sentence. Thus, a subject heard a sentence followed by the word list and he was to repeat first the sentence, then as many of the words as possible. It was reasoned that a more transformationally complex sentence would require more space in temporary memory than a less transformationally complex one, and this difference would be related to the number of words a person could remember in addition to the sentence. Presumably, the fewer words a person could remember, the more temporary memory space had been taken up by the transformational "tags" associated with the sentences. Savin and Perchonock's results were supportive of their hypothesis—the more transformationally complex the sentences, the fewer words recalled by subjects.

A number of experiments have been carried out using variations of the Savin and Perchonock technique. As a result, several explanations other than the coding hypothesis have been put forward to explain differences in word recall. Epstein (1969) suggests that the observed results can be accounted for by differential difficulty in retrieving the words from short-term memory. Foss and Cairns (1970), however, suggest that the difficulty lies in the initial storage of the words in short-term memory. Glucksberg and Danks (1969) and Matthews (1968) found the length of delay between sentence and word list to be a more salient variable than sentential complexity. The results of this subsequent research demonstrate that although the Savin and Perchonock results are compatible with the coding hypothesis, they do not constitute strong evidence for that hypothesis.

Counterarguments to the complexity thesis

The hypotheses advanced in the studies described above have subsequently been described as special cases of a *derivational theory of complexity* (Fodor and Garrett, 1967). This theory states that each transformation represents a psychological unit in sentence processing; hence, as already mentioned, a sentence containing more of such units should place more demands upon processing than one containing fewer such units.

In addition to the uncertainty of the explanations presented in the early studies, there was also the problem that certain types of transformations had not been studied under the complexity thesis. The following study represents the type of counterevidence raised against the derivational theory of complexity.

Based upon generative grammar, it can be argued that a sentence containing adjectives such as (1a) below, should be more difficult to understand than an identical sentence (1b) without adjectives.

(1a) The young prince rescued the beautiful princess.
(1b) The prince rescued the princess.

The difference in complexity is predicted because the grammar of English would first generate an underlying structure for sentence (1a) that included three sentences: "The prince was young." "The prince rescued the princess." "The princess was beautiful." From this underlying structure containing three sentences, a phrase marker is produced by transformational rules which could be read as "The prince who was young rescued the princess who was beautiful." Subsequently in the generation of sentence, the adjectives are rearranged to produce the form shown as sentence (1a).

Research has indicated that sentences such as (1a) are not, in fact, psycholinguistically more complex than sentences such as (1b). Evidence of this comes from a study by Fodor and Garrett (1967) in which subjects were required to paraphrase experimental sentences, and where speed and accuracy of paraphrase (properly quantified) served as the measure of psycholinguistic complexity. Sentences containing adjectives were paraphrased with even greater speed and accuracy than were matching sentences with the adjectives deleted.

It is fair to say, then, that the psychological status of transformational rules remains in question. On the one hand, it does not appear that every transformational rule has a corresponding psychological unit in behavior. On the other hand, however, certain transformations (such as the passive and the question transformations) seem to differentiate types of sentences which vary in terms of their demands upon processing behavior. Although evidence of the latter type may indicate general differences in processing complexity and the relation of this to grammatical complexity, it is not direct evidence of the psychological reality of individual transformations. A subsequent, and possibly more productive, approach to the studies of the correspondence between competence and performance is found in research that has attempted to gain evidence of the psychological reality of the level of deep structure in generative theory. The claim that deep structure (or any linguistic variable, for that matter) has psychological reality means simply that in dealing with language the human cognitive system performs an analysis which utilizes essentially the same kind of information as that provided by linguistic theory. Thus, linguistic levels (or variables) can be said to have psychological reality in the same way that the frequency of a tone is said to have psychological reality. That is, there is a psychological analog of tonal frequency, i. e. pitch. A demonstration of the psychological reality of deep structures, then, is the discovery of psychological analogs to various aspects of deep structures.

The Psychological Reality of Deep Structure

As described in Chapter 10, deep structures are those phrase markers generated by the phrase structure rules of the grammar. It may be recalled also that in linguistic theory deep structures are assumed to contain all the information necessary to derive a semantic interpretation for a sentence. Since comprehension is the process of deriving a semantic interpretation for a sentence and production is the process of expressing a semantic interpretation, it seems quite likely that deep structures would have psychological reality. This reasoning has led to psycholinguistic studies where the aim has been to find evidence of the psychological reality of various components contained in deep structures. This aim is in contrast to the studies just described which were focused upon finding psychological correlates for individual transformational rules. In the present focus, the question is whether psychological processes can be shown to refer to the linguistically-described elements of deep structure. The research strategy in this case has been to attempt to ascertain whether linguistic behavior can be elicited which will differentiate among elements described by the grammar as appearing in deep structure.

Words in deep structure

As was discussed in Chapter 10, the transformational component of the grammar frequently rearranges the elements of a sentence so that they have a different order in surface than in deep structure. An example of this is a sentence (2) which has undergone the passive transformation. Although "the letter" appears as the apparent subject of this sentence, "John" is the subject in deep structure in a way illustrated in sentence (3).

(2) The letter was sent by John.
(3) John sent the letter.

Now consider sentences (4) and (5) which have a superficial correspondence to (2) and (3):

(4) The letter was sent by mail.
(5) *(The) mail sent the letter.   * denotes unacceptable.

Upon closer consideration, it can be shown that sentence (4) does not have the same type of deep structure as sentence (2). One way of illustrating this is to show that if we assumed that sentence (4) incorporated a passive transformation, removing this transformation would result in the unacceptable sentence (5). As illustrated in the contrast between sentences (2) and (4), the words "John" and "mail" serve quite different syntactic functions in these sentences. "John" is the subject of the underlying sentence (deep structure) in example (2); whereas "mail" is part of an adverbial structure in sentence (4). Although sentences (2) and (4) have apparently the same surface structure, our knowledge of their differences in deep structure is presumably a basis for knowing that "John" is the subject of sentence (2), but "mail" is not the subject of sentence (4). The challenge for psycholinguistic research was to determine how to obtain evidence of the psychological existence of this deep structure knowledge.

One line of research into this problem involved the assumption that in sentences such as (2) and (4), a word such as "John," being the subject of a sentence, is a more salient part of the deep structure of a sentence than the word "mail," which is only a modifier. Accordingly it was reasoned that if subjects were required to learn and recall sentences such as (2) and (4), a word such as "John" would be a better prompt word for sentence recall than a word such as "mail" because the former was a more integral part of the deep structure of the sentence. The results of a study conducted by Blumenthal (1967) supported this hypothesis. He found that words which were subjects in deep structure were more effective memory probes than were adverbials. In a subsequent experiment (Blumenthal and Boakes, 1967), it was demonstrated that deep structure subjects are more effective memory probes than deep structure objects, even when they hold similar positions in surface structure (see, for instance, sentences (12) and (13) later in this chapter). In all, these experiments represent support for the hypothesis that lexical elements which play a role in the grammatical relations described by deep structures do have psychological correlates.

Underlying sentences

Another line of research on the psychological reality of deep structure has focused upon underlying sentences rather than individual lexical items. When a generative grammar is used to describe the derivation of many of the sentences that we observe in everyday language behavior, we find that most sentences, except very simple ones, are made up in deep structure of several smaller sentences. For example, sentence (6) has a deep structure which includes sentences (6a) and (6b):

(6)   The boy kissed the girl who ran home.

(6a)   The boy kissed the girl.

(6b)   The girl ran home.

In the generative account of sentence (6), sentence (6b) becomes the relative clause in sentence (6a) by the application of two transformational rules. The point to be emphasized here is that the psychological representation of the deep structure of sentence (6) should reflect the two smaller sentences (6a) and (6b). There are additional kinds of sentences that reflect multiple underlying sentences, as for example sentences (7) and (8):

(7)   The boy kissed the girl and she ran home.

(8)   The boy said that the girl ran home.

Several experiments (Fodor and Bever, 1965; Garrett et al., 1966) have yielded evidence of the psychological reality of multiple underlying sentences in deep structure. The research strategy common to these studies is based upon the following perceptual phenomenon. If the attention of one's perceptual mechanisms at a given instant is devoted to the processing of a particular stimulus, the perception of other stimuli occurring simultaneously may be delayed by the perceptual mechanisms. Thus, two events which occur at the same time may be perceived as occurring in series because the perception of one of the two events is delayed slightly. For the studies of underlying sentences, audible clicks were placed somewhere in the surface structure of a complex sentence. Each subject was required to listen to the sentences and indicate where in the sentence he thought the click had occurred. It was found that when the clicks were located near the boundaries of what would be the underlying sentences in the deep structure of a sentence, subjects tended to report the clicks as having occurred at these boundaries. These results indicated that the clicks were perceptually (and subjectively) displaced from their objective locations. The experimenters assumed that perception of the clicks was delayed because the perceptual mechanisms were engaged in processing the clause as a unit. This was interpreted as evidence that the clause in surface structure—which corresponds to the underlying sentence in deep structure—constitutes a unit of perceptual processing. For an example of this technique consider sentences (9) and (10) where parentheses indicate underlying sentence boundaries:

(9)   (In her hope of marrying) (Anna was surely impractical.)

(10)   (Your hope of marrying Anna) (was surely impractical.)

When a click is placed within the word "Anna" in sentences (9) and (10), it will be perceived as occurring between the words "marrying" and "Anna" for sentence (9) and between the "Anna" and "was" if the subject hears sentence (10). In short, the same click in the same word ("Anna") will be perceived as occurring either before or after this word, depending upon the syntactic context in which it occurs. If the earlier sentence, "The boy kissed the girl and she ran home," were used in such an experiment, a click located in "girl" would be perceptually displaced to the right (between "girl" and "and") and a click objectively located in "she" would be displaced to the left.

In all of these experiments there was a strong implication that the perceptual bias of locating the click was a function of the psychological reality of the underlying sentences as they were relevant to the perception of the surface structure of the more complex overall sentence. It should be added that materials for these experiments were prepared by dubbing and splicing critical segments of the experimental sentences so the locations of clicks were not influenced by additional perceptual cues such as stress and intonation.

One criticism of the above studies is that the perceptual displacement of the clicks is perhaps evidence only of the psychological reality of divisions among surface clauses rather than divisons among the underlying sentences in deep structure (Bever et al., 1969). A study by the researchers who raised this criticism attempted to overcome the problem as follows.

Clicks were used in sentences where the separate underlying sentences did not appear as separate clause units in the corresponding combined surface structure. An example of this is sentence (11):

(11)   The reporters (assigned to George) drove to the airport.

The grammatical derivation of the above sentence represents two underlying sentences ("The reporters were assigned to George." "The reporters drove to the airport."), which are first transformed into the relative clause structure: "The reporters (who were assigned to George) drove to the airport." A further transformation then modifies this form of the sentence to reflect the example shown in (11). According to this grammatical derivation, there exists no clause boundary in the surface structure between the words "George" and "drove." However clicks located in "George" are in fact perceptually displaced to the right between "George" and "drove." Accordingly, this example provides evidence of a perceptual division between underlying sentences where that division is not represented by a clause separation in surface structure.

As in the interpretation of studies investigating the psychological reality of linguistic rules, caution is necessary in interpreting the generality of results of the above studies. Although it has been implied by the perceptual displacement of clicks that language users have some type of an awareness of divisions among the underlying sentences, this does not necessarily mean that *all* underlying sentences have a psychological reality. For example, the grammatical derivation of the insertion of adjectives within a surface structure initially involves underlying sentences for those adjectives. There is no experimental evidence that the click displacement phenomenon holds for the division among adjectives in a surface structure (Bever et al., 1969).

Although questions about the psychological reality of deep structure remain an important area for psycholinguistic research, current psycholinguistic studies have moved toward the development of sentence processing models which, while incorporating concepts of deep and surface structure, are envisaged as relatively separate from the grammatical rules of linguistic theory. At this point it might be useful to recall (Chapter 10) the analogy of linguistic competence and performance as compared with the rules of chess and the way one uses these rules. What seems important for the psycholinguist is that he develop accounts of the kinds of *operational strategies* that would be necessary in using the rules to create and understand sentences. It may be that in many cases these strategies are not directly related to the rules of grammar. This type of theorizing is illustrated next in terms of a discussion of sentence comprehension.

Toward a Theory of Sentence Comprehension

Assumptions

The minimal (although possibly not sufficient) information which the hearer must recover when comprehending a sentence is information about (a) the meanings of the lexical items contained in the sentence and (b) the grammatical relations expressed by the sentence. One of the key problems faced by the hearer is that the speech signal arrives in a left-to-right sequence—or word by word, as it were—while relationships among the words are dependent upon hierarchial structuring. Consider, for example sentences (12) and (13):

(12) John is easy to please.

(13) John is eager to please.

The left-to-right surface structure order of the above sentences is identical, but the critical difference between them is that at the level of deep structure "John" is the object of the verb "please" in sentence (12), while it is the subject in sentence (13). Since in comprehension the structural information must be recovered from this serially presented information, it is impossible to have a theory of sentence comprehension such that the structure of an entire sentence can be predicted with certainty by perception of its first few words. It seems important to assume, therefore, that as a sentence is comprehended in a sequential order, the perceptual mechanisms may project hypotheses (which may be subsequently modified) about the lexical interpretations of the words and about the structural relations among them. In brief, even though the structure of a sentence cannot usually be determined from its first few words, the perceptual operation may involve the attempt to formulate hypotheses as soon as there is sufficient information.

Another alternative suggestion, but an unlikely one, is that hypotheses concerning lexical interpretations and structural relations are not formed until all of the sentence is received by the hearer. The problem with this formulation is that if the hearer made no syntactic hypotheses, it would be difficult to explain how it is possible to recognize sentence units as a whole. When we mention hypotheses pertaining to structural relations, this refers to predictions about the deep structure of the sentence, as guided by cues in its surface structure. The hearer must use these cues as they occur serially in the sentence input, and must accordingly adjust his comprehension hypotheses about the lexical and structural information intended by the speaker.

As suggested elsewhere (Cairns, 1971) it may be the case that hypotheses about the meaning of individual lexical items are projected immediately upon the serial receipt of these items by the hearer. Structural hypotheses, by contrast, are probably deferred until approximately one word beyond the main verb of a clause. This is because it is that point in the typical sentence construction at which there has been a sufficient sequence of information to make the most complete types of structural hypotheses. These hypotheses thus project expectations mainly about the structure of the predicate of each incoming clause.

It seems reasonable to assume that hypotheses concerning the interpretation of lexical items must be made prior to structural hypotheses because the lexical interpretations of a sentence item necessarily constrain the kinds of structural hypotheses that might be projected. Consider, for example, a sentence beginning "Paul slept. . . ." Since the verb "sleep" is a pure intransitive verb (i. e., it never takes a direct object), the interpretation of this word thus provides a basis for a structural hypothesis about the predicate construction. Typically, it is the case that the verb of a sentence severely constrains the possible syntactic forms of the post-verbal portion of that sentence. Thus, knowledge of the verbal element allows the hearer to formulate predictions about the structure of the remainder of the predicate.

Some predictions

The assumptions presented above lead to a number of testable predictions. For example, if it is necessary to induce the deep structure of a sentence from surface structure cues, then the more that a surface structure represents a distortion of any underlying structure of a sentence, the more difficult that sentence should be to comprehend—that is, the more demands it should place upon psychological-processing mechanisms. Also, if cues of deep structure are omitted from the surface structure, a sentence should be more difficult to comprehend. Finally, we would expect structural hypotheses to be more difficult to formulate, and, accordingly, sentences more difficult to comprehend, if the lexical items of a sentence can fit into a variety of different syntactic structures. We will next discuss some observations of language behavior which reflect upon these conditions.

A clear example of a situation in which surface structure is different from deep structure is the passive sentence, in which the object of the verb in deep structure has been moved to subject position in surface structure. As mentioned earlier in this chapter, a number of researchers have found that passive sentences are, in general, more difficult for persons to deal with in experimental tasks (learning and recall, comprehension, sentence matching, and so on) than are the corresponding active forms. The explanation for these results, which is compatible with the present discussion, is that the passive surface structure is a distortion of its underlying structure.

The two sentences given below illustrate an example of the omission of cues in surface structure to relations that exist in deep structure:

    (14)   The man the dog bit died.

    (15)   The man whom the dog bit died.

Sentence (15) contains the relative pronoun "whom" which signals the presence of an embedded sentence in the deep structure of the sentence being perceived. In sentence (14) the relative pronoun cue is absent. Thus, it is not until he processes the verb "bit" that the hearer knows he is processing a relative clause. In one study (Fodor and Garrett, 1967) involving sentences of the above types, it was found that people were typically more accurate in their paraphrases of sentences which contained relative pronouns, as opposed to the same sentence with the relative pronoun deleted. An experiment by Hakes and Cairns (1970) using a different measure of processing difficulty replicated Fodor and Garrett's finding. Thus, there is good experimental evidence that the deletion of relative pronouns makes comprehension more difficult. All of the investigators cited above attribute this increased difficulty to the loss of surface structure cues to deep structure with the deletion of the pronoun.

    The fact that verbs differ in the number of different structures which they may precede leads to the *verb complexity hypothesis*. There are some verbs (e. g., "cut") in English known as pure transitive verbs, which may be followed by a direct object, but which can never be followed by a sentential complement. By contrast, there are other verbs (e. g., "feel") which may take either a direct object or a complement sentence. Following are three sentences which illustrate differences in the verbs:

    (16)   The woman cut the fabric.

    (17)   The woman felt the fabric.

    (18)   The woman felt the fabric was a bargain.

    Upon receipt of a complex verb such as "feel," the hearer must hypothesize (or predict) two possible predicate structures. A simple verb like "cut," however, necessitates fewer structural hypotheses. According to the verb complexity hypothesis, the prediction is that sentences such as (17) or (18), because their verbs offer more structural alternatives than does the verb of sentence (16), would place more demands on the sentence comprehension process. Experimental support for the verb complexity hypothesis has been reported by Fodor, et al. (1968) and Cutrona (1968).

    The above research strategies illustrate a current trend in psycholinguistics to deal with the kinds of cues in surface structure which facilitate the discovery of information contained in deep structure and, hence, the comprehension of sentences. In contrast with the types of studies discussed earlier in this chapter, this trend also illustrates the move away from psycholinguistic studies that attempt to develop the details of a psychological model of sentence processing directly from the details of generative linguistic theory. This contemporary psycholinguistic approach, although incorporating the concepts of deep structure and surface structure, as well as the concept of linguistic knowledge, stresses the discovery of the language user's strategies for reconstructing deep structure from cues in surface structure; or for creating surface structure from deep structure. This focus is in contrast to the psychological account of grammatical rules such as formed the basis for many of the earlier studies. Another view of this same trend in psycholinguistic research can be seen in the current approach to the study of child language acquisition, which is discussed in the following section.

A Current Perspective on Language Acquisition

The last decade has seen the emergence of a body of literature on language acquisition which has been stimulated by generative linguistic theory and by the cognitive view of language behavior.[2] An introduction to the cognitive approach to language acquisition must include current approaches to the following questions: What is attained when a child acquires language? How does this acquisition take place? What are the research methods for studying language acquisition?

Biological and experiential factors

Elsewhere in this chapter, as well as in Chapter 10, the theoretical differences between linguistic competence and linguistic performance have been explained. Considering the competence-performance distinction, it is assumed that a child must acquire a formal grammar of his language. It is also assumed that he must acquire the psychological processes that allow him to use his linguistic knowledge in the production and comprehension of sentences of his language. Relative to linguistic competence, it is probably more accurate to say that the child must acquire the epistomological (or cognitive) structures which may be described symbolically by the formal grammar of his language.

One of the crucial assumptions of the cognitive approach to language acquisition is that there is a large biological component to language development. This assumption (Lenneberg, 1967) holds that a child is genetically predisposed to develop language, just as he is genetically predisposed to develop upright posture, to use his opposed thumb, and to engage in various types of feeding and sexual behaviors.

---

[2] Earlier research on language acquisition was of two basic types. Many studies simply listed samples of the speech of children, with no attempt at theoretical explanation or analysis (e.g., McCarthy, 1930; Templin, 1957). Another type was generally concerned with the application of the principles of traditional psychological learning theory. This latter approach will be mentioned in the section of this chapter entitled "The Learning Theory Approach."

Recall that in the last chapter the existence of linguistic universals was discussed. Again, linguistic universals are those aspects of language which are common to all the world's languages. For example, all languages have nouns and verbs, consonants and vowels, and subjects and objects. All languages can be described by generative grammars which are organized according to the principles discussed in the preceding chapter. It is assumed that these common properties of language result from the species-specific organization of the human brain. A newborn baby is assumed to possess the neurological organization responsible for the existence of universals of human language. Thus, it can be said that when the human is born, he "knows" the universal features of human language, just as a newborn baby hummingbird "knows" how to build a hummingbird nest.

The genetic predisposition of the human child to acquire language has two major components. One is the child's innate knowledge of linguistic universals. The second is the human child's possession of a set of strategies which enable him to construct a description of his particular language. The two components are certainly not independent. Part of the child's strategy for learning his particular language will involve his analyzing the speech around him into subjects and objects, nouns and verbs, and so on. As he attempts to discover how his particular language is organized, his early hypotheses involve, for example, transformational rules.

Given his genetic predisposition to develop language, a child then experiences the language of his environment and develops competence and performance capabilities that eventually allow him to become an adult speaker-listener within his speech community.

Obviously, the child is typically reared among a group of people who all speak the same language—that is, a group whose members have internalized essentially identical grammars.[3] In his social milieu, then, the child hears many utterances in his native language. The vast majority of those utterances are unique. Many of them are complete sentences, but others are bits and pieces of sentences exchanged in normal conversation. The one thing all the utterances he hears have in common is that underlying them is a common organizational system, or grammar. It is this basic organization that the child must decipher and eventually internalize if he is to be able to construct his own unique well-formed utterances.

Several contemporary theorists have likened the child's task to that of a linguist attempting to construct a generative grammar of a new language.

[3] There is always some individual variation among the grammars of individual speakers in a language community. Some of these differences are dialect-based and as such are studied in sociolinguistics (see the section of this chapter entitled "A Sociolinguistic Approach"). Differences among individual members of a language community, however, are very slight, involving the pronunciation of individual words, the presence or absence of one or two transformational rules, or the use of a particular lexical item. This is what is meant by the term "essentially identical."

This is a good analogy if it is not carried too far. Both the child and the linguist have data (sentences in the language) and both must somehow construct a system of rules which will generate the sentences which are found in these data. Additionally, these rules must generate novel sentences which are grammatical in the language of the speech community. However, the situation of a linguist is much more advantageous than that of the child. For example, the linguist usually has access to a native speaker (*informant*) of the language to whom he can direct questions about what is admissible in that language. Additionally, the linguist typically has assistance in the form of tape recorders, pencil and paper, and the like, for recording his experiences.

The child or infant, by contrast, hears many imperfect, often ill-formed and incomplete sentences, and has no informant nor recording assistance readily at hand. Thus the linguist's data are a great deal more accurate and better organized than are the child's. The child and the linguist both seek to identify the relationship that exists between the data (linguistic examples) and the grammar (the rules which could generate all of the well-formed sentences of the examples and of the language as a whole). Neither of them has available well-defined formulae for deriving the rules of the grammar from the details of the data. Presumably, such rules can only be hypothesized, based upon principles suggested by linguistic universals and principles which appear to be needed in order to generate sentences having the characteristics of sentences in the particular language. As discussed in Chapter 10, the linguist attempts to construct such hypotheses, then to test them upon the intuitions of the native speaker. By the same token, current theories suggest that the development of the infant's grammar is similarly *constructive*, rather than imitative.

The constructive character of the emerging linguistic knowledge of children is demonstrated by the uniqueness of most of their early sentences. Young children produce sentences which are markedly different from those of the adult speech which he hears (e. g., "Why not me careful?"). The most reasonable explanation for these novel utterances is that children construct their sentences not as direct imitations of adult sentences but upon the basis of their own grammars. Although the child's grammar differs from the adult's, it appears that the child's grammar is constantly being modified in the direction of becoming increasingly more complex. Eventually, such increases in complexity result in the child's having an internalized grammar essentially identical to those of the adults in his language community.

We should be careful to note that the claim that the child "forms hypotheses" is almost metaphorical. Neither the form nor the content of children's thought processes are known. However, most researchers agree that the language acquisition processes are largely unconscious in the sense that the child has no explicit knowledge of his language-learning strategies. The unconscious nature of his efforts is another aspect of the process of language acquisition which differentiates the child from the linguist.

It is important to note that as the child is developing language he is also developing a wide variety of other cognitive skills and strategies (Hayes, 1970).

Research methods

The most popular research strategy (e. g., Brown et al., 1969) in the last decade of studying language development has been to record utterances produced by individual children at fixed time intervals. Typically, researchers constructed linguistic descriptions of the child's utterances at each interval. They then compared each linguistic description to those of the same child at different periods and of other children at the same period. Research of this type has demonstrated that it is possible to describe the organization of children's linguistic output using phrase structure rules and transformations very similar to the rules discussed in Chapter 10. If such rules are regarded as only *production* rules describing the child's linguistic output, no theoretical problems ensue. However, if they are regarded as grammars in the sense of being a description of the child's linguistic competence, difficulties arise. It is well known and has been experimentally demonstrated (Brown et al., 1963) that children can understand much more complicated sentences than they can produce. This is also true of adults to some degree; the typical passive vocabulary substantially exceeds the active one. Moreover, in children the production-comprehension gap appears to be much larger than for adults. Since we assume that a speaker's linguistic competence underlies his ability to understand as well as to produce sentences, and since children comprehend more complex sentences than they produce, it follows that the complexity of a child's linguistic competence is not revealed by the sentences which he produces. For this reason, researchers are moving toward investigation of children's comprehension of linguistic structures (Chomsky, 1969; Kessel, 1969; Shipley et al., 1969). A central question is whether developmental stages which characterize language production will correspond to stages in language comprehension.

The preceding remarks may foster the incorrect conclusion that it is more important theoretically to understand the development of linguistic competence than of linguistic performance. The theoretical goal is to understand how the structures of competence interact with the processes of performance. To realize this goal, however, it is necessary to describe competence as fully as possible for the child as well as for the adult. This issue, of course, points to the overall problem of attempting to describe factors of performance as they may exist separate from the details of linguistic rules described in theories of competence. Just as the early psycholinguistic studies attempted to develop a performance model based upon the psychological reality of individual rules of a generative grammar, many studies of child language acquisition have assumed a close correspondence between linguistic rules and performance. As in the move to effect a clearer distinction between psychological descriptions of performance and formal descriptions of competence for the adult, the current trend in theories of child language acquisition incorporates more careful distinctions between competence and performance.

An example of grammatical development

To conclude this section, the stages theorized for the development of negative utterances will be briefly summarized. This topic is treated in great detail by Klima and Bellugi (1966) and McNeill (1970).

When the child first begins to utter words, he appears to do so one word at a time, and is said to be in the *holophrastic* stage of linguistic development. This term is a reflection of the fact that the child's single words seem to represent whole sentences. Thus "shoe" might mean that the child sees a shoe or that he wants his shoe on or off. There is no negation at this stage, with the possible exception of head-shaking.

Following the holophrastic stage, the child begins producing two and sometimes three-word sentences. It is at this time that the first stage of linguistic negation seems to emerge. The negative element, usually "no" but sometimes "not," is simply prefixed or suffixed to the child's short sentence. It is never inserted inside the sentence itself. The child will produce "no me fall," or "me fall no," but never "me no fall." McNeill (1970) states that this first type of negation, referred to as *external sentential negation*, might well be a developmental universal, as there is evidence that Russian, French, and Japanese children all use similar structures in the first stage of negation production.[4]

At a next stage the child moves the negative element into the sentence itself, producing such utterances as "me no fall." New negative elements are also added to the child's repertoire as he begins to use "don't" and "can't" in such sentences as "Me can't fall." An interesting point about "don't" and "can't" at this stage is that the child never uses "do" and "can" without the negative contraction appended to them. Thus "don't" and "can't" at this stage do not have the structure of an auxiliary verb plus a negative element as they do in the adult grammar. Since the child does not use auxiliary verbs ("do" or "can") at this stage, "don't" and "can't" are described as *holistic*

---

[4] It should be noted that Bloom (1970) has a different analysis of those forms which we have referred to as external sentential negation. She claims that the negative element in utterances of this type are "anaphoric," that is, they refer to some previous event (linguistic or otherwise) and do not negate the utterance of which they are a part. While it is unquestionably true that such anaphoric negation does take place, it is the position of most researchers that the majority of negative utterances of this form should be analyzed as external sentential negation.

negative elements in the child's speech. Also, at this stage the child has not yet learned that he should use the article "any" in negative sentences. He generalizes his use of the article "some" to produce sentences such as "I don't want some milk."

At a third stage, the child begins to use auxiliary verbs in his affirmative sentences, so "don't" and "can't" can be analyzed as auxiliary verb plus a negative element as found in the adult grammar. It appears that at this period the child has recognized his error in overgeneralizing his use of "some" and realizes that some sort of negative marker should replace it. He has not, however, mastered the use of "any." This situation results in a short period of the production of double negatives, such as "I don't want no milk." By the fourth stage the child has simple negation well in hand and produces well-formed sentences such as "I don't want any milk."

The development of negation throughout these stages illustrates the step-by-step nature of linguistic development. Most children seem to go through stages similar to those described, although the ages at which individual children occupy each stage varies widely. The preceding examples also demonstrate the constructive nature of grammatical development; children produce linguistic structures which they never hear. It is clear also that children do differ from adults both in terms of the internalized grammar which they construct and in the performance rules by which they produce sentences. The exact nature of these differences is a major topic for research.

THE LEARNING THEORY APPROACH

The traditional psychological views of linguistic performance, particularly prior to the advent of the cognitive approach, incorporated extensions of the basic concepts of learning theory. Such concepts are used to explain how man acquires new patterns of behavior, and language is treated as one of these patterns. In contrast to the cognitive view, man is not seen as having any special inborn inclination to speak; he is seen simply as a superior learner. If learning capacity is taken as the key factor underlying language capability, then it is logical to assume that any psychological theory of language will also be a learning theory. Thus researchers who take this point of view turn to learning theory for their hypotheses about verbal behavior, and their objective is to characterize the capabilities of the language user in terms of the concepts of human learning.

Learning theory views of verbal behavior are based upon research which follows the behavioristic or mediational approaches in psychological studies. As will be discussed, some of these theories attempt to say as much as possible about verbal behavior but at the same time try to avoid generalizations about anything that is not susceptible to observation, manipulation, and measurement under laboratory conditions. No matter what position a person takes regarding a theory of linguistic performance, it is important to know the contrast between the cognitive and learning theory views to be able to understand the issues that are reported in the research literature.

Learning Theory: Some Early Views

Some of the early approaches to theories of human learning are helpful as a basis for understanding how learning theory has been expanded to incorporate linguistic performance. We can only superficially review several of these early approaches. However, the student with detailed interest in learning theory can find copious literature on the topic elsewhere (e. g., Dixon and Horton, 1968).

Classical conditioning

As shown in Figure 11-1, classical conditioning describes a situation where some formerly neutral stimulus (the conditioned stimulus) comes to elicit a response (the conditioned response) that approximates the response to another stimulus (the unconditioned stimulus). In simplest terms, the learning process is described as follows: The unconditioned stimulus is assumed to be some object or event that is already known to elicit a particular pattern of response. A well-known example is Pavlov's use of meat powder as the unconditioned stimulus to elicit a dog's salivation as the unconditioned response. The repeated presentation of an additional stimulus (e. g., a light or bell) either preceding or simultaneous with the presentation of the meat powder results in the new stimulus becoming a conditioned stimulus, with the ability to elicit salivation even when the meat powder is not present. Learning (*or conditioning*) in this case can be viewed as a process of stimulus substitution. What was formerly a neutral stimulus comes to elicit the response which was essentially the same as that evoked by the unconditioned (original) stimulus. In this sense the formerly neutral stimulus becomes conditioned.

The situation depicted in Figure 11-1 also provides the basis for discussing further variables that can be studied in the classical conditioning process. For example, if bell ringing were the conditioned stimulus, the experimenter could study whether variations in the type of ringing or even the ringing of

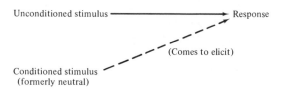

Figure 11-1   A diagram of classical conditioning.

bells with different tone quality would elicit the same conditioned response; this is the study of *stimulus generalization*. The opposite of this is the study of *stimulus discrimination*. If the dog salivated as a conditioned response to one bell but not to another, he would be discriminating among the stimuli. Another aspect involves *reinforcement*, the reward which comes from the stimulus-response association. In this example, meat powder is the reward.

Instrumental conditioning

In contrast to classical conditioning, instrumental conditioning puts the emphasis upon response conditions rather than upon stimulus conditions. This type of conditioning is described as follows (Figure 11-2): The organism is placed in a stimulus situation where a variety of responses ($R_1 \ldots R_4$) might occur. Suppose that the organism is a hungry rat and the stimulus situation is a cage containing a feeding apparatus which can be activated by the rat pressing on a lever. The rat's hunger is regarded as *internal stimulation;* this is the motivational aspect of the situation. The rat may make a variety of responses—e. g., running, scratching, squealing, toying with the lever. These are *emitted responses* (or *operants*), rather than responses which are particularly elicited (as in classical conditioning) by the experimenter. Eventually the rat will find that one of these responses (i. e., lever pressing) will lead to his receiving a morsel of food. Under these conditions such a response (e. g., R_2) is said to be rewarded (or *reinforced*) because it is appropriate to a need state. The consequence is that the rewarded response will increase in frequency over the other responses; this response is said to be a learned *instrumental* response. It is also possible to consider instrumental conditioning from a non-reward or even from a *punishment* point of view. Emitted responses which result in no reward or in some type of punishment (e. g., electrical shock) will decrease in frequency or simply be avoided.

Both classical and instrumental conditioning have been useful in portraying aspects of learning behavior. Moreover, it is not difficult to envisage examples of their general application to verbal behavior. For example, the pairing of the word "water" with the presentation of a glass of water over a period of time would lead to a case of stimulus substitution. That is, by classical

Figure 11-2   A diagram of instrumental conditioning.

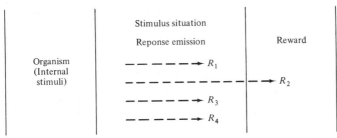

Stimulus situation

Reponse emission

Reward

Organism
(Internal
stimuli)

R_1

R_2

R_3

R_4

conditioning, it is predicted that the word "water" would come to stimulate response in the organism similar to those responses stimulated by the water itself. Similarily, learning theorists believe that instrumental conditioning can account for a person's calling for "water" in a general condition where he is thirsty. It is easy under laboratory conditions to demonstrate examples of classical or instrumental conditioning involving words or sounds as stimuli or responses, or to demonstrate phenomena of stimulus discrimination or generalization. Such experiments, however, are limited to relatively simple verbal materials in highly-structured learning situations. This type of verbal learning behavior lacks the *constructive* characteristics of human language acquisition. Another important point is that the foregoing learning models constrain the researcher to only theorize about that which he can directly manipulate and observe under rigorously controlled conditions.

Skinner's Operant Conditioning Theory

Some of the best-known applications of instrumental conditioning as a theory of verbal behavior are associated with the work of Skinner (1957). He argues that the greatest shortcomings in prior attempts to create adequate theories of verbal behavior has been the consequence of trying to describe internal states of cognitive or meaning behavior in man. Skinner argues for a theoretical framework which will accommodate an interaction of observable stimulus and response relationships in the description of verbal behavior. His theorizing represents the attempt to do this while staying within the methodological constraints of behaviorism.

Framework of the theory

The theoretical framework which Skinner proposes for analysis of the verbal act is the paradigm for instrumental conditioning, which was shown in Figure 11-2. Only here, a *verbal* response that is emitted and reinforced in a particular stimulus situation will eventually lead to the emission of the same response in future cases of the same stimulus situation. Such a response, in Skinner's theory, is called a *verbal operant*. We picture the initiating organism (Speaker) to be in some motivational state. In Skinner's conception, this state can range all the way from physical needs (e. g., thirst, hunger) to a generalized social need of simply gaining approval or avoiding disapproval. The discriminative stimulus or stimuli in the situation are phenomena relevant to satisfaction of this motivational state. For example, the speaker is thirsty; relevant stimuli (discriminative) are the presence of water and someone to provide him a glass of it. The verbal operant is the request for water. A more subtle situation might involve a mother speaking a word to her child. Both the mother and her utterance are discriminative stimuli. The need state is the child's motivation to gain approval from his mother. The operant could be the child's repetition of the word. Reinforcement is provided by the mother's overt approval (e. g., smile) of the repetition. In contexts such as these, language usage is viewed by Skinner as a conditioned response in a verbal situation. In the course of language development the language user will gain a repertoire of such responses, or verbal operants, as a function of his conditioning history. The elaboration of Skinner's theory entails the description of the types of operants and eventually their complex manifestation as verbal behavior.

Verbal operants

Skinner divides operants into classes in terms of how each represents some basic functional form of response. He has coined original terms to name some of these classes. Some verbal operants function directly as a consequence of the need state of the organism; in fact it is useful to note that such operants specify their reinforcement. Skinner calls these operants, *mands* (consider the similarity to the word command). Such utterances as questions, requests, and the like, are examples of mands. Whereas the mand is an utterance that has a close relation with its reinforcement, a *tact* operant is closely related to its stimulus. A tact is an utterance that is conditioned by reinforcement during co-occurrence with a particular object or event, or a property of an object or an event, as a stimulus. That a child has been conditioned to utter "ball" when a ball is a stimulus is an example of tact conditioning. It is misleading to say that a tact "refers to" a stimulus; no such implication is intended in Skinner's definition. Instead, a tact is a response that simply has a high probability of occurrence solely as a function of conditioning with particular features of the controlling stimulus. Like the tact, the *echoic, textual*, and *intraverbal* operants are responses controlled by particular features of external stimuli. Whereas the tact is considered as a response to an object or event, or features of same, echoic, textural, and intraverbal operants are responses to verbal stimuli. Echoic behavior occurs when the response is a sound pattern approximating an acoustic stimulus. In textural behavior the response is under the control of some nonauditory verbal stimulus. Reading aloud would be an example of this type of response behavior. Intraverbal operants are verbal responses highly associated with some verbal stimulus in sequence, as when saying "Washington," and this has a high probability of being followed by "D.C."

Operants and the language user

What we have discussed so far has centered upon a relationship between individual stimulus conditions and individual response behaviors. Little has been said about the contributions, if any, of the human in these situations.

The definition of the basic operants does seem to lessen the contribution of the human speaker, other than his being the locus of the individual stimulus-response relationships. However, if we were to consider verbal behavior solely in terms of individual operants, we would not be able to explain much of the verbal behavior we witness in our everyday lives. Most human discourse comprises complex production sequences as well as often lengthy periods of nearly continuous perception. It is difficult indeed to conceive of any but the most rudimentary situations of verbal behavior which can be adequately described in terms of a simple operant.

Skinner explains that typical verbal behavior is a combination of operants, and that operants are only the "raw material out of which sustained verbal behavior is manufactured" (p. 312). The role of the speaker emerges when we consider him as the center of a complex interaction among stimulus variables, listener variables, and his own conditioning history. In short, it is the organism that is the synthesizer of the multiple causal and response variables that make up so many of the everyday situations of verbal behavior.

Although we have only been able to sketch a few of the main points of Skinner's theory, the form of the theory has been accurately portrayed. In brief, this theory attempts to identify situations in which particular types of verbal behavior may be described, predicted, or even manipulated. It is important to see, however, that the types of verbal behavior compatible with operant conditioning theory show very little correspondence with any of the details of linguistic theory. All types of verbal behavior in Skinner's theory are defined relative to their stimulation conditions; they are never defined in terms of particular linguistic units. Accordingly, there is no productive relation between the details of linguistic theory and the details of Skinner's theory. The lack of such a relationship, as well as the shortcomings of behaviorism, were the topic of an essay-review of Skinner's theory (Chomsky, 1959) which outlined many of the fundamental distinctions between traditional learning theory approaches to verbal behavior, and the philosophy and objectives of the cognitive view.

A Mediational Theory

The main distinction between behavioristic and mediational theories is that the mediational approach makes theoretical statements about the internal states of the organism. This type of theoretical account depends upon inferring the existence of internal states from what is observed in overt stimulus-response relationships. One mediational account of verbal behavior that is frequently encountered in the research literature is Osgood's (1963) *representational mediation* process.

Representation-mediation hypothesis

A major premise of Osgood's theory is that organisms are capable of a specialized type of internal behavior called *sign-behavior*. In general terms, signs are stimuli which come to "stand for" other stimuli. Figure 11-3 illustrates how Osgood represents a mediational account of sign behavior. For purposes of discussion, consider an example where meat powder and a bell are the unconditioned stimulus and the conditioned stimulus, respectively. This situation fits readily into the diagram presented above. As an unconditioned stimulus, the powder ($\dot{S}$) elicits a pattern of total behavior (R_t)—e. g., attention, hunger, wanting to eat, and so on. After conditioning, the formerly neutral stimulus ($\boxed{S}$), the bell, now comes to elicit a response (R_x) that is somehow related to the original response (R_t). A main point in Osgood's theory, as contrasted with classical conditioning, is that the response (R_x) to the conditioned stimulus need only be a part of the original response (R_t). What Osgood proposes is that the initial response (r_m) to the stimulus ($\boxed{S}$) is internal behavior "detached" from the original total response (R_t). This internal behavior, called a *mediating reaction* (r_m), is conceived as an increment of the total behavior (R_t) elicited by the unconditioned stimulus.

Unconditioned stimulus   Total response

Conditioned stimulus   Response

Mediating   Self
reaction   stimulation

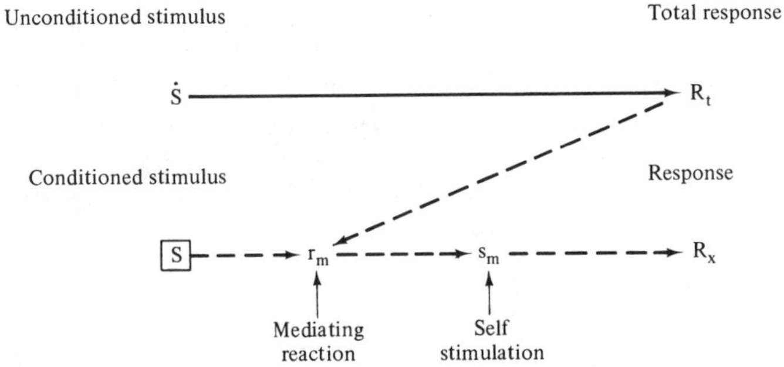

Figure 11-3   The representation—mediation process. [*From C. E. Osgood, G. J. Suci, and P. H. Tannenbaum,* The Measurement of Meaning (*Urbana, Ill.: University of Illinois Press, 1957*), *p. 7. (Reprinted by permission of the authors and the publisher.*]

This internal mediating reaction (r_m) then leads to an internal stimulus (s_m) which produces an overt response (R_x). Osgood describes the initial response (r_m) as *representational* of some total response behavior. The basis for such representation is in the conception that r_m is some increment of R_t (hence the arrow from R_t to r_m). Because of this representational quality, Osgood proposes that this mediating behavior serves as a basis for the symbolizing process. Hence, the conditioned stimulus ($\boxed{S}$) is taken as a *sign* of the unconditioned stimulus because it prompts, in the organism, an internalized response which is an increment of the external response which would result if the unconditioned stimulus were indeed present. In formal terms this is how the bell comes to "represent" the meat powder. Osgood (1963, p. 740) states the representational-mediational hypothesis as follows:

> Whenever some originally neutral stimulus (sign-to-be), S, is repeated contiguous with another stimulus (significate), $\dot{S}$, which regularly and reliably elicits a particular pattern of total behavior, R_t, the neutral stimulus will become associated with some portion, r_m, of this total behavior as a representational-mediational process.

As in the previous examples, it is not hard to imagine how the learning of a word would be explained in terms of Osgood's representation-mediation process. Suppose, for example, that the unconditioned stimulus ($\dot{S}$) were an apple and the response to this (R_t) is the totality of all of a person's reactions upon perceiving a real apple. During the process of sign-learning, the organism becomes aware of the association between the word "apple" as a sign ($\boxed{S}$) and its association with the referent known as an apple. The representational-mediational hypothesis attempts to explain the meaning of the word "apple" by assuming that, as a response to the word, there is an internal mediating reaction (r_m) that represents some internal increment of overall behavior to apples. In turn, this mediating reaction is capable of producing an internal stimulus (S_m) which in turn elicits some type of overt response in the organism. The overt response might be the disposition to ask for an apple, reaching out for it, and so on.

A three-stage mediation-integration model

In subsequent theorizing, Osgood (1963) incorporated the basic representation-mediation process within a three-stage mediational model of the human learner. It is this model that has been Osgood's main basis for theorizing about linguistic performance.

As shown in Figure 11-4, the three stages of this model postulate three different types or levels of association which may take place in the organism between stimulus inputs and response outputs. The first of these stages, the *projection* level, represents the kinds of involuntary stimulus-response behaviors that are assumed to be innate. For example, if a hot stove is a stimulus and your hand touches it, the jerking away of your hand is an unlearned response. A second level of association between stimulus and response behaviors is one Osgood conceives as comprising learned stimulus-response relationships; this is called the *integrational* level. An example of association on the integrational level would be if someone yells "duck" at you, and you immediately ducked. Although at some time it was necessary for you to learn a response to "duck," it is so well known that you can respond almost unconsciously. Finally, Osgood envisages a third level of association as the representation-mediation process which has already been discussed. This is the most flexible level of association between stimulus inputs and response outputs. It is on this level that meaning presumably exists.

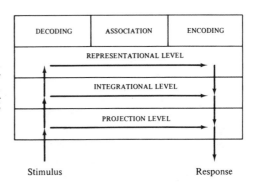

Figure 11-4 Three-stage model. [*After C. E. Osgood, "On understanding and creating sentences,"* Amer. Psychol., *18 (1963), 740. Copyright 1963 by the American Psychological Association. Reproduced by permission.*]

When considering the three-stage model as a description of verbal behavior, Osgood posits a dynamic relation among the three levels just discussed. The process of *decoding*, for example, would involve first the organism's sensing a stimulus on the projection level. This stimulus internally elicits highly learned verbal responses on the integrational level. Finally, these internal verbal responses stimulate meaning on the representational level. Similarily, the process of *encoding* involves an intended message as meaning initially existing on the representational level. This meaning stimulates verbal encoding units on the integrational level, and these in turn stimulate the movement of the speech articulators on the projection level.

Although a detailed discussion of Osgood's three-stage model as it applies to verbal behavior is beyond the scope of this chapter, we can summarize several of the main points here. For one thing, as already implied, the projection, integrational, and representational levels of association are meant to represent different internal stages of human verbal behavior. Thus, for example, the projection level is where one could incorporate the operation of the auditory mechanism as well as the neural mechanism of the speech articulators. The integrational level, by contrast, would incorporate one's knowledge of his language, or in learning theory terms, his verbal habits. As already discussed in some detail, the representational level is a theoretical account of the meaning component in verbal behavior. According to Osgood's theorizing, verbal units are "meaningless" until they are interpreted on the representational level. He speculates that the immediate relation between form and meaning in decoding is when *word* units are meaningless stimulus inputs on the integration level but become meaningful responses on the representational level. What we have then is a picture of the organism which says that linguistic performance on the projection and integrational levels consists of behavioral mechanisms and skill processes dealing with the stimuli of expression. On the representational level, by contrast, the organism is dealing with meaning.

Arguments Concerning the Learning Theory Approach

Although this section has not presented an exhaustive review of learning theory models of language acquisition and use, it has described the general form of such theories. Mediational accounts, of which Osgood's theory is an example, have also been put forth by a number of theorists (see esp., Jenkins, 1965; Braine, 1963). Mediational theories represent the most elaborate attempts to apply learning models as a theory of linguistic performance. At the same time, however, even the most elaborate learning theory represents a fundamentally different view of verbal behavior than that found in the cognitive approach. In short, if it is not already apparent, the learning theory and cognitive views of language behavior are drastically different schools of thought on the nature of linguistic performance.

Close to the heart of the differences between these approaches is whether linguistic knowledge shall be formally represented in performance models as internalized response sequences (akin to learned verbal skills) or as a competence component (linguistic knowledge describable by generative grammar). The former requires the assumption that verbal skills can be conditioned from environmental experiences—that is, that they are patterned from units of external experience. The cognitive view requires the assumption that the human organism is biologically endowed with a capacity to develop a grammar.

Even closer to the heart of the differences are the assumptions which one makes about the nature of linguistic knowledge itself. That is, apart from whether it is best represented as mediational skill sequences or a competence component, what is it that one has to know in order to create and understand sentences? The answer to this question is one of the fundamental assumptions of generative linguistic theory, and consequently, fundamental to the cognitive approach to performance theory. A grammar is what one has to know in order to perform the processes of sentence creation and comprehension. By contrast, in learning theory accounts, it is the answer to this question that is an immediate focus for study. What environmental experiences cause a child to become conditioned so as to have the skills for sentence processing? The answer is sought in the conditioning operation: What external phenomena become internalized as verbal skills?

If one accepts the generative theory of language, there is little alternative to espousing the cognitive approach to the study of performance. This is because most of what is postulated about grammar within generative theory is very difficult, if not impossible, to explain by a learning theory. For example, a concept such as deep structure cannot be identified with environmental experiences that could become internalized through conditioning processes. Nor, for another example, can one easily explain, within a learning theory account, how a child comes to associate deep and surface structures. Even a child's capacity for differentiating the phonetic features from the total acoustic spectrum of speech stimuli is an extremely challenging matter for the learning theory viewpoint.

On a less abstract and more practical level, much of what we can observe and deduce about the natural aspects of child language acquisition belies a learning theory explanation. As already discussed, children seldom utter things exactly as they hear them. Most child utterances, being structurally different from those of the adult, show a definite *constructive* quality as compared with an *imitative* quality which would be most symptomatic of a learning theory account. Moreover, learning theory analyses must incorporate reinforcement as a factor in conditioning. Systematic observation (e. g., Brown and Hanlon, 1970) shows that parents typically reward their children for accurate (i. e., "true") utterances, even if these utterances are ungrammatical from the point of view of adult grammar. This is in addition to the fact that much of the language that a child hears is grammatically imperfect or incomplete in the first place. Finally, there is the most practical argument (Miller, 1965) that children know almost infinitely more language by the age of five years than would ever be possible to experience, let alone be conditioned to use, in their short lives.

Most research which is supportive of the learning theory view, as previously mentioned, has involved the acquisition of very simple verbal units. Although these studies are typically quite accurate in their accounts of learning under such very restricted conditions, it is the generalization of this account to the language acquisition process as a whole that is most suspect. The brief history of the development of the cognitive approach to linguistic performance and the generative theory of linguistic competence is filled with lengthy and detailed arguments between cognitive theorists and learning theorists. Although it should be obvious that the sympathies of the present authors lie with the cognitive approach, the interested reader is urged to explore in more detail the discussions available in the psycholinguistic literature. Most of the major papers on the issue can be found in such collections as edited by De-Cecco (1967), Jakobovits and Miron (1967), and Dixon and Horton (1968).

A SOCIOLINGUISTIC APPROACH[5]

In much of the research into language behavior that has been discussed so far, the attempt has been to make generalizations that transcend individual speaker differences. Such differences are assumed to be negligible when one is attempting to draw generalizations about the language of a speech community or the language processes in the human species. By contrast, however, there are formal lines of study into the nature of individual differences among speakers of the same language. There is, for example, a rich research tradition in the area of *dialectology* (see Allen and Underwood, 1971) in which intra-language variations are the subject of linguistic study. This tradition has been more linguistically than psychologically or sociologically oriented. Recently there has evolved a more social-psychological, or *sociolinguistic*, approach which focuses upon linguistic variations within speech communities, and which attempts to relate such variation to social variables. In somewhat the same way that psycholinguistics represents a working combination of the tools of the psychologist and linguist, research of this type illustrates a combination of the tools of sociologist and linguist. Characteristic of this new line of research are the urban language studies (Labov, 1966; Shuy et al., 1967, 1968; Wolfram, 1969) conducted in the United States.

Urban Language Research

Essentially, the task in urban language research has been to find relationships between linguistic variations and social variables. The concept of *free* or *random* variation of phonetic features serves as a useful introduction to the types of linguistic variables studied in this research. Free variation is that aspect of phonetic variation that cannot be predicted upon the basis of phonologic context. Such variation is assumed to vary randomly and is thus uninteresting for any type of linguistic generalizations. In contemporary research into urban dialects, however, free variation has typically been a focus for study. This is because much of what has been relegated to free variation can be accounted for in terms of social variables relating to the speaker, his social group, and the nature of the speech situation. In the theoretical view, the interest is not so much upon only the language found in urban areas, as it is that urban areas have social stratification, and such

---

[5] As the heading of this section implies, there are several approaches that mark sociolinguistic study. The approach reviewed here was selected because of its generality to most types of sociolinguistic inquiries, and because it introduces the contrast between socially conditioned and linguistically conditioned variation. For other viewpoints on sociolinguistics see Fishman (1968) or Ervin-Tripp (1969).

stratification has its correlates in differences in verbal behavior. In these studies, social stratification refers to group differences in terms of such social variables as income, education, occupation, dwelling area, and the like.

Several characteristics illustrate the major contrast between urban language research and more traditional approaches in linguistic research. For one thing, this research has incorporated procedures for gathering representative samples of social variables as well as associated linguistic variables. Social variables, such as those already mentioned, are used to define samples of socially stratified and often ethnically different populations. Groups of informants are selected because they are representative of larger segments of the population. So too are situations of speech sampled. Here it is presumed that under specifically designated speech conditions, the language usually used by a particular segment of the population in those situations can be elicited.

Language is sampled in regard to identification of the *linguistic variable* and its *variation*. The linguistic variable is a definition of the particular linguistic feature to be studied. Its variation is a definition of the differences expected for that feature relative to differences in speech situations, speakers, or both. For example, the -ing [ŋ] ending is often pronounced as -in [n] in informal speech situations. The variable in this case would be the /ŋ/ phoneme and the variation would be articulations varying between [n] and [ŋ]. Behavior involving this variation would be studied by sampling groups of people whose speech may be characteristic of one or the other or both of these variations and also sampling situations in which these different phonetic realizations are predicted to occur.

A further characteristic of research of this type is the use of quantitative data. Whereas the traditional linguist is more interested in making qualitative types of decisions, the urban language researcher typically deals with frequency data. It is usually the case, for example, that the realization of the /ŋ/ phoneme does not vary *totally* one way or the other relative to variation in the speech situation or the speaker. In this example, it would be the relative frequency of using [n] or [ŋ] under different conditions that would be the index of differences. Thus it is necessary for the urban language researcher to observe a variety of instances where the predicted linguistic variation is expected to occur, then to tabulate the frequency of such occurrence in order to make the comparisons among groups of people, different situations, or both. This approach to quantification is another contribution of the sociological aspect of this research. Frequency data, when gathered on samples of people and situations, can be incorporated into the use of inferential statistics which allow findings, based upon samples, to be tested for generality relative to statements about the populations from which the samples were drawn. Some samples of research of this type will be next discussed.

Pronunciation of /r/ in New York City

Among a number of features of New York City speech studied by Labov (1966), the pronunciation of /r/ was hypothesized to correlate with the social stratification of speakers from the city. More specifically, the hypothesis was (p. 64): "If any two subgroups of New York City speakers are ranked in a scale of social stratification, then they will be ranked in the same order by their differential use of /r/." In this case, the linguistic variable /r/ had a defined variation between a (usual) pronunciation as [r], as against an unconstricted glide, lengthening of vowels, or no phonetic representation.

As an initial test of this hypothesis, Labov obtained samples of the pronunciation of /r/ from sales personnel in three large Manhattan department stores representative of the top, middle, and bottom of the fashion and price scales. The assumption underlying this choice was that the employees of a store attempt to share in the status of the clientele and will therefore emulate the speech of the store's customers rather than the speech of New York sales persons in general. The speech situation was thus defined as the type of speech expected in these different stores.

Labov gathered his speech samples by visiting the stores in the guise of a customer. Upon encountering a sales person he would ask for the location of a store item which he knew to be located on the fourth floor. Accordingly, when he was answered by a clerk, this elicited the utterance "fourth floor" in a natural conversational style. He then typically followed the sales person's reply with the question "Excuse me?" to elicit the same reply but in a stressed utterance. The four occurrences of /r/ in the typical responses of the clerk uttering "fourth floor" served as the realizations of the linguistic variable. These data were then divided into the [r] and non-[r] categories mentioned earlier. The results revealed a stratification of the pronunciation of /r/ similar to the social stratification of the department stores. The employees of the highest ranked store also were ranked highest in their use of /r/ pronounced as [r] in both casual and emphatic situations. Speech from the lower status stores had, by contrast, a relatively greater incidence of non-[r] pronunciations. This evidence then tended to confirm the thesis that certain detailed variations in the pronunciation of /r/ could be predicted on the basis of social stratification. In a more traditional linguistic view these variations in pronunciation would be relegated to free variation. Here, however, it could be seen that the variation was predictable from social factors.

In a more formal study of variations in New York speech, Labov (1966) again included /r/ among other phonologic variables. In this case, speech was elicited in linguistic interviews which were manipulated to gain speech samples under conditions of casual speech, careful speech, and particularly careful speech as elicited from a word list. This was an attempt to vary the circumstances of speech so as to elicit language variations according to

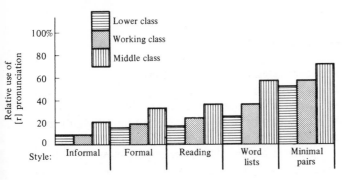

Figure 11-5 Variations of /r/ pronunciation in New York City. [After W. Labov, The Social Stratification of English in New York City (Arlington, Va.: Center for Applied Linguistics, 1966), p. 222. Copyright W. Labov. Reprinted by permission of the author and the publisher.]

stylistic differences. The speakers in this study were a sample drawn from the New York City population, identified along lines of a sociologic study done in the city several years earlier. In the description of each person who served as an informant, a particular variable of interest was a social status index based upon factors of occupation, income, and education. These factors enabled Labov to divide his speakers into categories defined as lower class, working class, and middle class. Casual speech was identified, for example, as that speech obtained during informal sessions of an interview. Careful speech was identified as that elicited in the formal interview situation where the speaker realized that his language was being recorded for subsequent study. Additionally, there were situations where speech was obtained while reading aloud continuous text, where the speaker was reading aloud lists of individual words, and where some of these words represented minimal pairs (e. g., "bared-bad"). Presumably these latter conditions represented increasingly careful speech. Figure 11-5 illustrates the results of the study of the /r/ variable.

The vertical continuum represents the relative degree to which /r/ was pronounced as [r]; the horizontal continuum differentiates styles. Note, for example, that in informal speech the speakers from all classes had less than a 20% relative frequency of [r] pronunciation, but that this increased as speech ranged from informal to formal, and also increased from the condition of reading aloud to the articulation of words in lists, and to minimum pairs. Note also, that the middle class had a generally higher use of [r] than the other groups, and that this difference had generality across speech styles. It can also be seen here how quantitative data are used in a sociolinguistic study. Unlike a more traditional phonological analysis of the speech in this case, there is a concern with the relative frequency of the phonetic realizations of /r/. Social class differences did not involve a total contrast in terms of the articulation of /r/; instead this was in terms of the relative frequency of usage.

489

An Example from Detroit Speech

A sociolinguistic project conducted by Shuy and his colleagues (Shuy et al., 1967) involved gathering language samples from a population sample of approximately 700 residents in the city of Detroit. Similar to Labov's research, this sample of informants was drawn according to sociological criteria. Social status of the informants was classified so as to form the basis for defining four groups: upper- and lower-middle class and upper- and lower-working class. Language samples were gathered in interview situations located in the informants' homes. Among many linguistic variables available for study within the context of the overall investigation, was the occurrence of *multiple negation*, such as found in the utterance "He can't hit nobody." As reasoned in this research, grammatical variations such as multiple negation are thought to be socially stratified in the urban population. That is, the higher the person's social status the less multiple negation will be observed. In this case, multiple negation is treated as a linguistic variable, and its occurrence as against nonoccurrence is treated as the linguistic continuum.

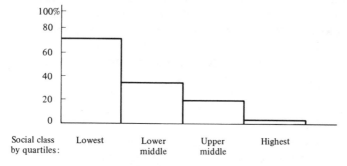

Figure 11-6 Use of multiple negation in Detroit adult speech. [*After R. W. Shuy, "Linguistic correlates of social stratification in Detroit speech,"* U.S. Office of Education Cooperative Research Project No. 6-1347, *Michigan State Univ.*]

Figure 11-6 summarizes the relationship found between the relative frequency of multiple negation found in adult language samples and the different social status groups with which the adults were identified. These results clearly indicate that as one moves (left to right in Figure 11-6) from the speech of the lowest class group to that of the highest class group, the incidence of multiple negation has a corresponding and substantial decrease.

It should be noted in passing that all of the linguistic variables studied in urban language research do not have the clear-cut correlation as shown in the last two figures. There are a number of variables both in the research by Labov and by Shuy that show only a slight contrast or even no contrast across different social classes. A further note is that some of the variation in urban language studies has its source in ethnic differences rather than, or in addition to, social stratification. For example, in most major cities of the United States, different ethnic groups exercise particular dialects of English. Hence, in addition to the variables of social stratification, one finds a number of subcultural and ethnic group variables which will also account for linguistic variation.

Attitudinal Correlates of Language Features

Urban language research has also incorporated some investigation of how social class differences in language features may serve as cues in a person's impressions of, general attitudes toward, or expectations of a speaker. It stands to reason that if certain features of language are socially stratified, then these features should serve as cues as to a person's social status. Research by Labov (1966) as well as by Shuy and his colleagues (Shuy et al., 1969) illustrate this type of investigation.

Labov, for example, took selected phonological variables from his New York City study, transcribed them into individual recorded segments, then presented them to listeners who were asked to judge a suitable occupation for the person whose speech they had heard. As anticipated, listeners typically assigned speech samples to occupations that were socially stratified in ways similar to the status of original speakers. For example, the pronunciation of /r/ as [r] would be associated with a "television personality," whereas the alternative form of this linguistic variable (e. g., [ə]) was associated with occupations such as "factory worker."

In Detroit research, brief (roughly 30 sec) tape samples of speech were presented to individuals who answered questions about the likely social status of the speakers. On the average, approximately 30 % of speakers from the upper-middle class group were correctly identified by listeners. By contrast, some 41 % of the upper-working class speakers and 61 % of the lower-working class speakers were correctly identified with their original groups. One generalization drawn by Shuy and his colleagues was that the cues for social class identification were probably more in the direction of grammatical or phonetic nonstandardizations that marked lower social status, rather than any types of speech cues which marked higher status.

The notion of linguistic variation being related to the social prestige of speech has been described by Stewart (1965) as the differentiation between *basilect* (low prestige) and *acrolect* (high prestige). Presumably most persons' speech varies somewhere within this continuum. Moreover, this continuum not only can be found in the social stratification of linguistic variables, but seems also to exist in listeners' attitudes. That is, the above studies indicate that the social stratification of linguistic variables exists not only in speech behavior, but in peoples' attitudes and expectations associated with variations in speech behavior. Such attitudes, as well as the notion of a linguistic continuum varying between basilect and acrolect, have their bases in social values rather than linguistic ones. That is to say, it is because of social values, not objective linguistic criteria, that one dialect becomes more prestigious than another. Linguists have long argued that no language is really more "complex" than another (Williams, 1970).

Prospects for Sociolinguistics

Because sociolinguistics is a relatively new and burgeoning area of research, we lack a sufficient body of knowledge to suggest major theory. Even within the existing knowledge there is considerable inconsistency in assumptions, research strategies, and terminology. On the other hand, one emerging benefit of sociolinguistic research activities is that they are attracting the joint cooperation of linguists, psycholinguists, sociologists, anthropologists, and speech scientists in several problem areas. This is not to claim that sociolinguistics is the wave of the future in language research but that there are many language researchers who are coming to hold major expectations about its development.

REFERENCES

ALLEN, H. A. and UNDERWOOD, G. N. 1971. (eds.) *Readings in American Dialectology*. New York: Appleton-Century-Crofts.

BEVER, T. G., LACKNER, J. and KIRK, R. 1969. The underlying structure sentence is the primary unit of speech perception. *Percept. Psychophys.* 5: 225–34.

BLOOM, L. 1970. *Language Development: Form and Function in Emerging Grammars*. Cambridge, Mass.: M.I.T. Press.

BLUMENTHAL, A. L. 1967. Prompted recall of sentences. *J. Verbal Learning Verbal Behav.* 6: 203–6.

BLUMENTHAL, A. L. and BOAKES, R. 1967. Prompted recall of sentences. *J. Verbal Learning Verbal Behav.* 6: 674–76.

BRAINE, M. D. S. 1963. On learning the grammatical order of words. *Psychol. Rev.* 70: 332–48.

BROWN, R., and HANLON, C. 1970. Derivational complexity and the order of acquisition in child speech. *In* John R. Hayes (ed.). *Cognition and the Development of Language*. New York: John Wiley & Sons, Inc. Reprinted in Roger Brown (ed.). 1970. *Psycholinguistics*. New York: The Free Press.

BROWN, R., CAZDEN, C. and BELLUGI, U. 1969. The child's grammar from I to III. *In* John P. Hill (ed.). *Second Annual Minnesota Symposium on Child Psychology*.

Reprinted in Roger Brown (ed.). 1970. *Psycholinguistics.* New York: The Free Press.

BROWN, R., FRASER, C. and BELLUGI, U. 1963. Control of grammar in imitation, comprehension, and production. *J. Verbal Learning Verbal Behav.* 2: 121–35. Reprinted in Roger Brown (ed.). 1970. *Psycholinguistics.* New York: The Free Press.

CAIRNS, H. S. 1971. Ambiguous sentence processing. Paper presented at the Midwestern Psychological Association Convention.

CHOMSKY, C. S. 1969. *The Acquisition of Syntax in Children from 5 to 10.* Cambridge, Mass.: M.I.T. Press.

CHOMSKY, N. 1959. A review of B. F. Skinner's *Verbal Behavior, Language.* Reprinted in J. A. Fodor and J. J. Katz (eds.). 1964. *The Structure of Language: Readings in the Philosophy of Language.* Englewood Cliffs, N.J.: Prentice-Hall, Inc.

CUTRONA, L. J., JR. 1968. Preliminary investigation of a forced-choice sentence construction task. Unpublished manuscript.

DeCECCO, J. P. 1967. (ed.). *The Psychology of Language, Thought, and Instruction.* New York: Holt, Rinehart and Winston, Inc.

DIXON, T. R. and HORTON, D. L. 1968. *Verbal Behavior and General Behavior Theory.* Englewood Cliffs, N.J.: Prentice-Hall, Inc.

EPSTEIN, W. 1969. Recall of word lists following learning of sentences and of anomalous and random strings. *J. Verbal Learning Verbal Behav.* 8: 20–25.

ERVIN-TRIPP, S. 1969. *Sociolinguistics. In* L. Berkowitz (ed.). *Advances in Experimental Social Psychology.* Vol. 4. New York: Academic Press.

FISHMAN, J. A. 1968. (ed.). *Readings in the Sociology of Language.* The Hague: Mouton.

FODOR, J. and BEVER, T. 1965. The psychological reality of linguistic segments. *J. Verbal Learning Verbal Behav.* 4: 414–21.

FODOR, J. A. and GARRETT, M. 1967. Some syntactic determinants of sentential complexity. *Percept. Psychophys.* 2: 289–96.

FODOR, J. A., GARRETT, M. and BEVER, T. 1968. Some syntactic determinants of complexity. II: Verb structure. *Percept. Psychophys.* 3: 453–61.

FOSS, D. J. and CAIRNS, H. S. 1970. Some effects of memory limitation upon sentence comprehension and recall. *J. Verbal Learning Verbal Behav.* 9: 541–47.

GARRETT, M., BEVER, T. G., and FODOR, J. 1966. The active use of grammar in speech perception. *Percept. Psychophys.* 1: 30–32.

GLUCKSBERG, S. and DANKS, J. H. 1969. Grammatical structure and recall: A function of the space in immediate memory or of recall delay? *Percept. Psychophys.* 6: 113–17.

HAKES, D. T. and CIARNS, H. S. Do relative pronouns affect sentence comprehension? *Percept. Psychophys.* 8: 5–8.

HAYES, J. R. 1970. (ed.). *Cognition and the Development of Language*. New York: John Wiley & Sons, Inc.

JAKOBOVITS, L. A. and MIRON, M. S. 1967. (eds.). *Readings in the Psychology of Language*. Englewood Cliffs, N.J.: Prentice-Hall, Inc.

JENKINS, J. J. 1965. Mediation theory and grammatical behavior. *In* Sheldon Rosenberg (ed.). *Directions in Psycholinguistics*. New York: The Macmillan Company.

KESSEL, F. S. 1969. The development of children's comprehension from 6 to 12. Unpublished doctoral dissertation. University of Minnesota.

KLIMA, E. S. and BELLUGI, U. 1966. Syntactic regularities in the speech of children. *In* J. Lyons and R. Wales (eds.). *Psycholinguistic Papers*. Edinburgh: Edinburgh University Press.

LABOV, W. 1966. *The Social Stratification of English in New York City*. Washington, D.C.: Center for Applied Linguistics.

LENNEBERG, E. H. 1967. *Biological Foundations of Language*. New York: John Wiley & Sons, Inc.

McCARTHY, D. 1930. *The Language Development of the Preschool Child*. Institute of Child Welfare Monographs Series, No. 4. Minneapolis: University of Minnesota Press.

McNEILL, D. 1970. *The Acquisition of Language: The Study of Developmental Psycholinguistics*. New York: Harper & Row, Publishers.

MATTHEWS, W. A. 1968. Transformational complexity and short-term recall. *Lang. Speech* 11: 120–28.

MEHLER, J. 1963. Some effects of grammatical transformations on the recall of English sentences. *J. Verbal Learning Verbal Behav.* 2: 346–51.

MILLER, G. A. 1962. Some psychological studies of grammar. *Amer. Psychol.* 17: 748–62.

MILLER, G. A. 1965. Some preliminaries to psycholinguistics. *Amer. Psychol.* 50: 15–20.

MILLER, G. A., and McKEAN, K. 1964. A chronometric study of some relations between sentences. *Quart. J. Exper. Psychol.* 16: 297–308.

OSGOOD, C. 1963. On understanding and creating sentences. *Amer. Psychol.* 18: 735–51. Reprinted in L. A. Jakobovits and M. S. Miron (eds.). 1967. *Readings in the Psychology of Language*. Englewood Cliffs, N.J.: Prentice-Hall, Inc.

SAVIN, H. B. and PERCHONOCK, E. 1965. Grammatical structure and the immediate recall of English sentences. *J. Verbal Learning Verbal Behav.* 4: 348–53.

SHIPLEY, E. F., SMITH, C. S. and GLEITMAN, L. R. 1969. A study in the acquisition of language. *Language* 45: 322–42.

SHUY, R. W., BARATZ, J. C. and WOLFRAM, W. A. 1969. Sociolinguistic factors in speech identification. National Institutes of Mental Health Research Project No. MH-15048-01. Center for Applied Linguistics.

SHUY, R. W., WOLFRAM, W. A. and RILEY, W. K. 1967. Linguistic correlates of social stratification in Detroit speech. U.S. Office of Education Cooperative Research Project No. 6-1347. Michigan State University.

SHUY, R. W., WOLFRAM, W. A. and RILEY, W. K. 1968. *Field Techniques in an Urban Language Study.* Washington, D.C.: Center for Applied Linguistics.

SKINNER, B. F. 1957. *Verbal Behavior.* New York: Appleton-Century-Crofts.

STEWART, W. A. 1965. Urban Negro Speech: Sociolinguistic factors affecting English teaching. *In* R. W. Shuy (ed.). *Social Dialects and Language Learning.* Champaign, Ill.: National Council of Teachers of English.

TEMPLIN, M. C. 1957. *Certain Language Skills in Children, Their Development and Interrelationships.* Institute of Child Welfare Monographs Series, No. 26. Minneapolis: University of Minnesota Press.

WILLIAMS, F. 1970. Language, attitude, and social change. *In* F. Williams (ed.). *Language and Poverty: Perspectives on a Theme.* Chicago Ill.: Markham.

WOLFRAM, W. A. 1969. *A Sociolinguistic Description of Detroit Negro Speech.* Washington, D.C.: Center for Applied Linguistics.

INDEX

A

Abdomen, 75
Abdominal aponeurosis, 77
Abdominal hydraulics, 110
Abscissa, 346
Acceleration, particle, 25
Acoustic, 2
  coupler, 368
  cues, 397–98
  energy, 7
  free field, 367
  reactance and resistance, 291, 296
  resonator, 278, 370
  volume velocity, 57
  waveform, 213
Acoustical:
  filter (vocal tract), 274
  filtering, 262
  phonetics, 3
  resonances, 262
Acoustics, 1, 5

Adaptation, 400
Aerodynamic:
  coupling force, 142
  events, 80, 114
Aerodynamic-myoelastic theory of voice
      production, 140
Afferent auditory system, 326
Afferent system, 332
Affricates, 272
Air conduction, 306
Airflow, 127, 139, 216
  laminar, 82
  turbulent, 82, 143, 144
Airway:
  lower, 77
  resistance, 216
  upper, 77, 222
Allophones, 194, 237
Allophonic variation, 199
Alpha motor system, 122
Alveoli, 77
Amplification, 63

Amplifier, 66–67
Amplitude, 5, 14–15, 17, 19
Ampulae, 298
Annular ligament, 288
Antinode, 39, 43, 46
Antiresonances, 279
Aphasia, 3
Articulation, 6–7
Articulation targets, 197
Articulators, 170
Articulatory, 6
  behavior, 280
  positions, 6
  processes, 6
Aspiration, 422
Audiogram, 372
Audiometric zero, 372
Auditory adaptation, 407
  mechanism, 3, 6
  nerve, 301, 315
  pathway, 314
  perception, 5
  short-term memory, 329
  system, 7, 11, 329
Aural harmonics, 388, 390, 392
Axon, 310

B

Basilar membrane, 301, 303, 411
  movement, 305
Beats, 386
  best beats, 391
Békesy audiometer, 401
Bel, 27
Bernoulli effect, 213
Bernoulli's law, 141
Bone conduction:
  compressional, 306
  inertial, 306
  osseotympanic theory, 307
  stimulation, 306
Bony spiral lamina, 299
Breathy voicing, 144

C

Capacitance, 51
Cartilage:
  arytenoid, 13, 133, 134

  costal, 75
  cricoid, 129, 133
  thyroid, 129, 133
Cathode ray oscilliscopes, 63
Cell body, 310
Central nervous system, 212
Cerumen, 286
Characteristic frequency, 320
Classical conditioning, 476
Clavicles, 75
Closure duration, 266
Coarticulation, 6, 7, 201, 269, 276, 279
  mechano-inertial timing, 203
  neurally programmed, 204
Cochlea, 298, 309
Cochlear:
  function, 310
  microphonic, 307, 324
  nucleus, 316
  response, 324
  responses (to stimuli), 309
  structures, 44
Coding hypothesis, 459, 461
Cognitive behaviors, 4
  processes, 2, 4
  psycholinguistics, 457
Competence, 421, 452, 474
Competence-performance distinction, 470
Competence-performance relationship, 458
Compliance, 57
Comprehension, 462
  of sentences, 469
Concha, 286
Condensation, 23
Conduction of nerve impulses, 313
Consonant, 219, 237
Consonant sounds, 189
  voiced and voiceless, 257
Consonants:
  affricates, nasals, laterals, semi-
    vowels, 191
  stop, aspirated, fricative, 190
Constituent, 443
Constituents, discontinuous, 445
Contraction:
  isometric, 106
  miometric, 106
  pliometric, 106

Corda tympani, 290
Cortex, 320, 323, 328
Cortical auditory system, 330
Cortical lesions, 329
Coxal bones, 77
Cricoarytenoid joint, 35
Critical band concept, 382
Critical bandwidth, 381
Crystals piezoelectric, 59
Current, 48, 49
    alternating, 48
    direct, 48
    electrical, passive, 55
    oscillatory, 52
Cycle, 14

D

Damping, 37, 46, 52
Decibel, 26, 27, 28
Decoding, 483
Delayed auditory feedback, 213
Dendrites, 310
Density, 29
Dependent variable, 345
Derivational theory of complexity, 461
Detection, 347
Dialectology, 486
Diaphragm, 75, 78, 85
Diaphragms, 44
Diaphramatic activity, 111
Differential threshold, 353, 355
Diphthongs, 193, 277
Discrimination, 347, 353, 373
    duration, 377
    frequency, 375
    functions, 330
    intensity, 375
Distortion, 69
Ductus reuniens, 298
Duration of stimuli, 385
Duty cycle, 242
Dynamic range, 69
Dyne, 25

E

Ear canal, 9
Efferent system, 331, 332

Effort:
    expiratory, 163
    inspiratory, 103
Elasticity, 29
Electrical potential, 48
Electrical potentials, 311
Electroacoustics, 5
Electrodynamic earphone, 67
Electromagnet, 71
Electromyography, 106, 119
Electrostatic field, 51, 53, 57
Emitted responses, 477
Encoding, 483
Endolymph, 298
Endolymphatic duct, 298
Energy:
    acoustic, 3, 56, 62
    electrical, 56
    inertial, 56
    kinetic, 25
    neural, 3, 7
    potential, 25, 48, 57, 142
Epiglottis, 162
"Error," 349
    constant, 349
    variable, 349
Esophagus, 77
Eustachian tube, 180, 288
Exhalation, 88
Experiment, 345
Experimental method, 345
Expiration, 88
    active, 90
    passive, 89
    quiet, 89
External auditory meatus, 286, 290, 370

F

False vocal fold, 163
Fatigue, 400
Features:
    distinctive, 423
    nondistinctive, 423
    phonetic, 422, 423, 427, 449
        random variation, 486
    redundant, 423
Feedback, 213
    tactile, proprioceptive, 183
Filter function, 268, 279

Filters:
  electrical, 54
  fixed, 65
  sweeping, 64
Force, 25
Forces:
  aerodynamic, 141
  Bernoulli, 239
  damping, 33
  electromotive, 48
  inspiratory, 83
  muscular, 96, 216
  nonmuscular, 96, 216, 218
  recoil, 118
  respiratory, 101, 117
Formant, 248, 254, 269, 277
  amplitudes, 278
  bandwidths, 278
  frequency patterns, 274
    amplitude, bandwidths, fre-
      quency, 254
  structures, 264
  transitions, 257
Fourier analysis, 18, 19, 240
Frequency, 5, 10, 14, 15, 17, 19, 20, 58
    384
  coding, 318
  discrimination, 329, 394
Fricatives, 258, 260
Friction, 49
Function, 346
Fundamental, 40
Fundamental frequency, 18, 41, 147,
    413

G

Gamma-loop system, 121
Gamma motor system, 122
Generative, 450
Generative grammar, 8
Glides, 273
Glottal:
  articulations, 145, 148
  fricative, 149
  friction, 269
  resistance, 239
  sound source, 274
  stop, 148
  wave, 240

Glottis, 138, 139, 238, 270
Grammar, 422, 429, 432, 450, 451, 471
  general theory, 453
Grammatical development, 475
Grammatical rules, 453
Graphs, 346

H

Habenula perforata, 301, 316
Hair cells, inner, outer, 301
Hard palate, 175
Harmonic, 18
Harmonics, 39, 47
Hearing loss, 373
Helicotrema, 298
Helmholtz resonator, 35, 53, 247
Helmholtz's theory of hearing, 411
Holophrastic stage, 474
Hyoid bone, 163

I

Identification, 347
Impedance, 32, 52, 295
  acoustic, 31, 291
  measurement, 297
Imperfect unisons, 387
Incudostapedial joint, 294
Incus, 288
Inductance, 49, 57
Inductive reactance, 50
Inertance, 57
Inferior colliculus, 317, 322
Inner ear, 291
Inspiration, 80, 82
  forced, 86
  quiet, 84, 89
Instrumental conditioning, 477, 478
Instrumental response, 477
Insular cortex, 317
Intensity, 5, 25, 147, 149, 150, 409
Intensity discrimination, 394
Interaural intensity difference, 398
  phase, 395
  phase difference, 398
  time differences, 398
Internal stimulation, 477

International Phonetic Alphabet, 190, 236, 427
Interration level, 482
Intonation, 224, 225
Intonation contour, 227
Inverse square law, 26
Isometric contraction, 184
Isotonic contraction, 184

K

Kernel sentences, 459

L

Language, 2, 8, 421
　acquisition, 470
　　biological component, 470
　　cognitive approach, 470
　　genetic predisposition, 471
　behavior:
　　cognitive view, 484
　　development, 473
　　generative theory, 485
　　performance, 2, 8
Laryngeal actions, 145
Laryngeal ventricle, 163
Laryngealization, 145
Larynx, 6, 77, 127, 128, 222
Lateral lemniscus, 317
Lateralization, 397
Learning, 476
Learning theory, 475, 484
Lexical elements, 464
Lexical interpretations, 467, 468
Limbus, 299
Linguistic, 1
　competence, 8, 282, 429, 431
　development, 475
　meta-theory, 453
　performance, 429
　planning, 2
　theory, 429, 452, 454
　universals, 453, 471
　　formal, 453
　　substantive, 453
　variation, 491
Linguistic negation, 474
　development of, 475

external sentential, 474
holophrastic, 474, 475
multiple, 490
Lip rounding, 245, 276
Lips, 174
Localization, 397, 398
Logarithm, 27, 28
　characteristic, 27
　mantissa, 27
Logarithms, 26
Loudness, 382, 394
　adaptation, 405
　　short-term, 407
　balance, 383
　contour, 383
Loudspeaker, 67
Lung capacities, 94–95
　functional residual, 95–96
　inspiratory, 95, 96
　total lung, 95–96
　vital, 95–96
Lung volume, 97, 109, 108, 115
Lung volumes, 94
　expiratory reserve, 94, 96
　inspiratory reserve, 94, 96
　residual, 95–96
　tidal, 94, 96
Lungs, 77

M

Magnetic field, 50
Magnetic field strength, 71
Magnetization potential, 72
Malleo-incudal joint, 294
Malleus, 287
Mandible, 175
Manubrium, 287
Masker, 378
Masking, 378, 410
　effective, 382
　narrow band, 380
　pure tone, 379
Masking level difference (MLD), 395
Mass, 56
Medial geniculate, 317, 322, 329
Mediating reaction (r_m), 481
Mediational model, 482
Mels, 408
Membranes, 44

Meter, 62
Meters, DC, 63
Microphone, 71
  carbon, 58, 62
  condenser, 62
  crystal, 59, 62
  dynamic, 61
Middle ear function, 292
Middle ear muscles, 297
Minimal pairs, 422
Minimum audible field technique, 367
Minimum audible pressure technique, 368
Mistuned consonance, 387
Modiolus, 315
Morpheme, 427
Morphemes:
  grammatical, 428
  lexical, 428
Mouth, 77
Mucoviscoelastic aerodynamic theory, 143
Muscle:
  abdominal, 93, 108
    external oblique, 93
    internal oblique, 94
    rectus abdominis, 93
    transversus abdominis, 94
  accessory, 86
  cricopharyngeus, 165
  expiratory, 110
  external intercostal, 85, 107, 111, 120
  extrinsic laryngeal, 164
    sternohyoid, 164
    sternothyroid, 164
    thyrohyoid, 164
  extrinsic tongue, 176
    genioglossus, 178
    hyoglossus, 178
    palatoglossus, 178
    styloglossus, 178
  inspiratory, 107
  internal intercostal, 92, 108, 120
  intrinsic laryngeal, 155
    lateral cricoarytenoid, 156, 158
    oblique arytenoid, 157, 158
    posterior cricoarytenoid, 156
    thyroarytenoid, 159, 160
    transverse arytenoid, 156, 158
    vocalis, 160
  intrinsic tongue, 176

  inferior longitudinal, 177
  superior longitudinal, 177
  transverse, 177
  vertical, 176
  latissimus dorsi, 88, 93, 108
  levatores costarum, 88
  orbicularis oris, 185
  palatal levator, 180
  palatal tensor, 180
  palatoglossus, 171
  palatopharyngeus, 173, 180
  pectoralis major, 87
  pectoralis minor, 88
  pharyngeal constrictors, 182, 266
  quadratus lumborum, 93
  scalenus:
    anterior, 86
    medius, 86
    posterior, 86
  serratus:
    anterior, 88
    posterior inferior, 93
    posterior superior, 88
  stapedius, 288
  sternocleidomastoid, 86
  subclavius, 87
  subcostal, 93
  tensor tympani, 288
  thoracic, 85
  thyropharyngeus, 165
  transversus thoracis, 92
Muscle effort:
  expiratory, 97
  inspiratory, 97

N

Nasal:
  cavities, 174
  murmur, 279
  perception, 279
  septum, 174
  sounds, 278
Nasalization, 279
Nervous system, 327
  auditory, 7
Neural coding, 7
Neural-rate theory, 321
Neural-rate theory of frequency coding, 323

Neurons, 310
  afferent, 315
  bipolar, 311
  efferent, 315
Nodal positions, 41
Node, 46
Nodes, 39, 43
Noise, 21, 66
  gaussian, 21
  random, 21
  source, 143
  spectrum, 268
  thermal, 21
  white, 21
  wide-band, 21, 378
Nonlinear systems, 388, 389
Nose, 77
Number systems, 361
  nominal, 362
  ordinal, 362

O

Observational method (of scientific observations), 345
Occlusion release, 268
Ohm, 49
Ohm's law, 49
Olivocochlear bundle, 317, 331
Operant conditioning theory, 478
Operants, 477, 479
  echoic, 479
  intraverbal, 479
  mands, 479
  tact, 479
  textual, 479
  verbal, 478
Oral cavity, 171
Ordinate, 346
Organ of Corti, 301
Organic disorders, 4
Organismic variables, 372
Oscillation, 46
  frequency of, 32
Oscillators, 66
Ossicles, 288, 293

P

Pars flaccida, 287
Partials, 43, 47

Particle:
  acceleration, 24
  displacement, 23, 24
  velocity, 23, 25
Passive sentence, 468
Pattern discrimination, 329
Pectoral girdle, 75
Pelvic girdle, 77
Perception, 2, 3, 5, 264, 277, 324, 344
  of beats, 387, 464
Perceptual cues for stops, 271
Performance, 452, 474
Perilymph, 298
Period, 14, 15
Periodicity pitch, 415, 417
Pharynx, 127, 173
  laryngopharynx, 127, 173
  nasopharynx, 173
  oropharynx, 127, 173
Phase, 14, 17
  starting, 15
Phonation, 6, 7, 28
Phoneme identification, 272
Phonemes, 193, 236, 423
Phonemic level, 427
Phones, 185
Phonetic:
  context, 200
  features, 220
  level, 425
  redundancy, 272
  representation, 423
  transcription, 427
Phonetics, 193
Phonological:
  component, 452
  level, 428
  representation, 423
  rules, 3, 423, 448, 449
  theory, 428
Phonology, 193, 423
Phons, 383
Phrase markers, 435, 436, 443
Phrase-structure rules, 448
Physics of sound, 25
Physiologic, 2
Physiological process, 1
Physiology, 1, 5, 7
  articulatory, 7
  auditory, 7
  laryngeal, 6

Pinna, 286, 290
Piroform sinuses, 163
Pitch, 10, 154, 241, 407
Pitch measurement:
  direct, 407
  indirect, 408
Pitch perception, 318, 411, 413, 414, 418
Place theory of hearing, 318, 411
  frequency coding, 323
Plates, 44
Pleura:
  parietal, 78
  visceral, 78
Pleural linkage, 79, 80
Point of objective equality (POE), 348
Point of subjective equality (PSE), 348,
  355
Postures:
  supine, 112, 116
  upright, 111, 116
Power, 25, 49
Power summation hypothesis, 393
Presbycusis, 372
Pressure, 25
  abdominal, 80
  acoustic, 31
  air, 141, 216
  alveolar, 80, 81, 82, 89, 97, 101, 104,
    106, 109, 120
  expiratory, 98
  inspiratory, 98
  intraoral, 265, 270
  muscular, 101, 102, 103, 104, 106,
    108, 113, 117
  negative, 98
  negative muscular, 111
  oropharyngeal, 265
  pleural, 80, 111
  positive, 98
  relaxation, 97, 101, 102
  subglottal, 149, 164
  supraglottal, 164
Pressure-transformation ratio, 295
Pressure wave, 292
Probe tone technique, 369, 391
Probe tube technique, 370
Production, 462
Production-comprehension gap, 473
Projection level, 482
Projection rules, 451

Prosodic:
  aspects, 223
  features, 224
  function, 145
  parameters, 147
Prosodies, 224
Psychoacoustics, 3, 5, 343
Psycholinguistic, 2, 8, 452
  theories, 4
Psychological reality:
  linguistic rules, 466
  transformational rules, 460
  underlying sentences, 465
Psychometric function, 355
Psychophysical index, 356
Psychophysical methods, 355, 363, 371
  adjustment, 350, 356
  constant stimuli, 353, 355
  limits, 352, 355
Psychophysical methods (adaptive pro-
    cedures), 356, 357
  Békésy tracking, 358
  BUDTIF (Block Up Down Temporal
    Interval Forced Choice) method,
    360
  PEST (Parameter Estimation of Se-
    quential Testing) procedure, 359
    double rule, 359
    halving rule, 360
  Up and down method (of adaptive
    procedures), 357
Psychophysical methods (rating scales),
    363
  direct magnitude estimation, 363
  direct magnitude production, 363
  equal interval, 363
Psychophysical procedures, 345
Psychophysics, 343
Pulmonary subdivisions, 97
Pulmonary system, 75, 77
Pulsation, 145, 146

R

Radial fibers, 315
Rarefaction, 23
Rate of neural discharge theory, 416
Reactance, 31
  capacitive, 52
  inductive, 52

Receiver, 12
Recoding hypothesis, 460
Recording:
    disk, 69
    magnetic, 71
    optical, 70
    sound, 68
Recursiveness, 445
Reflective surfaces, 36
Reinforcement, 477
Reissner's membrane, 301
Representational mediation process, 480
Resistance, 31, 48, 52, 56, 141, 291
    acoustic, 32
    electrical, 53
Resonance, 5, 7, 32, 52, 56, 248, 268
    curve, 35
    system, 268
    tube, 36
Resonant characteristics of air-filled
        cavities, 34
Resonant frequency, 34, 52, 53
Resonators:
    Helmholtz, 34
    multiple, 247
    simple, 247
Respiration, 6, 73
Respiratory:
    airways, 77
    function, 98
    system, 221
Resting expiratory level, 80
Reverberation time, 36
Reynold's number, 258
Rhythm, 227, 228
Ribs, 75
Round window, 308

S

Saccule, 298
Scala:
    media, 298
    tympani, 298
    vestibuli, 298
Scalae, 298
Scaling (re: problems in psycho-
        acoustics), 348
Scapulae, 75
Segmental features, 220

Semantic rules, 8
Semicircular canals, 298
Semi-vowels, 273, 278
Sensation level, 298
Sensitivity, 348
    differential, 348
Sentence comprehension, 467
Sequence discrimination, 329
Shearing principle, 310
Short-term memory, 461
Sign-behavior, 481
Simple harmonic motion, 13, 14, 15, 23
Singing, 138
Sociolinguistics, 492
    acrolect, 491
    basilect, 491
    social prestige (of linguistic variation),
        491
    social stratification of linguistic vari-
        ables, 491
"Sodium-pump" hypothesis, 312
Soft palate, 180
Sones, 382
Sound, 11
    complex, 15
    conducting medium, 11
    energy, 292
    power, 28
    pressure, 27, 58
    pressure level, 365, 367, 373
    pressure measurements, 370
    shadow, 398
    source, 11, 36, 37
        turbulent, 258, 259
    spectrograph, 5, 66
    transmission, 29
    wave, 25, 32
Source-filter theory, 257
Spectra, 21
Spectral characteristics, 264, 267
Spectral distribution, 276
Spectrum, 19, 20, 261
    analyzer, 64
    glottal, 241, 243
    harmonic, 243
Speech:
    acoustics, 5
    perception, 281, 282
    physiology, 3
    production, 1, 5
    reception, 333

Speech: (*continued*)
  respiration, 99
  sounds, 170, 185, 195
Speech and hearing science, 1
Spike and slow-wave responses, 313
Spiral ganglion, 316
Spiral ligament, 301
Spiral tracts, 315
Spirogram, 94, 97
Stapedial motion, 295
Stapes, 288
Stapes displacement, 295
Sternum, 75
Stimulation:
  dimensions, 374
  discrimination, 277
  duration, 410
  stimulus frequency, 408
  stimulus generalization, 477
  stimulus intensity, 383, 392
Stop sounds, 265
  alveolar, 265, 268, 269
  aspirated, 267
  bilabial, 265, 268, 269
  explosive, 266
  implosive, 266
  unaspirated, 267
  velar, 265, 268
Strain, 29
Stress, 29, 226
  syllable, 29
Stria of Held, 316
Stria of Monakow, 316
Structural:
  hypotheses, 468
  information, 467
  relations, 467
Structure:
  deep, 437, 441, 448, 462, 468
  surface, 347, 441, 448
  syntactic, 441
Subarachnoid space, 298
Summation tone, 392
Superior olivary complex, 316, 326, 327
Suprasegmental feature, 224
Suprasegmental parameters, 281
Syllable, 219
Synapse, 311
Syntactic ambiguity, 435, 437
Syntactic rules, 435

T

Tectorial membrane, 301, 305
Teeth, 175
Telephone theory, 416
Temporal bone, 286
Temporal change detection, 377
Temporal sequencing, 277
Temporary threshold shift
  (TTS), 401
Temporomandibular joint, 175
Tense-lax (fortis-lenis), 270
Theory (definition of), 454
  meta-theory, 455
  universal linguistic theory, 455
Thoracic cavity, 78
Thoracic volume, 82
Thorax, 75, 77
Threshold, 373, 393
  absolute, 348, 374, 376
  differential, 348, 373
  estimates, 367
  fatigue, 400, 403
  feeling, 366
  performance, 365
Throat, 77
Time delay pitch, 415
Time separation pitch, 415, 417
Tone-noise discrimination, 329
Tongue, 6, 175
  height, 6
  position, 6
  root, 266, 274
Tonotopic organization, 320
Torso, 74
Trachea, 77
Transducer:
  acousticoelectric, 58
  electroacoustic, 62
  electrostatic, 62
Transformational rules, 437, 445, 448,
  458, 460, 462
Transformer action, 295
Transverse temporal gyri, 317
Trapezoid body, 316, 330
Traveling wave, 309, 324
Tuning curve, 320
Tympanic membrane displacement, 295
Tympanic membrane (ear drum), 44,
  287, 292, 369

U

Umbo, 287
Underlying sentences, 464, 466
Uniform circular motion, 13, 14, 22
Urban language research, 486
Urban language studies, 491
Utricle, 298

V

Vacuum tubes, 55
Variable:
  independent, 345
  irrelevant, 345
Velocity, 13, 39, 86, 141
  propagation, 29, 31
Velopharyngeal port, 180, 278
Velum, 180
Verb complexity hypothesis, 469
Verbal behavior, 477, 480, 483, 487
  linguistic variables, 487
  social stratification, 488
  social variables, 487
  theory, 478
  variations in New York speech, 488
Vertebrae:
  cervical, 75
  coccygeal, 75
  lumbar, 75
  thoracic, 75
Vertebral column, 75
Vestibular labyrinth, 298
Vestibule, 298
Vibration, 11, 12
  amplitude, 40
  frequency, 33, 38, 39, 41, 42, 43
  longitudinal, 40, 46
  periodic, 12, 270
  random, 20, 21
  torsional, 40
  transient, 20
  transverse, 37, 40
Vibration patterns, 40, 45
Vibratory motion:
  aperiodic, 12
  periodic, 12
Vital capacity, 116

Vocal:
  fry, 145
  ligament, 137
  tract, 169, 243, 246, 249, 277
Vocal effort, 231
Vocal fold, 138, 139
  longitudinal tension, 140, 151
  mechanical coupling, 140
  medial compression, 152
  vibration, 143
Vocalic transitions, 264, 269
Voice registers, 153
Voice-onset-time, 270
Voiced sounds, 238
Voicing, 138
Volley theory, 321, 416
Volleying, 417
Voltage, 48, 49
Volume flow, 81
Volume velocity, 31, 242
  glottal, 239
Vowels, 185, 186, 192, 219, 237, 256, 280

W

Wave motion, 22, 30
Waveform, 5, 15, 58, 172, 390
  aperiodic, 20
  complex, 17, 18, 19, 240
  generator, 66
  periodic, 20
Wavelength, 29, 31, 40
Wever-Bray effect, 307
Waves:
  plane acoustic, 22
  reflected, 46
  sawtooth, 66
  simple, 240
  sine, 15, 17, 321, 386
  spherical, 21
  square, 17, 66
  standing, 32, 35, 36, 86
  transverse, 39
  traveling, 303
  triangular, 66
Whispering, 143, 144
Word recall, 461
Work, 25